Vitamins and Minerals

Vitamins and Minerals
Fact versus Fiction

Myrna Chandler Goldstein
and Mark A. Goldstein, MD

GREENWOOD™

An Imprint of ABC-CLIO, LLC
Santa Barbara, California • Denver, Colorado

Copyright © 2018 by ABC-CLIO, LLC

All rights reserved. No part of this publication may be reproduced, stored in a retrieval system, or transmitted, in any form or by any means, electronic, mechanical, photocopying, recording, or otherwise, except for the inclusion of brief quotations in a review, without prior permission in writing from the publisher.

Library of Congress Cataloging-in-Publication Data

Names: Goldstein, Myrna Chandler, 1948– author. | Goldstein, Mark A. (Mark Allan), 1947– author.
Title: Vitamins and minerals : fact versus fiction / Myrna Chandler Goldstein and Mark A. Goldstein, MD.
Description: Santa Barbara, California : Greenwood, an imprint of ABC-CLIO, LLC, [2018] | Includes bibliographical references and index.
Identifiers: LCCN 2017055237 (print) | LCCN 2017059581 (ebook) | ISBN 9781440852107 (ebook) | ISBN 9781440852091 (alk. paper)
Subjects: LCSH: Vitamins in human nutrition—Encyclopedias. | Minerals in human nutrition—Encyclopedias. | Minerals in the body—Encyclopedias. | Vitamins—Encyclopedias. | Nutrition—Encyclopedias.
Classification: LCC QP771 (ebook) | LCC QP771 .G65 2018 (print) | DDC 612.3/9903—dc23
LC record available at https://lccn.loc.gov/2017055237

ISBN: 978-1-4408-5209-1 (print)
978-1-4408-5210-7 (ebook)

22 21 20 19 18   1 2 3 4 5

This book is also available as an eBook.

Greenwood
An Imprint of ABC-CLIO, LLC

ABC-CLIO, LLC
130 Cremona Drive, P.O. Box 1911
Santa Barbara, California 93116-1911
www.abc-clio.com

This book is printed on acid-free paper ∞

Manufactured in the United States of America

This book discusses treatments (including types of medication and mental health therapies), diagnostic tests for various symptoms and mental health disorders, and organizations. The authors have made every effort to present accurate and up-to-date information. However, the information in this book is not intended to recommend or endorse particular treatments or organizations, or substitute for the care or medical advice of a qualified health professional, or used to alter any medical therapy without a medical doctor's advice. Specific situations may require specific therapeutic approaches not included in this book. For those reasons, we recommend that readers follow the advice of qualified health care professionals directly involved in their care. Readers who suspect they may have specific medical problems should consult a physician about any suggestions made in this book.

We dedicate this book with love to our five grandchildren:
Aidan Zev Goldstein, born February 8, 2008
Payton Maeve Goldstein, born December 4, 2009
Milo Adlai Kamras, born August 9, 2011
Erin Abigail Goldstein, born December 29, 2011
Zoe "Scout" Eames Kamras, born February 16, 2014

Contents

Preface	ix
Acknowledgments	xi
What Are Vitamins and Minerals?	xiii
What Are Dietary Supplements?	xv
Determining Vitamin and Mineral Intake Levels	xvii
Boron	1
Calcium	6
Choline	14
Chromium	20
Copper	26
Fluoride	32
Iodine	39
Iron	46
Magnesium	53
Manganese	61
Molybdenum	69
Phosphorus	74
Potassium	80
Selenium	89
Sodium	98
Vitamin A	105
Vitamin B1 (Thiamin)	114

Vitamin B2 (Riboflavin)	122
Vitamin B3 (Niacin)	130
Vitamin B5 (Pantothenic Acid)	137
Vitamin B6 (Pyridoxine)	145
Vitamin B7 (Biotin)	153
Vitamin B9 (Folate)	157
Vitamin B12 (Cobalamin)	164
Vitamin C	173
Vitamin D	182
Vitamin E	193
Vitamin K	201
Zinc	206
Appendix: Recommended Intake Levels of Key Vitamins and Minerals for Different Populations	215
Glossary	225
Index	229
About the Authors	249

Preface

Many health claims have been made about a variety of vitamins and minerals, whether obtained from food or in supplement form. The objective of this book is to help readers evaluate these claims for themselves by providing key information and summaries of peer-reviewed scientific studies that take a critical look at the potential health benefits—and dangers—of these substances.

Each entry begins with an overview of the vitamin or mineral, followed by a list of top food sources and types of supplements available. Next, intake recommendations are provided, explaining exactly how much people should be ingesting based on their age, gender, and other factors. The next section describes the symptoms associated with a deficiency or excess intake of each vitamin or mineral. That information is especially important for those at increased risk for deficiencies, such as those with eating disorders or malabsorption problems, and those who tend to take higher amounts of certain types of supplementation.

The majority of each entry focuses on the findings of various published peer-reviewed, scientific studies. We explore the actual scientific proof—or lack thereof—that specific vitamins and minerals may have wide-ranging impacts on the human body. Although obviously not every study could be included, the ones summarized in this book represent a broad cross-section of the research available.

It was not possible to include every single vitamin and mineral, as credible research on some of these is lacking, and it is beyond the scope of this project to discuss the many other nonvitamin/nonmineral substances critical to human health. Still, we hope that this volume will prove an invaluable resource for those interested in learning more about their health.

Acknowledgments

We would like to thank our editor Maxine Taylor, who has edited several of our more recent books. Tirelessly dedicated, Maxine has repeatedly offered excellent suggestions and advice. She is one of the primary reasons that we continue to write books for ABC-CLIO.

What Are Vitamins and Minerals?

Vitamins and minerals are substances your body needs to grow and develop normally. In most cases, the body requires only very small quantities (although these needs may increase or decrease based on sex, age, and certain life events such as pregnancy). Without vitamins and minerals, your body is unable to complete the countless tasks it conducts each day; in short, vitamins and minerals are an integral part of your body's functioning. Most (but not all) vitamins and minerals cannot be manufactured by the body and must be absorbed from food and/or consumed in a supplement.

There are a few subtle differences between vitamins and minerals. Since they are organic—made by plants and animals—vitamins are somewhat fragile. Many may be broken down by heat, light, or acid. The very act of processing food can reduce the amount of many vitamins; they may lose potency or be destroyed by cooking, storage, or exposure to air. On the other hand, minerals are inorganic—from the soil and water—and are more stable.

Vitamins are classified as either water soluble or fat soluble. Water-soluble vitamins fill the watery portions of foods and are quickly and easily absorbed. The kidneys regulate the amount of water-soluble vitamins in the body; when the body has excess amounts, the kidneys remove them in the urine. On the other hand, fat-soluble vitamins usually must join with a protein to travel throughout the body. Fat-soluble vitamins may be stored in the body for extended periods of time. That is why it is important to avoid high levels of fat-soluble vitamin supplementation, which may become toxic.

Minerals are often categorized as macrominerals or trace minerals. Found in larger amounts in the body, the body needs to take in larger amounts of macrominerals. Calcium and phosphorous are two common macrominerals. Trace minerals are found in smaller amounts in the body; the body requires only tiny amounts. Iron and zinc are examples of trace minerals. In the body, minerals work in two ways. Many support body cells and structures. For instance, calcium and phosphorus help to build bones, and iron is an integral part of red blood cells. In addition, minerals may help to regulate body processes. Chromium, for example, is needed to normalize blood glucose levels.

Long before people knew anything about vitamins and minerals, they did recognize an association between diet and health. For example, sailors on long voyages, who did not have access to fresh foods, were prone to an illness known as scurvy. Scurvy had a host of different symptoms, including bleeding gums, poor wound healing, and severe pain, and could eventually lead to death. People at the time understood that scurvy was caused by the absence of something in fresh fruits and vegetables, so sailors were given lemon or lime juice to prevent illness. It was not until the early 20th century that researchers determined that scurvy was actually caused by a vitamin C deficiency.

Sailors also suffered from another ailment known as beriberi, which was characterized by mental confusion, muscle wasting, fluid retention, high blood pressure, walking problems, and heart disturbances. The rates of beriberi rose further when manufacturers began processing rice in the mid-1880s, which removed the vitamin-rich outer layer. Although the cause of beriberi eluded scientists for decades, eventually, it was determined that the condition was caused by a severe deficiency of vitamin B1. In 1912, the Polish-born biochemist Casimir Funk called the compound in the outer layer of rice "vital amine." Later, this was shortened to vitamin. By the 1930s, researchers had determined how to isolate and concentrate vitamins and minerals in pill form to supplement dietary intake.

Over the decades, researchers have devoted a great deal of time and energy to determining the medical and psychological problems associated with insufficient or excessive amounts of vitamins and minerals. And, this body of evidence continues to grow today.

People who tend to eat a wide variety of foods, including whole grain products, fresh fruits, lots of different vegetables, dairy products, nuts, seeds, eggs, and meats, may well obtain all the vitamins and minerals that they require. But people who skip meals, diet frequently, and have a less-than-ideal diet, may wish to consult a health-care provider about supplementation.

What Are Dietary Supplements?

Dietary supplements are products intended to add nutritional value to the diet. They are sold in many forms, including tablets, softgels, capsules, gelcaps, liquids, energy bars, or powders. All products labeled as dietary supplements have a "Supplement Facts" panel that lists the contents, amount of active ingredients per serving, and other added ingredients, such as flavorings, fillers, and binders. While the manufacturer-recommended serving size is also noted, health-care providers may suggest different serving sizes.

Most adults in the United States take some form of dietary supplements; in many cases, they take these supplements every day. The most commonly taken dietary supplement is a daily multivitamin. In other instances, individuals may take dietary supplements only when they experience certain symptoms, or they may intend to take a supplement regularly but frequently forget.

SUPPLEMENT SAFETY AND REGULATION

People may assume that the ingredients found in supplements are always safe. That is not true. Supplements sometimes contain active ingredients that may have a strong effect on the body. For example, it has been suggested that antioxidant supplements, such as vitamins C and E, may reduce the effectiveness of certain types of chemotherapy. Furthermore, supplements may interact with prescription medications. For instance, Coumadin, a blood-thinning medication should not be combined with vitamin E, which tends to thin the blood. Taking them together increases the risk of internal bleeding and stroke. Often, people are asked to stop taking supplements before a surgical procedure. Medical providers worry that there may be an interaction between anesthesia and supplements that might alter heart rate, blood pressure, and/or bleeding.

While the U.S. Food & Drug Administration (FDA) must approve prescription drugs before they are sold, no such requirement exists for dietary supplements. Dietary supplements are not considered drugs. Manufacturers are permitted to say that a dietary supplement addresses specific nutrient deficiencies or is linked to a body function, but the label must note that the statement has not been evaluated by the FDA, and the product is not intended to diagnose, treat, cure, or prevent any disease. Still, the FDA does have the ability to take action if a product is found to be unsafe or unfit for human consumption. It may force the removal of the product from the marketplace or compel the manufacturer to order a recall. In addition, the FDA monitors the labeling information of supplements. The agency attempts to ensure that the labeling information, including any package inserts, is accurate and not misleading. This information is also reviewed by the Federal Trade Commission, which oversees advertising.

Consumers should be wary of any vitamins and minerals that are sold with unrealistic and exaggerated claims or offer miraculous improvements in physical and/or psychological well-being. No vitamin or mineral supplement should be considered a cure for any disease; people who are quoted or appear in videos claiming that a supplement offered an astonishing cure should be ignored. Most medical and psychological problems are not easily solved with a vitamin or mineral supplement.

The supplement industry emerged about a century ago and has grown exponentially since then. The fact that the FDA has limited control of the supplement industry has made this growth relatively easy. The FDA views supplements as food rather than drugs; manufacturers do not need to prove that they are effective. In some instances, this lack of regulation has led to a number of problems. Sometimes, supplements do not contain the specified vitamins or minerals. Instead, they have cheap fillers. Or, they may have more or less than the indicated amount of vitamins or minerals. People, especially those taking supplements from brands that may be less reputable, are at risk for negative outcomes. There are reports of people seeking emergency medical care after consuming certain supplementation. As has been noted, supplements may react with other supplements and/or prescription medications. Unlike prescription medications, which take years to develop and receive FDA approval, supplements may be readily manufactured and quickly sold. It is important to purchase vitamins and minerals from companies that have sound reputations. It may be a good idea to ask a medical provider for recommendations.

It is important to remember that vitamin and mineral supplementation is not a substitute for a healthful diet. People should always strive to eat the most healthful diet possible. Still, certain people are considered to be at higher risk for dietary deficiencies. These include people who eat fewer than two meals per day, people on a restricted diet, vegetarians and vegans, people who take three or more prescriptive drugs per day, people with gastrointestinal disorders such as Crohn's disease that may interfere with nutrient absorption, and people who drink large amounts of alcohol.

Determining Vitamin and Mineral Intake Levels

For decades, the Recommended Dietary Allowances (RDAs), which was designed by the Food and Nutrition Board of the National Academy of Sciences—National Research Council, has been used as a guide for determining the amount of vitamins the body needs to prevent deficiency diseases. The RDA has been an estimate of the average requirements of dietary components such as calories, vitamins, minerals, and proteins that help prevent deficiency. Requirements varied based on gender and age.

But the Food and Nutrition Board RDA has been replaced by a new standard known as the Dietary References Intakes (DRI or DRIs), which is a fairly general term that describes the types and amounts of nutrients that healthy people require. The DRIs have four types of nutrient reference values; each one of these has a different use. These designations, which are used in the United States and Canada, are intended for the general public and health professionals:

Estimated average requirement (EAR)—The EAR is the amount of a nutrient that is estimated to meet the requirements of half of all healthy individuals in a given age and gender group. This value is obtained through a comprehensive review of the scientific literature, including experimental and clinical studies.

Recommended Dietary Allowance (RDA)—The RDA now means the average daily dietary intake of a nutrient that is sufficient to meet the requirement of 97 to 98 percent of all healthy people. This is intended to serve as a goal for people to try to meet. It is calculated from the EAR.

Adequate intake (AI)—AI is used only when the data are not sufficiently clear—making it impossible to determine an EAR (and RDA). AI figures are based on experimental data or are determined by taking an estimate of the amount of a nutrient eaten by a group of people.

Tolerable upper intake level (UL)—The UL is the highest daily intake level of a nutrient that is likely to pose no risks of having an adverse effect for most people. When people consume more than this amount, they have an increased risk of an adverse effect.

In addition to the DRIs, the acceptable macronutrient distribution range (AMDR) was developed for macronutrients. The AMDR is the percentage range of protein, fat, and carbohydrate intake that is associated with a reduced risk of chronic disease while also providing adequate intake of essential nutrients.

Today, food and supplement labels normally list the daily value. This is the amount of nutrients that experts believe people require in their daily diet. On food labels, this is based on a serving size for one person who consumes 2,000 calories per day.

HISTORY OF RDA AND DRI

The RDAs and DRIs actually have a noteworthy history. The early years of dietary standards are described in an article published in 1985 in the *American Journal of Clinical Nutrition*. The author observed that it often seems that the RDAs emerged "out of thin air." But, of course, that is not true. In fact, dietary standards have a long history that may be traced to the passage in Britain of the Merchant Seamen's Act of 1835. To help prevent scurvy, the act required that lime or lemon juice be available "in the rations of the mercantile service." A few years later, in 1847, a researcher examining the rations of the Dutch army recommended 100 g of protein per day for laborers and 60 g of protein per day for sedentary people. This researcher considered protein to be "the fuel of muscular activity."[1]

By the early 1860s, in an effort to prevent starvation and disease during a period of industrial dislocation and unemployment, Britain established dietary standards. The goal was to define a diet that maintained health at the lowest cost. Still, the focus during the 19th century remained on energy sources and protein.

With the arrival of the 20th century came an increased interest in calories and essential nutrients. Then, in 1918, the British Royal Society appointed a Food Committee that began to direct attention to protective foods. From the mid-1920s to the mid-1930s, other countries devoted time and attention to foods and nutrition, and several conferences were held. In 1933, the U.S. Department of Agriculture proposed the first set of standards for several vitamins and minerals. "These were the first recommendations designed for maintenance of health, rather than maintenance of work capacity." During the next decade, there was greater movement in the United States toward the development of standards. The printed version of the first edition of the RDAs appeared in 1943. Soon, other countries were creating their own dietary standards. At the end of the article, the author summarized the history of dietary standards by quoting the French proverb, "The more things change, the more they stay the same."[2]

Over the decades, there were numerous revisions of the RDAs. But, eventually, people were ready to transition to the DRIs. The DRI framework was conceptualized in 1994, and the first reports were issued from 1997 to 2004.

According to an article published in 1998 in the *Journal of the American Dietetic Association*, the DRIs offered a new approach that "included current concepts about the role of nutrients and food components in long-term health, going beyond deficiency diseases."[3] Still, the process has been far from smooth. In fact, it has presented an array of challenges. In a 2016 article in the journal *Advances in Nutrition*, researchers from Hawaii, Washington, DC, Maryland, Massachusetts, and Canada commented that "numerous conventions, challenges, and controversies were encountered during the process of defining and setting the DRIs." But, thanks to the DRIs, it is now possible "to estimate both the prevalence of inadequate intake and the prevalence of potentially excessive intake within a group." The DRIs have strongly influenced national nutrition policies, such as those concerning dietary guidance, food labeling, and nutrition monitoring.[4] It has certainly been a long road from those first lime and lemon juice requirements in Britain.

NOTES

1. Harper, A. E. "Origin of Recommended Dietary Allowances—An Historic Overview." *The American Journal of Clinical Nutrition* 41, no. 1 (January 1985): 140–148.

2. Ibid.

3. Yates, Allison A., Sandra A. Schlicker, and Carol W. Suitor. "Dietary Reference Intakes: The New Basis for Recommendations for Calcium and Related Nutrients, B Vitamins, and Choline." *Journal of the American Dietetic Association* 98, no. 6 (June 1998): 699–706.

4. Murphy, Suzanne P., Allison A. Yates, Stephanie A. Atkinson, et al. "History of Nutrition: The Long Road Leading to the Dietary Reference Intakes for the United States and Canada." *Advances in Nutrition* 7 (January 2016): 157–168.

REFERENCES

Harper, A. E. "Origin of Recommended Dietary Allowances—An Historic Overview." *American Journal of Clinical Nutrition* 41, no. 1 (January 1985): 140–148.

Murphy, Suzanne P., Allison A. Yates, Stephanie A. Atkinson, et al. "History of Nutrition: The Long Road Leading to the Dietary Reference Intakes for the United States and Canada." *Advances in Nutrition* 7 (January 2016): 157–168.

Yates, Allison A., Sandra A. Schlicker, and Carol W. Suitor. "Dietary Reference Intakes: The New Basis for Recommendations for Calcium and Related Nutrients, B Vitamins, and Choline." *Journal of the American Dietetic Association* 98, no. 6 (June 1998): 699–706.

Boron

A vital trace mineral that is found in foods and the environment, people may also take boron as a supplement. Boron is thought to be useful for building strong bones and muscles, treating osteoarthritis, increasing levels of testosterone in the blood, and improving cognitive skills and muscle coordination.

Women have used capsules containing boric acid, the most common form of boron, to treat vaginal yeast infections. They place the capsules directly in the vagina. People sometimes apply boric acid to the skin as an astringent or to prevent infections. In addition, it has been used as an eye wash.

Boron supplementation appears to interact with magnesium and reduce the amount of magnesium that is eliminated in the urine. This may result in elevated levels of magnesium in the blood. Among older women, this tends to occur in those who consume small amounts of magnesium. In young women, this happens more often among individuals who rarely exercise. It is not known if this occurs in men. In some people, supplemental boron may reduce blood phosphorus levels.

FOOD SOURCES AND SUPPLEMENTS

Boron is found in some fruits, such as apples, oranges, red grapes, pears, plums, kiwis, dates, and avocados. Other sources of boron are soybeans, nuts, chickpeas, peanut butter, red kidney beans, tomatoes, lentils, olives, and onions.

Supplements are readily available. Boron is sold in single-ingredient tablets and capsules; boron may also be combined with other vitamins and minerals such as calcium and magnesium. There are a few types of liquid boron. Small amounts of boron are often included in most multivitamins. However, there is no general agreement that boron supplementation is needed. Boric acid should never be taken by mouth; when ingested, it has poisonous properties.

INTAKE RECOMMENDATIONS

According to the U.S. National Library of Medicine at the National Institutes of Health, the average man or woman 19 years or older should consume no more than 20 mg of boron per day. All adolescents between the ages of 14 and 18 years, including those who are pregnant or breast-feeding, should have no more than 17 mg per day. Higher doses may be unsafe while pregnant or breast-feeding. Higher doses in pregnant women have been linked to birth defects. Children between the ages of 9 and 13 years should have no more than 11 mg per day; children between the ages of four and eight years should have no more than 6 mg per day; and children between one and three years should have no more than 3 mg per day.[1]

For most women, intravaginal boric acid is considered safe to use for up to six months. However, when used during the first four months of pregnancy, it has been associated with an increased risk of birth defects.

Women who have been diagnosed with hormone-sensitive conditions, such as breast cancer, uterine cancer, ovarian cancer, endometriosis, or uterine fibroids, should avoid boron supplementation or excess amounts of boron-rich foods. Boron may act like estrogen, which has the potential to exacerbate these conditions. People who have kidney problems should avoid boron supplements. Weakened kidneys may be unable to flush out boron. Excessive amounts could then build up in the heart, kidneys, and brain as well as other parts of the body.

There is no Recommended Dietary Allowance for boron supplementation. This may be a result of the limited research on boron.

DEFICIENCY AND EXCESS

With so many food sources of boron, deficiency is rare and not fully understood. It is believed that boron deficiency would result in the abnormal metabolism of calcium and magnesium. Other boron deficiency symptoms include hyperthyroidism (overactive thyroid gland), sex hormone imbalance, osteoporosis, arthritis, and neural malfunction. Excessive amounts of boron may cause a type of poisoning characterized by skin inflammation and peeling, irritability, tremors, convulsions, weakness, headaches, depression, nausea, diarrhea, and vomiting.

KEY RESEARCH FINDINGS

Boron May Be Useful for Dysmenorrhea, Painful Menstrual Cramps without Pelvic Pathology

In a study published in 2015 in the journal *Complementary Therapies in Clinical Practice*, researchers from Iran noted that dysmenorrhea or menstrual cramps is a common condition among women and negatively impacts their quality of life. They wanted to learn if boron, which has anti-inflammatory properties, would reduce the severity and duration of pain associated with this medical problem. The researchers recruited 113 university students; 58 were placed in an intervention group and 55 in a control group. At baseline, the two groups had no significant differences in severity and duration of pain. The students in the intervention group were told to take 10 mg per day of boron from two days before the menstrual flow until the third day of the flow. The members of the control group took capsules that appeared to be the same, but they were actually placebos. The students took these capsules for two consecutive menstrual cycles. Pain severity and duration measurements were taken at baseline and during the two cycles. Following the intervention, the students taking boron had significantly less pain and a significantly shorter duration of pain than the students taking the placebos. The researchers concluded that "boron supplementation can reduce the severity and duration of menstrual pain through exerting anti-inflammatory effects." And boron appeared to have no side effects.[2]

There May Be an Association between Boron and Reductions in Body Weight

In a prospective, observational study published in 2013 in the journal *Biological Trace Element Research*, researchers from Turkey evaluated the levels of boron in the blood of normal, overweight, obese, and morbidly obese subjects. Based on their body mass index, a total of 80 subjects were placed in one of these four groups; each group had 20 subjects. The researchers found a significant inverse relationship between body mass index and blood boron levels. As a result, when compared to the nonobese subjects, the heavier subjects had lower levels of boron in their blood. The researchers commented that while it is evident that boron supplement does not lower the body mass index, "the effect of boron on energy substrate utilization and mineral metabolism in causing reduction in body weight should be regarded as an important step for prevention and medical treatment of obesity."[3]

In a study published in 2011 in the *International Journal of Medical Sciences*, researchers from Turkey investigated the use of boric acid to reduce weight in mice. The researchers divided 20 mice into two groups of 10 each. The mice in the intervention group drank water treated with boric acid. On average, the mice in the intervention group received about 0.2 mg/kg per day of boric acid. The mice in the control group drank standard tap water. At the end of five days, the mice were sacrificed, and the researchers determined that the mice drinking the boric acid–treated water experienced "serious body weight reduction."[4]

A Supplement Containing Boron, Calcium, and Fructose Appears to Be Useful for Osteoarthritis

In a placebo-controlled, randomized, double-blind study published in 2011 in the journal *Biological Trace Element Research*, researchers from Romania wanted to learn if calcium fructoborate, a supplement containing boron, calcium, and fructose, would be useful for people dealing with primary osteoarthritis, a medical problem that occurs when cartilage between the joints breaks down and causes pain, stiffness, and swelling. The initial cohort consisted of 72 subjects, who were divided into four groups. For two weeks, the subjects in three of the groups took varying doses of calcium fructoborate. The subjects in one group took no calcium fructoborate and served as controls. Sixty people completed the study. The researchers determined that compared to the placebo group, all the treatment groups demonstrated reduced markers of inflammation. With less inflammation, there should be reduced pain and stiffness. "This study suggests that short-term (2 weeks) calcium fructoborate supplementation in patients with osteoarthritis symptoms has a favorable prognosis on inflammation diseases."[5]

The Supplement with Boron, Calcium, and Fructose Appears to Be Useful for Knee Discomfort

In a study published in 2014 in the journal *Clinical Interventions in Aging*, researchers from Irvine, California, wanted to learn if calcium fructoborate would be useful for people with self-reported knee discomfort. The cohort of 60 men and women, between the ages of 35 and 65 years, was randomly placed in a group to receive the supplement or a group to receive a placebo. Pain evaluations were conducted at the beginning of the study, after 7 days, and after 14 days. Beginning two weeks before the study and then during the study, participants were not allowed to consume any medications or other supplements. The researchers found that supplementation with calcium fructoborate at a dose of 110 mg twice per day significantly improved knee discomfort. The members of the placebo group did not experience any changes in their pain scores. No one reported any adverse side effects from the treatment. "Overall the result supported significant activity for CFB (calcium fructoborate) in reducing reported discomfort due to joint pain during the two-week course of the study."[6]

Boron Appears to Kill Prostate Cancer Cells

In a study published in 2014 in the journal *Tumour Biology*, researchers from Turkey wanted to determine if a compound found in boron would be useful for killing prostate cancer cells in the laboratory setting. As a result, they treated hormone-independent human prostate cancer cells with a boron agent known as disodium pentaborate decahydrate for 24, 48, and 72 hours. The researchers learned that the boron agent disrupted the normal functioning of the actin filaments of the prostate cancer cells. The threadlike actin filaments are an essential component of the building blocks of the cells. In addition, the researchers observed that the boron agent had other cell-killing effects. The researchers concluded that "DPD could be an important agent for its therapeutic potential in the treatment of prostate cancer by inducing apoptosis or cell death."[7]

NOTES

1. Medlineplus. "Boron." December 27, 2017. U.S. National Library of Medicine, National Institutes of Health. https://medlineplus.gov/druginfo/natural/894.html.

2. Nikkhah, Somayeh, Mahrokh Dolation, Mohammad Reza Naghii, et al. "Effects of Boron Supplementation on the Severity and Duration of Pain in Primary Dysmenorrhea." *Complementary Therapies in Clinical Practice* 21 (2015): 79–83.
3. Hasbahceci, Mustafa, Gokhan Cipe, Huseyin Kadioglu, et al. "Revere Relationship between Blood Boron Level and Body Mass Index in Humans: Does It Matter for Obesity?" *Biological Trace Element Research* 153, nos. 1–3 (June 2013): 141–144.
4. Aysan, Erhan, Fikrettin Sahin, Dilek Telci, et al. "Body Weight Reducing Effect of Oral Boric Acid Intake." *International Journal of Medical Sciences* 8, no. 8 (2011): 653–658.
5. Scorei, Romulus, Paul Mitrut, Iulian Petrisor, and Iulia Scorei. "A Double-Blind, Placebo-Controlled Pilot Study to Evaluate the Effect of Calcium Fructoborate on Systemic Inflammation and Dyslipidemia Markers for Middle-Aged People with Primary Osteoarthritis." *Biological Trace Element Research* 144 (2011): 253–263.
6. Pietrzkowski, Zbigniew, Michael J. Phelan, Robert Keller, et al. "Short-Term Efficacy of Calcium Fructoborate on Subjects with Knee Discomfort: A Comparative, Double-Blind, Placebo-Controlled Clinical Study." *Clinical Interventions in Aging* 9 (2014): 895–899.
7. Korkmaz, Mehmet, Cigir Biray Avci, Cumhur Gunduz, et al. "Disodium Pentaborate Decahydrate (DPD) Induced Apoptosis by Decreasing hTERT Enzyme Activity and Disrupting F-Actin Organization of Prostate Cancer Cells." *Tumour Biology* 35 (2014): 1531–1538.

REFERENCES AND FURTHER READINGS

Aysan, Erhan, Fikrettin Sahin, Dilek Telci, et al. "Body Weight Reducing Effect of Oral Boric Acid Intake." *International Journal of Medical Sciences* 8, no. 8 (2011): 653–658.

Hasbahceci, Mustafa, Gokhan Cipe, Huseyin Kadioglu, et al. "Reverse Relationship between Blood Boron Levels and Body Mass Index in Humans: Does It Matter for Obesity?" *Biological Trace Element Research* 153, nos. 1–3 (June 2013): 141–144.

Korkmaz, Mehmet, Cigir Biray Avci, Cumhur Gunduz, et al. "Disodium Pentaborate Decahydrate (DPD) Induced Apoptosis by Decreasing hTERT Enzyme Activity and Disrupting F-Actin Organization of Prostate Cancer Cells." *Tumour Biology* 35 (2014): 1531–1538.

Medlineplus. "Boron." December 27, 2017. U.S. National Library of Medicine, National Institutes of Health. https://medlineplus.gov/druginfo/natural/894.html.

Nikkhah, Somayeh, Mahrokh Dolation, Mohammad Reza Naghii, et al. "Effects of Boron Supplementation on the Severity and Duration of Pain in Primary Dysmenorrhea." *Complementary Therapies in Clinical Practice* 21, no. 2 (May 2015): 79–83.

Pietrzkowski, Zbigniew, Michael J. Phelan, Robert Keller, et al. "Short-Term Efficacy of Calcium Fructoborate on Subjects with Knee Discomfort: A Comparative, Double-Blind, Placebo-Controlled Clinical Study." *Clinical Interventions in Aging* 9 (2014): 895–899.

Scorei, Romulus, Paul Mitrut, Iulian Petrisor, and Iulia Scorei. "A Double-Blind, Placebo-Controlled Pilot Study to Evaluate the Effect of Calcium Fructoborate on Systemic Inflammation and Dyslipidemia Markers for Middle-Aged People with Primary Osteoarthritis." *Biological Trace Element Research* 144 (2011): 253–263.

Calcium

Calcium is the most abundant mineral found in the human body. And almost all of the calcium—about 99 percent—is stored in the bones and the teeth. The remaining calcium may be found in the blood, muscles, and fluids between the cells. Without calcium, the body is unable to function. It uses calcium to help muscles and blood vessels contract and expand, and to secrete hormones and enzymes. The various components of the nervous system require calcium to communicate with one another, and the brain needs calcium to communicate with other parts of the body.

Meanwhile, bones are continuously remodeling, with the constant reabsorption and depositing of calcium into new bones. Vitamin D is an essential part of this process. Without the intake or supplementation of vitamin D, this remodeling may not take place. When people are younger, more calcium is absorbed into the bones. During mid-adulthood, there is about the same amount of bone absorption and depletion. As people age closer to their senior years, more calcium is depleted from the bones. This is especially true for postmenopausal women, and it increases their risk for osteoporosis.

FOOD SOURCES AND SUPPLEMENTS

Many foods have excellent and very good amounts of calcium. These include dairy products such as milk, yogurt, and mozzarella and cheddar cheese. Other foods with higher amounts of calcium include soymilk, sardines, fortified orange juice, tofu, fortified cereal, kale, and turnip greens. Still, many people do not obtain a sufficient amount of calcium from food. For them, taking daily supplementation is normally recommended. Calcium is usually sold as calcium carbonate or calcium citrate. In order to be absorbed, calcium carbonate requires stomach acid. Therefore, it needs to be consumed with food. Calcium citrate may be taken with or without food. Calcium citrate is a better choice for people with low levels of stomach acid, inflammatory bowel disease, or gastrointestinal absorption problems. Other types of calcium in supplements or fortified foods include gluconate, lactate, and phosphate. Calcium citrate malate is found in some fortified juice. In supplements, calcium is frequently combined with magnesium. Magnesium is a key element in the body's proper assimilation of calcium. Calcium supplementation may be purchased as tablets, capsules, a chewable, or a liquid.

People who take calcium supplementation sometimes complain of side effects such as gas, bloating, and/or constipation. Calcium carbonate appears to be more associated with these problems than calcium citrate. People who are experiencing these side effects may wish to try another form of calcium and to take their supplements with meals.

INTAKE RECOMMENDATIONS

The Food and Nutrition Board has established the following Recommended Dietary Allowances for calcium: Males and females who are 71 years and older should take in 1,200 mg per day. Men between the ages of 51 and 70 years should take in 1,000 mg per day, while women between these ages should take in 1,200 mg per day. Men and women between the ages of 19 and 50 years should take in 1,000 mg per day, males and females between the ages of 9 and 18 years should take in 1,300 mg per day. Children between the ages of four and eight should take in 1,000 mg per day, while children between the ages of one and three years should take in 700 mg per day. Infants between the ages of 7 and 12 months should take in 260 mg per day, while infants between the ages of birth and six months should take in 200 mg per day.[1]

Absorption of calcium is best with doses that do not exceed 500 mg. As a result, a dose of 1,000 mg should be split into two doses and taken at two different times during the day.

DEFICIENCY AND EXCESS

In the short term, low levels of calcium have no apparent symptoms. Over a longer period of time, inadequate calcium intake may lead to osteopenia, low levels of bone density, which in turn may lead to osteoporosis, very low levels of bone density. Low levels of bone density increase the risk of bone fractures, especially hip fractures. A number of groups have an increased risk for having low calcium levels. These include males between the ages of 9 and 13 years, females between the ages of 9 and 18 years, postmenopausal women, people who avoid dairy products, people with an eating disorder, people who take medications for osteoporosis, and people who have parathyroid disorders, inflammatory bowel disease, or liver or kidney disease.

Higher intakes of calcium may cause constipation and interfere with the absorption of iron and zinc. High intake of calcium from supplements, but not food, has been associated with an increased risk of kidney stones. And a few studies have found an association between calcium supplement intake and a higher risk of cardiovascular disease.

KEY RESEARCH FINDINGS

Calcium Supplementation May Lower Diastolic Blood Pressure

In a double-blinded, placebo-controlled clinical trial published in 2015 in the *Journal of Education and Health Promotion*, researchers from Iran investigated the association between calcium supplementation and systolic (top number) and diastolic (bottom number) blood pressure. The initial cohort consisted of 75 healthy adult women between the ages of 18 and 30 years who had normal blood pressure. Almost all of the women consumed insufficient amounts of calcium. The women were randomly divided to receive 1,000 mg per day of calcium or a placebo. At the end of the 30-day trial, there were still 53 volunteers—27 in treatment and 26 in the control group. The researchers found no significant changes in the systolic readings, but there were significant reductions in the diastolic blood pressure readings. The researchers commented that their findings indicated that "calcium supplementation may be useful for people with increased diastolic blood pressure, especially for those who receive less calcium than recommended dietary allowance."[2]

There May Be an Association between Calcium Supplementation and Subclinical Cardiovascular Disease

In a study published in 2015 in the journal *Atherosclerosis*, researchers from Germany and Austria wanted to learn if supplementation with calcium placed people at increased risk for myocardial infarction and stroke. The cohort consisted of 1,601 people between the ages of 50 and 81 years, who participated in a German population-based cross-sectional study that had a seven-year follow-up. Supplemental calcium was consumed regularly by only 11.1 percent of the participants. But the regular use of calcium supplementation had a significant positive association with the presence of atrial fibrillation, an irregular, often higher, heartbeat that may be associated with a stroke. No other significant association was observed. Still, the researchers added, "The established associations do not necessarily indicate cause-effect relationships."[3]

Calcium Supplementation May Not Cause Constipation in Healthy Women

In a randomized, double-blind crossover pilot study published in 2016 in the *Canadian Journal of Dietetic Practice and Research*, researchers from Gainesville, Florida, wanted to test the common assumption that calcium supplementation is associated with constipation. The cohort consisted of 27 females with an average age of 43 years. After a two-week baseline period and separated by a two-week washout period, they each took 250 mg supplemental calcium twice daily with meals for two weeks. In addition, they completed questionnaires about capsule intake compliance and stool frequency. The researchers found no differences in stool frequency between the periods when the participants took or did not take the calcium supplements. The calcium did not appear to impact gastrointestinal mobility in the women studied. The researchers wondered if a higher dose might have yielded different results.[4]

Compliance Rates Vary in People Taking Calcium Supplementation for Osteoporosis

In an observational pilot study published in 2015 in the journal *Patient Preference and Adherence*, researchers from the Czech Republic analyzed the levels of compliance in 49 women placed on calcium and vitamin D supplementation for their osteoporosis. The women, who were all older than 55 years, were patients at one of three "osteocenters" in the Czech Republic between May 2013 and October 2014. Because they all had osteoporosis, they were at increased risk for fractures. Compliance was measured with the assistance of an electronic monitoring device. The researchers determined that the mean overall rate of compliance was 71 percent; good compliance was seen in 59 percent of the patients. As many as 71 percent of the women took "drug holidays," in which they went more than three days without taking supplementation. Interestingly, the women who took their supplementation in the afternoon or evening had a compliance rate of 82 percent, while the rate of the morning and night takers was 51 percent. The researchers commented that "consecutive supplementation-free days were common."[5]

Low-Dose Calcium May Be Useful in the Prevention of Preeclampsia

In a study published in 2014 in the journal *BJOG*, researchers from South Africa wanted to learn if low-dose calcium supplementation (less than 1 g per day) would be useful for the prevention of preeclampsia, a pregnancy complication characterized by high blood pressure and organ damage, usually the kidneys. The researchers reviewed nine trials that included a total of 2,234 women. They found that low-dose calcium supplementation in women at high risk of preeclampsia worked as well as high-dose calcium supplementation in reducing the risk of preeclampsia. The researchers commented that "the available evidence is consistent with a reduction in the risk of pre-eclampsia."[6]

Calcium-Fortified Food Does Not Appear to Alter Iron Status

In a randomized, double-blind, placebo-controlled trial published in 2016 in the *British Journal of Nutrition*, military researchers from Natick Massachusetts and Fort Eustis Virginia noted that during the early days of military training, calcium supplementation helps to maintain bone health and decreases the risk of stress fractures. They wanted to determine if adding 2,000 mg per day of calcium (as well as vitamin D) to a food product during the nine weeks of initial military training would alter the iron status of the soldiers. A total of 98 males and 54 females, who were enrolled in the U.S. Army Basic combat training program, received snack bars with or without the supplementation. They were told to consume two snacks bars between meals throughout their training; one bar in the mid-morning and a second bar in the mid-afternoon. Compliance rates were good: 88 percent in the placebo group and 81 percent in the calcium and vitamin D group. The researchers found that the supplementation did not affect the iron status of the soldiers. The researchers commented that "interventions to prevent bone injury, while improving and maintaining Fe [iron] status, are important for optimizing the health and performance of military trainees and for the successful completion of training and entry into the armed forces."[7]

Calcium Does Not Appear to Provide Protection from Colorectal Adenomas

In a randomized, multicenter, double-blind, placebo-controlled trial published in 2015 in The New England Journal of Medicine, researchers from multiple locations but based in Chapel Hill, North Carolina, wanted to test the prevailing belief that the higher intakes of calcium and vitamin D are associated with a reduced risk for colorectal adenomas or benign tumors. They initially recruited 2,259 participants, between the ages of 45 and 75 years, who had recently had adenomas removed during a colonoscopy. The participants were then assigned to take 1,200 mg calcium carbonate per day or vitamin D or calcium and vitamin D or a placebo. During follow-up colonoscopies, which were performed three to five years later, 43 percent of the 2,088 participants who were included in the analysis had one or more adenomas. The researchers determined that daily supplementation with calcium, vitamin D, or both did not reduce the incidence of colorectal adenomas. The researchers commented that the results were "contrary to our expectation." And they had "no ready explanation for the finding."[8]

There Is Some Evidence That Calcium Supplementation Improves Clinical Outcomes in Intensive Care Unit Patients

In a study published in 2015 in the journal SpringerPlus, researchers based in China wanted to determine if calcium supplementation could improve the 28-day survival rates of adult critically ill patients. They noted that electrolyte disturbance is frequently seen in critically ill patients, and calcium may play an important role in maintaining "biological homeostasis." The cohort consisted of a large clinical database of critically ill patients; it included 28,062 survivors and 4,489 nonsurvivors. The researchers found that calcium supplementation was independently associated with improved 28-day and 90-day mortality. The researchers commented that their findings "for the first time suggests that calcium supplementation may be helpful in reducing mortality in critically ill patients."[9]

Calcium and Vitamin D Supplementation Prevent Fractures

In a study published in 2016 in the journal *Osteoporosis International*, researchers from many different locations in the United States conducted a meta-analysis of randomized, controlled trials on the ability of calcium and vitamin D supplementation to reduce the incidence of total fractures and hip fractures in adults. They included eight trials with 30,970 participants, who had 2,231 total fractures and 195 hip fractures. The researchers learned that supplementation with both calcium and vitamin D produced a statistically significant 15 percent reduction in total fractures and a 30 percent reduction in hip fractures. Why is it so important to identify ways to reduce osteoporosis-related fractures? According to these researchers, it has been estimated that 53.6 million Americans aged 50 years and older have low bone mass or osteoporosis. And, every year, more than two million people in the United States experience an osteoporosis-related fracture. This accounts for more than $19 billion in annual health-care costs. The researchers noted that their findings "support the use of calcium plus vitamin D supplements as an intervention for fracture reduction in both community-dwelling and institutionalized middle-aged to older adults."[10]

The Intake of Dairy Products, Which Contain Calcium, Does Not Increase the Risk of Lung Cancer

In a meta-analysis published in 2016 in the journal *Scientific Reports*, researchers from China examined the association between the intake of dairy products, which contain calcium, and the risk of developing lung cancer. The meta-analysis consisted of 32 studies, including 12 cohort studies and 20 case-control studies. The vast majority of the studies were conducted in Europe and the Americas, and sample sizes ranged from 159 to 492,810. The lung cancer cases ranged from 56 to 4,278. The researchers found no evidence of an association between the consumption of dairy products, such as milk, cheese, yogurt, and low-fat milk and an increased risk for lung cancer. These foods were not "significantly associated with lung cancer risk."[11]

There Appears to Be an Association between Increased Consumption of High-Fat Dairy Products in Middle-Aged and Older Women and Better Weight Control

In a prospective study published in 2016 in the *American Journal of Clinical Nutrition*, researchers from Boston, Massachusetts, and Stockholm, Sweden, investigated the association between the consumption of dairy products in middle-aged and older women and weight change and obesity. The cohort consisted of 18,438 women 45 years and older from the Women's Health Study, whose initial body mass index (BMI) was between 18.5 and less than 25 or normal. Dairy intake was assessed using a 131-item food frequency questionnaire. Women who had BMI values between 25 and less than 30 were considered overweight; women who had BMI values over 30 were obese. During a mean follow-up of 11.2 years, 8,238 of the women became overweight or obese. Interestingly, greater intake of high-fat dairy products, but not intake of low-fat dairy products, was associated with less weight gain. The researchers concluded that the "greater consumption of total dairy products may be of importance in the prevention of weight gain in middle-aged and elderly women who are initially normal weight."[12]

NOTES

1. Office of Dietary Supplements, National Institutes of Health. "Calcium." December 27, 2017. https://ods.od.nih.gov.

2. Entezari, Mohammad Hassan. "The Effect of Supplementary Calcium on Blood Pressure in Healthy Adult Women Aged 18–30 Years in Tehran, Iran." *Journal of Education and Health Promotion* 4 (2015): 67+.

3. Thiele, Inke, Jakob Linseisen, Christa Meisinger, et al. "Associations between Calcium and Vitamin D Supplement Use as Well as Their Serum Concentrations and Subclinical Cardiovascular Disease Phenotypes." *Atherosclerosis* 241 (2015): 743–751.

4. Alyousif, Zainab, Amanda L. Ford, and Wendy J. Dahl. "Calcium Supplementation Does Not Contribute to Constipation in Healthy Women." *Canadian Journal of Dietetic Practice and Research* 77, no. 2 (June 2016): 103–105.

5. Touskova, Tereza, Magda Vytrisalova, Vladimir Palicka, et al. "Drug Holidays: The Most Frequent Type of Noncompliance with Calcium plus Vitamin D Supplementation in Persistent Patients with Osteoporosis." *Patient Preference and Adherence* 9 (2015): 1771–1779.

6. Hofmeyr, G.J., J.M. Belizán, and P. von Dadelszen. "Low-Dose Calcium Supplementation for Preventing Pre-Eclampsia: A Systematic Review and Commentary." *BJOG* 121, no. 8 (July 2014): 951–957.

7. Hennigar, S.R., E. Gaffney-Stomberg, L.J. Lutz, et al. "Consumption of a Calcium and Vitamin D-Fortified Food Product Does Not Affect Iron Status during Initial Military Training: A Randomized, Double-Blind, Placebo-Controlled Trial." *British Journal of Nutrition* 115, no. 4 (February 2016): 637–643.

8. Baron, John A., Elizabeth L. Barry, Leila A. Mott, et al. "A Trial of Calcium and Vitamin D for the Prevention of Colorectal Adenomas." *The New England Journal of Medicine* 373, no. 16 (October 15, 2015): 1519–1530.

9. Zhang, Zhongheng, Kun Chen, and Hongying Ni. "Calcium Supplementation Improves Clinical Outcome in Intensive Care Unit Patients: A Propensity Score Matched Analysis of a Large Clinical Database MIMIC-II." *SpringerPlus* 4 (2015): 594+.

10. Weaver, C.M., D.D. Alexander, C.J. Boushey, et al. "Calcium plus Vitamin D Supplementation and Risk of Fractures: An Updated Meta-Analysis from the National Osteoporosis Foundation." *Osteoporosis International* 27 (2016): 367–376.

11. Yang, Yang, Xu Wang, Qinghua Yao, et al. "Dairy Product, Calcium Intake and Lung Cancer Risk: A Systematic Review with Meta-Analysis." *Scientific Reports* 6 (February 15, 2016): 20624.

12. Rautiainen, Susanne, Lu Wang, I-Min Lee, et al. "Dairy Consumption in Association with Weight Change and Risk of Becoming Overweight or Obese in Middle-Aged and Older Women: A Prospective Cohort Study." *American Journal of Clinical Nutrition* 103, no. 4 (April 2016): 979–988.

REFERENCES AND FURTHER READINGS

Alyousif, Zainab, Amanda L. Ford, and Wendy J. Dahl. "Calcium Supplementation Does Not Contribute to Constipation in Healthy Women." *Canadian Journal of Dietetic Practice and Research* 77, no. 2 (June 2016): 103–105.

Baron, John A., Elizabeth L. Barry, Leila A. Mott, et al. "A Trial of Calcium and Vitamin D for the Prevention of Colorectal Adenomas." *The New England Journal of Medicine* 373, no. 16 (October 15, 2015): 1519–1530.

Entezari, Mohammad Hassan. "The Effect of Supplementary Calcium on Blood Pressure in Healthy Adult Women Aged 18–30 Years in Tehran, Iran." *Journal of Education and Health Promotion* 4 (2015): 67+.

Hennigar, S. R., E. Gaffney-Stomberg, L. J. Lutz, et al. "Consumption of a Calcium and Vitamin D-Fortified Food Product Does Not Affect Iron Status during Initial Military Training: A Randomized, Double-Blind, Placebo-Controlled Trial." *British Journal of Nutrition* 115, no. 4 (February 2016): 637–643.

Hofmeyr, G. J., J. M. Belizán, and P. von Dadelszen. "Low-Dose Calcium Supplementation for Preventing Pre-Eclampsia: A Systematic Review and Commentary." *BJOG* 121, no. 8 (July 2014): 951–957.

Office of Dietary Supplements, National Institutes of Health. "Calcium." December 27, 2017. https://ods.od.nih.gov/factsheets/Calcium-Consumer/.

Rautiainen, Susanne, Lu Wang, I-Min Lee, et al. "Dairy Consumption in Association with Weight Change and Risk of Becoming Overweight or Obese in Middle-Aged and Older Women: A Prospective Cohort Study." *American Journal of Clinical Nutrition* 103, no. 4 (April 2016): 979–988.

Thiele, Inke, Jakob Linseisen, Christa Meisinger, et al. "Associations between Calcium and Vitamin D Supplement Use as Well as Their Serum Concentrations and Subclinical Cardiovascular Disease Phenotypes." *Atherosclerosis* 241 (2015): 743–751.

Touskova, Tereza, Magda Vytrisalova, Vladimir Palicka, et al. "Drug Holidays: The Most Frequent Type of Noncompliance with Calcium plus Vitamin D Supplementation in Persistent Patients with Osteoporosis." *Patient Preference and Adherence* 9 (2015): 1771–1779.

Weaver, C. M., D. D. Alexander, C. J. Boushey, et al. "Calcium plus Vitamin D Supplementation and Risk of Fractures: An Updated Meta-Analysis from the National Osteoporosis Foundation." *Osteoporosis International* 27 (2016): 367–376.

Yang, Yang, Xu Wang, Qinghua Yao, et al. "Dairy Product, Calcium Intake and Lung Cancer Risk: A Systematic Review with Meta-Analysis." *Scientific Reports* 6 (February 15, 2016): 20624.

Zhang, Zhongheng, Kun Chen, and Hongying Ni. "Calcium Supplementation Improves Clinical Outcome in Intensive Care Unit Patients: A Propensity Score Matched Analysis of a Large Clinical Database MIMIC-II." *SpringerPlus* 4 (2015): 594+.

Choline

The National Academy of Sciences added choline to the list of required nutrients in 1998. While it is relatively new to the list of human vitamins, choline is considered to be a nutrient that should be part of everyone's everyday diet. Although it was previously thought that the body could make its own choline, that is no longer believed to be true. Researchers now advise people that choline should be obtained from an outside source, such as the diet or a supplement.

Choline, which is water soluble, plays a key role in the basic cellular functioning of the body. It is essential for liver function, normal brain development, nerve function, and muscle movement. It supports energy levels and helps maintain a healthy metabolism. Choline is a key nutrient in the production of phosphatidylcholine, an important structural building block of living cells, and it is an essential part of the process of methylation, which is needed to create DNA. Choline is also a crucial component of the neurotransmitter acetylcholine. Without acetylcholine, muscles cannot contract—the heart is unable to beat and the gastrointestinal track is unable to move along the food that has been consumed.

FOOD SOURCES AND SUPPLEMENTS

Excellent food sources of choline include shrimp, eggs (especially egg yolks), beef liver, and scallops. Other very good and good food sources of choline include chicken, turkey, tuna, cod, salmon, sardines, green peas, cabbage, soy products, quinoa, and beef. Vegetables with good amounts of choline include collard greens, Brussels sprouts, broccoli, Swiss chard, cauliflower, shitake and crimini mushrooms, green beans, bok choy, summer squash, and asparagus. Other sources are chickpeas, split peas, milk, nuts, and navy beans. In addition, choline is found in food additives such as soy lecithin, a widely used emulsifying agent that helps to keep oil and water-soluble ingredients from separating in packaged foods. Choline is sold in tablets and capsules by itself or, most often, with inositol, also known as vitamin B8. It may also be found in multivitamins.

INTAKE RECOMMENDATIONS

In 1998, the Food and Nutrition Board of the U.S. Institute of Medicine established adequate intake levels for choline. Lactating women and males who are 14 years old or older should take in 550 mg per day, while pregnant women should take in 450 mg per day. Females who are 19 years or older should take in 425 mg per day, while females who are between 14 and 18 years should take in 400 mg per day. Children between the ages of 9 and 13 years should take in 375 mg per day, while children between the ages of 4 and 8 years should take in 250 mg per day. Children between the ages of one and three years should take in 200 mg per day; infants between the ages of 6 and 12 months should take in 150 mg per day; and infants up to the age of six months should take in 125 mg per day. It also established a tolerable upper intake level of 3.5 g per day for most adults.[1]

DEFICIENCY AND EXCESS

While most people probably consume adequate amounts of choline in their diets, it may not be properly absorbed. And some people simply have higher requirements for choline. Symptoms of choline deficiency include nerve damage, learning problems, memory loss, cognitive decline, low energy levels, and mood changes. People with a condition known as "fatty liver," in which triglyceride fat accumulates in the cells of the liver, are at increased risk of choline deficiency. People who drink excessive amounts of alcohol and those who are obese or have types 2 diabetes are also at increased risk for choline deficiency. Some believe that choline deficiency may play a role in age-related cognitive decline, including Alzheimer's disease.

Excessive amounts of choline supplementation may be toxic. Symptoms of choline toxicity include changes in blood pressure, diarrhea, nausea, fatigue, excessive sweating, and a fishy odor of the skin.

KEY RESEARCH FINDINGS

Intake of Choline Does Not Appear to Be Associated with Cardiovascular Disease Mortality

In a study published in 2015 in *The Journal of Nutrition*, researchers from Japan examined the association between choline intake and cardiovascular disease mortality. The cohort consisted of 13,355 males and 15,724 females, 35 years or older, who were residents of Takayama City, Japan. Their diets were assessed using validated food frequency questionnaires. Deaths from coronary heart disease and stroke were identified from death certificates. During the 16-year follow-up, the researchers documented 308 deaths from coronary heart disease and 676 deaths from stroke. The researchers found no association between intake of choline and cardiovascular disease mortality.[2]

Choline Supplementation during Pregnancy May Reduce the Risk of the Later Development of Schizophrenia

In a randomized, placebo-controlled clinical trial published in 2013 in the *American Journal of Psychiatry*, researchers based in Colorado tested the ability of a dietary supplement known as phosphatidylcholine, which converts into choline in the body, to help prevent a child's future development of schizophrenia. While schizophrenia does not generally manifest symptoms until late adolescence or adulthood, it is believed to be caused by a combination of genes and the environment that are present during pregnancy. The researchers initially recruited

100 healthy pregnant women; at the beginning of their second trimester, they were placed on either the supplement or a placebo. Every day, the pregnant women on the supplement took the equivalent of the amount of choline in three large eggs. After delivery, the infants of the mothers on choline were placed on choline supplementation for 12 weeks. Neither the mothers nor the infants experienced any side effects from the choline. Although seven women dropped out of the study, the remaining 93 women had notable results. Testing administered after the infants were born found that the infants of the mothers on choline were far less likely to have physiologic factors associated with the future development of schizophrenia, such as responses to a pair of clicking sounds and the presence of a specific genotype. The researchers recommended the longer-term follow-up of the children who received the supplement.[3]

A Choline-Rich Diet Appears to Be Associated with a Sharper Memory

In a study published in 2011 in the *American Journal of Clinical Nutrition*, researchers based in Boston examined the association between dietary intake of choline and memory. The dementia-free cohort included 1,391 subjects between the ages of 36 and 83 years from the Framingham Offspring population. Between 1991 and 1995, the subjects completed food frequency questionnaires, and between 1998 and 2001, they had neuropsychological evaluations and brain MRIs. The researchers found that the men and women in the top quarter of choline intake performed better on the memory tests than those on the bottom quarter. And people who had lower intakes of choline were more likely to be on a pathway toward mental decline than their counterparts with higher intakes. Moreover, the subjects with higher choline intake at the outset of the trial were less likely to show areas of "white-matter hyperintensity" in their MRI scans. These areas are believed to be an indication of blood vessel disease, which may signal a heightened risk of stroke or dementia. The researchers concluded that "in this community-based population of nondemented individuals, higher concurrent choline intake was related to better cognitive performance."[4]

Intake of Choline Is Associated with a Reduced Risk of Breast Cancer

In a case-control study published in 2013 in the journal *Cancer Science*, researchers based in China investigated the association between intake of choline and risk of breast cancer among Chinese women. The cohort consisted of 807 women with confirmed breast cancer and 807 matched controls. To improve the statistical power of the study, the researchers recruited a second set of cases and controls. This time there were 369 cases and 369 controls. Dietary assessments were made with face-to-face interviews and validated food frequency questionnaires. The main sources of choline were eggs, chicken, and while milk. The researchers learned that the intake of total choline was inversely related to breast cancer in a dose-response manner. Thus, higher intakes of choline were associated with lower risks for breast cancer. "The mean dietary choline intake in the control group of the present study was 173 mg/day, which shows the potential deficiency of choline in the current study population."[5]

In a study published in 2008 in *FASEB Journal*, researchers from New York City and Chapel Hill, North Carolina, wanted to examine the association between intake of choline and incidence of breast cancer. The cohort consisted of a population-based study, the Long Island Breast Cancer Study Project, of 1,508 cases and 1,556 controls. The participants ranged in age from 20 to 98 years. The researchers found an association between the highest intake of choline consumption and a reduced risk of breast cancer. By eating high amounts of dietary choline, women reduced their risk of breast cancer by 24 percent. According to the researchers, "Choline metabolism may play an important role in breast cancer etiology."[6]

Prenatal Dietary Choline Appears to Improve Memory in Adult Rats

In a study published in 2013 in *Nutritional Neuroscience*, researchers from Spain noted that choline is an essential nutrient required for early development. They wanted to learn more about the effect a choline prenatal supplement would have on adult memory. As a result, the researchers divided pregnant Wistar rats into three groups. One group of five rats was fed a choline-deficient diet; a second group of seven rats was fed a standard rat diet; and a third group of five rats was fed a choline-supplemented diet. When the offspring were born, they were fed a standard rat diet. At the age of three months, the offspring were put through memory tests. By the second retention test, it became evident that the offspring whose mothers ate the supplemented food had better memory scores. The researchers noted that their findings "supported the notion of long-lasting beneficial effect of prenatal choline supplementation on object recognition memory which is evident when the rats reach adulthood."[7]

Higher Dietary Choline Intake Seems to Lower the Risk of Nonalcoholic Fatty Liver Disease

In a study published in 2014 in *The Journal of Nutrition*, researchers from Nashville, Tennessee, and China wanted to determine if there was an association between dietary intake of choline and nonalcoholic fatty liver disease in the general population. Nonalcoholic fatty liver disease is associated with several medical problems, including insulin resistance, dyslipidemia, cardiovascular disease, some cancers, and liver-related morbidity and mortality. The cohort consisted of 56,195 Chinese men and women between the ages of 40 and 75 years, who drank no alcohol or negligible amounts of alcohol. All of the participants completed food frequency questionnaires and had at least one liver ultrasound examination. Their primary sources of dietary choline were eggs, soy foods, red meat, fish and shellfish, and vegetables. The researchers learned that choline intake was inversely associated with fatty liver in middle-aged and older normal-weight women. This association did not exist for overweight or obese women.[8]

Choline May Help Prevent the Development of Pancreatic Cancer

In a study published in 2016 in the journal *Cancer Epidemiology, Biomarkers & Prevention*, researchers from Pittsburgh, Pennsylvania, and Singapore examined the association between the intake of several nutrients, including choline, and the risk of pancreatic cancer "among the most deadly malignancies in the world." The cohort initially consisted of 63,257 men and women, between the ages of 45 and 74 years, enrolled in the Singapore Chinese Health Study. All the participants were residents of Singapore. Nutrient assessments were made using a food frequency questionnaire. During an average follow-up of 16.3 years, there were 271 incident cases of pancreatic cancer. The mean age at cancer diagnosis was 72 years for males and 71.6 years for females. In the final analysis, which included 60,298 subjects, the researchers found that higher intakes of choline were associated with statistically significant decreases in the risk of developing pancreatic cancer. This association was more apparent in men than in women.[9]

NOTES

1. U.S. Institute of Medicine. "Choline." December 28, 2017. https://iom.nationalacademies.org.

2. Nagata, Chisato, Keiko Wada, Takashi Tamura, et al. "Choline and Betaine Intakes Are Not Associated with Cardiovascular Disease Mortality Risk in Japanese Men and Women." *The Journal of Nutrition* 145 (2015): 1787–1792.

3. Ross, Randal G., Sharon K. Hunter, Lizbeth McCarthy, et al. "Perinatal Choline Effects on Neonatal Pathophysiology Related to Later Schizophrenia Risk." *American Journal of Psychiatry* 170 (March 2013): 290–298.

4. Poly, Coreyann, Joseph M. Massaro, Sudha Seshadri, et al. "The Relation of Dietary Choline to Cognitive Performance and White-Matter Hyperintensity in the Framingham Offspring Cohort." *American Journal of Clinical Nutrition* 94 (2011): 1584–1591.

5. Zhang, Cai-Xia, Mei-Xia Pan, Bin Li, et al. "Choline and Betaine Intake Is Inversely Associated with Breast Cancer Risk: A Two-Stage Case-Control Study in China." *Cancer Science* 104, no. 2 (February 2013): 250–258.

6. Xu, Xinran, Marilie D. Gammon, Steven H. Zeisel, et al. "Choline Metabolism and Risk of Breast Cancer in a Population-Based Study." *FASEB Journal* 22 (2008): 2045–2052.

7. Moreno, Hayarelis C., Isabel de Brugada, Diamela Carias, and Milagros Gallo. "Long-Lasting Effects of Prenatal Dietary Choline Availability on Object Recognition Memory Ability in Adult Rats." *Nutritional Neuroscience* 16, no. 6 (2013): 269–274.

8. Yu, Danxia, Xiao-Ou Shu, Yong-Bing Xiang, et al. "Higher Dietary Choline Intake Is Associated with Lower Risk of Nonalcoholic Fatty Liver in Normal-Weight Chinese Women." *The Journal of Nutrition* 144 (2014): 2034–2040.

9. Huang, Joyce Y., Lesley M. Butler, Renwei Wang, et al. "Dietary Intake of One-Carbon Metabolism-Related Nutrients and Pancreatic Cancer Risk: The Singapore Chinese Health Study." *Cancer Epidemiology, Biomarkers & Prevention* 25, no. 2 (February 2016): 417–424.

REFERENCES AND FURTHER READINGS

The George Mateljan Foundation. "Choline." December 28, 2017. http://whfoods.com/genpage.php?tname=nutrient&dbid=50.

Huang, Joyce Y., Lesley M. Butler, Renwei Wang, et al. "Dietary Intake of One-Carbon Metabolism-Related Nutrients and Pancreatic Cancer Risk: The Singapore Chinese Health Study." *Cancer Epidemiology, Biomarkers & Prevention* 25, no. 2 (February 2016): 417–424.

Moreno, Hayarelis C., Isabel de Brugada, Diamela Carias, and Milagros Gallo. "Long-Lasting Effects of Prenatal Dietary Choline Availability on Object Recognition Memory Ability in Adult Rats." *Nutritional Neuroscience* 16, no. 6 (2013): 269–274.

Nagata, Chisato, Keiko Wada, Takashi Tamura, et al. "Choline and Betaine Intakes Are Not Associated with Cardiovascular Disease Mortality Risk in Japanese Men and Women." *The Journal of Nutrition* 145 (2015): 1787–1792.

Poly, Coreyann, Joseph M. Massaro, Sudha Seshadri, et al. "The Relation of Dietary Choline to Cognitive Performance and White-Matter Hyperintensity in the Framingham Offspring Cohort." *American Journal of Clinical Nutrition* 94 (2011): 1584–1591.

Ross, Randal G., Sharon K. Hunter, Lizbeth McCarthy, et al. "Perinatal Choline Effects on Neonatal Pathophysiology Related to Later Schizophrenia Risk." *American Journal of Psychiatry* 170 (March 2013): 290–298.

U.S. Institute of Medicine. "Choline." December 28, 2017. https://iom.nationalacademies.org.

Xu, Xinran, Marilie D. Gammon, Steven H. Zeisel, et al. "Choline Metabolism and Risk of Breast Cancer in a Population-Based Study." *FASEB Journal* 22 (June 2008): 2045–2052.

Yu, Danxia, Xiao-Ou Shu, Yong-Bing Xiang, et al. "Higher Dietary Choline Intake Is Associated with Lower Risk of Nonalcoholic Fatty Liver in Normal-Weight Chinese Women." *The Journal of Nutrition* 144 (2014): 2034–2040.

Zeisel, Steven and Marie A. Caudill. "Choline." *Advance in Nutrition* 1 (2010): 46–48.

Zhang, Cai-Xia, Mei-Xia Pan, Bin Li, et al. "Choline and Betaine Intake Is Inversely Associated with Breast Cancer Risk: A Two-Stage Case-Control Study in China." *Cancer Science* 104, no. 2 (February 2013): 250–258.

Chromium

It is very fortunate that the body requires only trace amounts of the mineral chromium. While chromium is found in many foods, such as vegetables, fruits, grains, legumes, nuts, seeds, seafood, meats, and dairy, these foods generally have only small amounts—1 to 2 mcg or less. Food sources with larger amounts of chromium are exceedingly rare.

It is known that chromium plays an essential role in helping the hormone insulin regulate blood sugar levels. People have been using brewer's yeast, which contains chromium, since the American Civil War to balance blood sugar levels. That is why there is some evidence that chromium supplements may be useful for people with type 2 diabetes.

It is known that vitamin C enhances the absorption of chromium. As a result, it is a good idea to take supplemental chromium with a vitamin C supplement or with a food that contains high amounts of vitamin C, such as berries and citrus fruits. In terms of chromium, the best food is broccoli; it contains high amounts of both chromium and vitamin C.[1]

FOOD SOURCES AND SUPPLEMENTS

While the only excellent source of chromium is broccoli, chromium is found in slightly better-than-average amounts in brewer's yeast, whole grain breads and cereals, lean meats, organ meats, grape juice, red wine, cheese, black pepper, and thyme. Other sources include barley, oats, green beans, tomatoes, molasses, prunes, orange juice, and romaine lettuce. As a supplement, chromium is most often sold as chromium picolinate in a tablet or capsule. But it may be purchased as a single ingredient or as chromium chloride, chromium nicotinate, chromium histidinate, high-chromium yeast, and chromium citrate. Since there are minimal data on the topic, it is not clear if some forms are preferable.

INTAKE RECOMMENDATIONS

The Food and Nutrition Board has established the following adequate intake levels of chromium. Adult men between the ages of 19 and 50 years should take 35 mcg per day, while adult men 51 years and older should take in 30 mcg per day. Adult women between the ages of 19 and 50 years should take in 25 mcg per day, while adult women 50 years and older should take in 20 mcg per day. Pregnant and breastfeeding females 19 years and older should take in 30 mcg per day. Pregnant teens between the ages of 14 and 18 years should take in 29 mcg per day, while breastfeeding teens between the ages of 14 and 18 years should take in 44 mcg per day. Male teens between the ages of 14 and 18 years should take in 35 mcg per day, while female teens between the ages of 14 and 18 years should take in 24 mcg per day. Boys between the ages of 9 and 13 years should take in 25 mcg per day, while girls between the ages of 9 and 13 should take in 21 mcg per day. Children between the ages of four and eight years should take in 15 mcg per day, while children between the ages of one and three years should take in 11 mcg per day. Infants between the ages of 7 and 12 months should take in 5.5 mcg per day, while infants from birth to six months should take in 0.2 mcg per day.[2]

DEFICIENCY AND EXCESS

While it has been estimated that as many as 90 percent of Americans have diets that are low in chromium, it is believed that true chromium deficiency is rare. The people most likely to be deficient in chromium are those who participate in excessive strenuous exercise, those who eat large amounts of sugary foods or highly refined foods, people on prolonged intravenous nutrition, women who are pregnant, and the elderly. People who have low levels of serum chromium may have elevated levels of blood sugar, triglycerides (a type of fat), and cholesterol, and they may be at increased risk for type 2 diabetes and cardiovascular disease.

Chromium from food is generally considered to be safe. On the other hand, very high doses of this mineral may reduce the ability of insulin to control blood sugar and may cause stomach irritation, itching, and flushing. There are a few anecdotal reports of high levels of chromium causing irregular heart rhythms and liver problems, and high levels of chromium picolinate supplementation may be associated with kidney damage. People with mental health problems should consult their health-care provider before taking chromium supplementation. While chromium may be useful for mental health conditions, the data are not definitive.

KEY RESEARCH FINDINGS

There Appears to Be an Association between Morbid Obesity and Serum Chromium Deficiency

In a study published in 2014 in the journal *Obesity Surgery*, researchers from Brazil wanted to learn more about the association between people who are extremely overweight and levels of serum chromium. The cohort consisted of 73 morbidly obese patients, mostly women, awaiting bariatric surgery (surgery to help people lose weight). Their mean age was 37.2 years, and their mean duration of obesity was almost 16 years. The researchers found that 64 of the patients (87.7%) had chromium deficiency. That is a notable number. Thus, while the patients were clearly eating large amounts of foods, they were not eating foods with sufficient amounts of chromium. The researchers commented that "early nutritional interventions are needed to reduce nutritional deficiencies."[3]

Chromium May Be Useful for Binge Eating Disorder and Other Psychiatric Problems

In a pilot study published in 2013 in the *Journal of Psychosomatic Research*, researchers from Chapel Hill, North Carolina, wanted to learn if there was an association between chromium and binge eating disorder and other psychiatric problems. Binge eating disorder was defined as the consumption of an unusually large amount of food coupled with a feeling of the loss of control over eating. The cohort consisted of 24 overweight adults with binge eating disorder. They were enrolled in a six-month double-blind, placebo-controlled trial and randomly assigned to receive either 1,000 mcg chromium per day (n = 8) or 600 mcg chromium per day as chromium picolinate (n = 9) or a placebo (n = 7). When compared to the placebo group, the researchers found that the fasting glucose of the members of the two chromium group was significantly reduced. Though the results were not statistically significant, the researchers found that the members of the chromium groups had reductions in binge frequency, weight, and the symptoms of depression. The researchers noted that as a result of their findings they believe that "further study of dietary chromium supplementation is warranted as the direction of effects indicates that it may help curb binge eating and related psychopathology, promote modest weight loss and reductions in symptoms of depression."[4]

It Is Not Clear If Chromium May Play a Role in Weight Loss

In a randomized, double-blind, placebo-controlled pilot trial published in 2010 in *The Journal of Alternative and Complementary Medicine*, researchers from Derby and New Haven, Connecticut, wanted to determine if chromium picolinate supplementation would be useful for weight loss. The initial cohort consisted of 80 overweight but healthy adults; there were 40 males and 40 females. The subjects were assigned to take two daily doses of 500 mcg of chromium picolinate or a placebo. All of the subjects received nutritional and weight loss education. At baseline, the body mass indices of both groups were similar; at the end of the 24-week study, the intervention and placebo groups, which included 58 subjects, still had similar body mass index readings. The chromium supplementation did not appear to promote weight loss in these overweight individuals. The researchers commented that there appears to be a "reduced enthusiasm for the use of chromium as a nutritional supplement for controlling weight."[5]

In a meta-analysis published in 2013 in *Obesity Reviews*, researchers from the United Kingdom wanted to learn if chromium supplementation was truly effective for weight loss in overweight and obese people. The meta-analysis included 18 randomized, placebo-controlled, double-blind trials that continued for at least eight weeks and included 978 subjects. In the majority of these trials, chromium supplementation resulted in statistically significant weight loss. But there was a good deal of variability. And there were reports of side effects, including watery stools, constipation, decreased appetite, vertigo, weakness, nausea, vomiting, dizziness, headaches, and hives. When the supplementation was discontinued, the side effects stopped, and they restarted if the supplementation was reintroduced. While the trials showed that chromium supplementation could generate statistically significant reductions in body weight, "the magnitude of the effect is small, and the clinical relevance is uncertain."[6]

Chromium May Improve Cognitive Functioning

In a double-blind, placebo-controlled study published in 2010 in the journal *Nutritional Neuroscience*, researchers from Cincinnati, Ohio, wanted to learn if chromium supplementation improved cognitive functioning in older adults. For 12 weeks, 12 men and 14 women from the greater Cincinnati area received either chromium picolinate or a placebo. Prior to the study, all of the participants, who were generally in their late 60s and early 70s, had experienced mild declines in memory. Assessments were made of memory and depression prior to the beginning of the supplementation and during the final week of supplementation. A subset of 13 subjects (9 from the treatment group and 4 from the placebo group) had magnetic resonance imaging scans. The subjects on the supplement did experience some degree of cognitive improvement, but the rate of learning and the level of retention were not enhanced. Still, the researchers concluded that "ultimately, chromium supplementation may be shown to be an effective intervention for older adults with early memory decline and metabolic disturbance factors that substantially increase risk for dementia."[7]

It Is Not Clear If Chromium Supplementation Is Useful for People with Type 2 Diabetes

In a study published in 2013 in the *Journal of Pharmacy & Pharmaceutical Sciences*, researchers from Iran wanted to determine if people with type 2 diabetes would benefit from chromium supplementation. They hoped to learn if chromium would be useful in controlling glucose levels and lipid profiles. As a result, they conducted a meta-analysis of seven trials. The researchers found that chromium supplementation significantly reduced fasting blood sugar, but it appeared to have no cholesterol-lowering benefit. Moreover, chromium failed to lower the body mass index. The researchers concluded that their findings did not find strong evidence that chromium supplement is useful for people with type 2 diabetes.[8]

Chromium Supplementation May Be Useful for Overweight and Obese People with Prediabetes

In a single-center, randomized, double-blind, placebo-controlled study published in 2015 in the online journal *PLoS ONE*, researchers from Paris wanted to learn if a supplement containing chromium, cinnamon, and carnosine (a protein building block that is naturally produced in the body) would be useful for overweight and obese people with prediabetes. Between November 2011 and April 2012, the researchers enrolled 62 overweight or obese subjects with prediabetes. For four months, the subjects, who were between the ages of 25 and 65 years, took the supplement or a placebo. After the trial ended, the 52 subjects who were still in the study were followed for up to six months. When compared to the subjects taking the placebo, the subjects on the supplement experienced significant reductions in fasting plasma glucose levels as well as significant increases in lean mass. The researchers noted that their findings "might open up new avenues in the prevention of diabetes."[9]

Chromium Supplementation Appears to Have Some Useful Properties for People with Diabetes

In a meta-analysis published in 2014 in the *Journal of Clinical Pharmacy and Therapeutics*, researchers from Thailand wanted to learn more about the effects chromium supplementation has on people with diabetes. The researchers included 25 randomized, controlled trials in their investigation. In 22 of these studies, the supplements contained only chromium. Duration of supplementation ranged from 3 to 24 weeks, and the doses of chromium varied from trial to trial. The researchers found that chromium supplementation improved the control of sugar levels. In addition, chromium supplementation reduced triglyceride levels and increased levels of HDL or "good cholesterol." Interestingly, the risk of adverse effects was the same for those taking chromium supplementation and those taking a placebo. The researchers concluded that "diabetic patients with inadequate glycaemic control may benefit from supplementation with chromium."[10]

Chromium Picolinate May Be Useful for Symptoms Associated with Polycystic Ovary Syndrome

In a double-blind, randomized, controlled trial published in 2016 in the journal *Obstetrics and Gynaecology Research*, researchers from Egypt wanted to learn if chromium picolinate supplementation would be useful for the symptoms associated with polycystic ovary syndrome, an endocrine disorder seen in women of reproductive age. Common symptoms include menstrual difficulties, excess weight, and insulin resistance. The cohort consisted of 85 women, between the ages of 20 and 35 years, who were diagnosed with polycystic ovary syndrome. For six months, the women were almost evenly divided into two groups. The participants in one group took chromium picolinate supplementation and those in the other group took a placebo. The women were encouraged to eat a healthy diet and exercise. By the end of the trial, the women on chromium experienced significant reductions in fasting serum insulin and body mass index. Chromium supplementation improved the rates of ovulation and regular menstruation. The researchers commented that "given the relative safety and low cost of chromium supplements, the benefit-to-risk ratio available so far still favors their use."[11]

NOTES

1. The George Mateljan Foundation. "Chromium." December 28, 2017. www.whfoods.com.

2. Office of Dietary Supplements, National Institutes of Health. "Chromium." December 28, 2017. https://ods.od.nih.gov.

3. Lima, Karla V.G., Raquel P.A. Lima, Maria C.R. Gonçalves, et al. "High Frequency of Serum Chromium Deficiency and Association of Chromium with Triglyceride and Cholesterol Concentrations in Patients Awaiting Bariatric Surgery." *Obesity Surgery* 24 (2014): 771–776.

4. Brownley, Kimberly A., Ann Von Holle, Robert M. Hamer, et al. "A Double-Blind, Randomized Pilot Trial of Chromium Picolinate for Binge Eating Disorder: Results of the Binge Eating and Chromium (BEACh) Study." *Journal of Psychosomatic Research* 75 (2013): 36–42.

5. Yazaki, Yuka, Zubaida Faridi, Yingying Ma, et al. "A Pilot Study of Chromium Picolinate for Weight Loss." *The Journal of Alternative and Complementary Medicine* 16, no. 3 (2010): 291–299.

6. Onakpoya, I., P. Posadzki, and E. Ernst. "Chromium Supplementation in Overweight and Obesity: A Systematic Review and Meta-Analysis of Randomized Clinical Trials." *Obesity Reviews* 14 (June 2013): 496–507.

7. Krikorian, Robert, James C. Eliassen, Erin L. Boespflug, et al. "Improved Cognitive-Cerebral Function in Older Adults with Chromium Supplementation." *Nutritional Neuroscience* 13, no. 3 (2010): 116–122.

8. Abdollahi, Mohammad, Amir Farshchi, Shekoufeh Nikfar, and Meysam Seyedifar. "Effect of Chromium on Glucose and Lipid Profiles in Patients with Type 2 Diabetes: A Meta-Analysis Review of Randomized Trials." *Journal of Pharmacy & Pharmaceutical Sciences* 16, no. 1 (2013): 99–114.

9. Liu, Y., A. Cotillard, C. Vatier, et al. "A Dietary Supplement Containing Cinnamon, Chromium and Carnosine Decreases Fasting Plasma Glucose and Increases Lean Mass in Overweight or Obese Pre-Diabetic Subjects: A Randomized, Placebo-Controlled Trial." *PLoS ONE* 10, no. 9 (2015): e0138646.

10. Suksomboon, N., N. Poolsup, and A. Yuwanakorn. "Systematic Review and Meta-Analysis of the Efficacy and Safety of Chromium Supplementation in Diabetes." *Journal of Clinical Pharmacy and Therapeutics* 39 (2014): 292–306.

11. Ashoush, Sherif, Amgad Abou-Gamrah, Hassan Bayoumy, and Noura Othman. "Chromium Picolinate Reduces Insulin Resistance in Polycystic Ovary Syndrome: Randomized Controlled Trial." *Obstetrics and Gynaecology Research* 42, no. 3 (March 2016): 279–285.

REFERENCES AND FURTHER READINGS

Abdollahi, Mohammad, Amir Farshchi, Shekoufeh Nikfar, and Meysam Seyedifar. "Effect of Chromium on Glucose and Lipid Profiles in Patients with Type 2 Diabetes: A Meta-Analysis Review of Randomized Trials." *Journal of Pharmacy & Pharmaceutical Sciences* 16, no. 1 (2013): 99–114.

Ashoush, Sherif, Amgad Abou-Gamrah, Hassan Bayoumy, and Noura Othman. "Chromium Picolinate Reduces Insulin Resistance in Polycystic Ovary Syndrome: Randomized Controlled Trial." *Obstetrics and Gynaecology Research* 42, no. 3 (March 2016): 279–285.

Brownley, Kimberly A., Ann Von Holle, Robert M. Hamer, et al. "A Double-Blind, Randomized Pilot Trial of Chromium Picolinate for Binge Eating Disorder: Results of the Binge Eating and Chromium (BEACh) Study." *Journal of Psychosomatic Research* 75 (2013): 36–42.

The George Mateljan Foundation. "Chromium." December 28, 2017. http://whfoods.com/genpage.php?tname=nutrient&dbid=51.

Krikorian, Robert, James C. Eliassen, Erin L. Boespflug, et al. "Improved Cognitive-Cerebral Function in Older Adults with Chromium Supplementation." *Nutritional Neuroscience* 13, no. 3 (2010): 116–122.

Lima, Karla V. G., Raquel P. A. Lima, Maria C. R. Gonçalves, et al. "High Frequency of Serum Chromium Deficiency and Association of Chromium with Triglyceride and Cholesterol Concentrations in Patients Awaiting Bariatric Surgery." *Obesity Surgery* 24 (2014): 771–776.

Liu, Y., A. Cotillard, C. Vatier, et al. "A Dietary Supplement Containing Cinnamon, Chromium and Carnosine Decreases Fasting Plasma Glucose and Increases Lean Mass in Overweight or Obese Pre-Diabetic Subjects: A Randomized, Placebo-Controlled Trial." *PLoS ONE* 10, no. 9 (2015): e0138646.

Office of Dietary Supplements, National Institutes of Health. "Chromium." December 28, 2017. https://ods.od.nih.gov/factsheets/Chromium-HealthProfessional/.

Onakpoya, I., P. Posadzki, and E. Ernst. "Chromium Supplementation in Overweight and Obesity: A Systematic Review and Meta-Analysis of Randomized Clinical Trials." *Obesity Reviews* 14 (June 2013): 496–507.

Suksomboon, N., N. Poolsup, and A. Yuwanakorn. "Systematic Review and Meta-Analysis of the Efficacy and Safety of Chromium Supplementation in Diabetes." *Journal of Clinical Pharmacy and Therapeutics* 39 (2014): 292–306.

Yazaki, Yuka, Zubaida Faridi, Yingying Ma, et al. "A Pilot Study of Chromium Picolinate for Weight Loss." *The Journal of Alternative and Complementary Medicine* 16, no. 3 (2010): 291–299.

Copper

Though it is normally found only in small amounts in the body, copper is a crucial mineral that is essential for many of the body's functions. Copper plays a key role in building strong tissue, maintaining blood volume, and producing energy in cells. Copper is needed to form an enzyme known as superoxide dismutase (SOD). The debilitating and ultimately fatal illness known as amyotrophic lateral sclerosis or Lou Gehrig's disease is believed to be associated with an underfunctioning SOD enzyme.

Copper is necessary for the body to make collagen, a major structural protein. It supports the incorporation of iron into red blood cells and helps to generate energy from the carbohydrates inside of cells. The body stores copper primarily in the bones and muscles, and the liver regulates the amount of copper in the blood.

FOOD SOURCES AND SUPPLEMENTS

There are many excellent sources of copper. These include liver, sesame seeds, cashews, soybeans, shitake mushrooms, beet greens, turnip greens, spinach, asparagus, Swiss chard, kale, mustard greens, and summer squash. Foods with very good amounts of copper include sunflower seeds, garbanzo beans, lentils, walnuts, pumpkin seeds, tofu, peanuts, kidney beans, shrimp, almonds, grapes, beets, raspberries, tomatoes, broccoli, cabbage, and eggplant. There are also many foods with good amounts of copper, including black beans, quinoa, barley, oats, potatoes, onions, bananas, cantaloupe, green beans, watermelon, carrots, celery, and apricots.

Copper supplementation is available in tablets, capsules, and liquids. Copper may be the only ingredient or combined with another mineral, such as zinc, or several other trace minerals.

INTAKE RECOMMENDATIONS

The Food and Nutrition Board has issued Recommended Dietary Allowances for copper for people over the age of one year and adequate intakes (AIs) for infants under one year. Pregnant women should take in 1.0 mg per day, while lactating women should take in 1.3 mg per day. Males and females 19 years and older should take in 0.9 mg per day, while teens between the ages of 14 and 18 years should take in 0.89 mg per day. Children between the ages of 9 and 13 years should take in 0.7 mg, while children between the ages of 4 and 8 years should take in 0.4 mg. Children between the ages of one and three years should take in 0.34 mg. An AI for infants between 6 and 12 months is 0.22 mg, while an AI for infants between birth and six months is 0.2 mg. For adult men and women, copper has a tolerable upper intake level of 10 mg per day.[1]

DEFICIENCY AND EXCESS

Many people have low and insufficient levels of copper. This is especially true for people who eat a good deal of refined and processed foods. However, because copper is available from so many different foods, serious copper deficiency is thought to be exceedingly rare. But it is known to appear in people who are severely undernourished or who have chronic diarrhea. People who have problems with the absorption of nutrients, such as those with Crohn's disease, may have a copper deficiency, as may people who have had intestinal bypass surgery or who are fed by feeding tubes. High dietary intake of iron or zinc may also trigger a deficiency. Symptoms of deficiency include bleeding under the skin, damaged blood vessels, hair loss, pale skin, and an enlarged heart. Copper deficiency may cause fatigue and an increased vulnerability to infection.

On the other hand, the high intake of copper is toxic. Symptoms of copper toxicity include nausea, vomiting, diarrhea, kidney damage, anemia, and death. People who have the rare inherited disorder known as Wilson's disease accumulate copper in the liver or brain. They should never take copper supplements and should be tested regularly to determine the levels of copper in their blood. In addition, the levels of copper in the blood may be altered by boron, vitamin C, selenium, manganese, and molybdenum. Since zinc is known to lower copper stores, people who take supplemental zinc should discuss taking copper supplements with their medical provider.

It should be noted that another source of excess copper is the leaching of copper from old pipes and fittings into drinking water. While replacing old pipes and fittings is the best solution, that is not always feasible. People who know that there is copper in their water should use the first gallon of water in the morning for a noncooking, nonconsuming function.

KEY RESEARCH FINDINGS

There May Be an Association between Serum Copper Levels and Autism Spectrum Disorders

In a study published in 2014 in the journal *NeuroReport,* researchers from China and Norway investigated the levels of copper and zinc in the blood in Chinese children with autism spectrum disorder. (Autism spectrum disorder is a group of neurodevelopmental disorders characterized by social and language deficits, stereotypic behavior, and abnormalities in motor functions.) The researchers assessed the serum copper and zinc levels of 48 males and 12 females with autism spectrum disorder and 60 healthy matched controls. Their mean age was 3.78 years. When compared to the children in the control group, the researchers found that the levels of serum copper were significantly higher in the children with autism spectrum disorder. At the same time, the zinc/copper ratio was significantly lower in the children with the disorder, and there was an association between this ratio and the level of severity of the disorder. The researchers suggested that the zinc/copper ratio could be considered a "biomarker" for autism spectrum disorders.[2]

Children Who Are Picky Eaters Tend to Have Lower Levels of Serum Copper

In a study published in 2015 in the journal *Appetite,* researchers from Los Angeles, China, and Finland wanted to learn more about factors associated with Chinese children who are picky eaters. A picky eater was defined as "as a child who consumes an inadequate variety and amount of food(s) through rejection of foods that were familiar (and unfamiliar)." The cohort consisted of 793 healthy children between the ages of 7 and 12 years, who were recruited from nine cities and rural areas in China. Using a structured questionnaire, researchers collected data between November 2011 and April 2012. Blood samples were taken for mineral analysis. According to the parents, 59.3 percent of the children were picky eaters. When compared to the nonpicky eaters, the picky eating children had a lower intake of a number of dietary minerals, including copper, and they had lower levels of serum copper. Over time, this may "have a major impact on the anthropometric parameters of children."[3]

Higher-Dose Zinc Supplementation May Trigger Copper Deficiency

In a study published in 2015 in the *Journal of Clinical Pathology*, researchers from the United Kingdom wanted to learn more about the side effects of high doses of zinc supplementation, which may be prescribed by medical providers. The cohort consisted of 70 subjects. The researchers learned that 62 percent of the patients were prescribed zinc at doses that may cause copper deficiency. The medical providers did not appear to be knowledgeable about copper deficiency, and plasma copper was measured in only two of the patients on prescription zinc. Both of those patients had low levels of copper. Nine percent of the patients developed unexplained anemia, and 7 percent had neurological symptoms, apparently from copper deficiency. The researchers commented that their findings "underline the lack of awareness of zinc-induced copper deficiency." The findings also "highlight the potential risk of developing zinc-induced copper deficiency as a result of such prescribing."[4]

Postmenopausal Women with Osteopenia or Osteoporosis May Have Low Levels of Copper in Their Blood

In a study published in 2015 in the journal *Clinical Cases in Mineral and Bone Metabolism*, researchers from Iran measured the levels of copper and other minerals in 23 postmenopausal women with osteoporosis and 28 postmenopausal women with osteopenia. The women ranged in age from 50 to 80 years; their mean age was 57.97 years. The researcher found that the mean serum levels of copper were significantly lower than normal. Because copper plays a role in supporting bone health, this is a disturbing finding. The researchers noted that it may be necessary to take supplemental minerals, including "perhaps" copper.[5]

People Who Eat Ultra-Processed Foods Consume Lower Amounts of Micronutrients, Including Copper

In a cross-sectional study published in 2015 in the journal *Revista de Saúde Púlica*, researchers from Brazil wanted to learn more about the impact of ultra-processed foods, which have been rapidly growing in sales, on the micronutrient content of the Brazilian diet. Copper was among the micronutrients they studied. According to the researchers, at least half of the world's population of children between the ages of six months and five years suffers from one or more micronutrient deficiencies. Though micronutrient deficiency may be caused by a number of factors, the primary cause is insufficient dietary intake.

The cohort consisted of 32,898 Brazilians aged 10 years or older. Food consumption data were collected through two 24-hour food records. The researchers found that 69.5 percent of the diet came from natural or minimally processed foods, 9 percent came from processed foods, and 21.5 percent came from ultra-processed foods. The more people consumed ultra-processed foods, the less their intake of copper. The amount of copper found in the ultra-processed foods was at least two times lower than that found in the natural or minimally processed foods. In fact, there was an inverse, significant association between consumption of ultra-processed foods and the amount of copper. The researchers advocated eating more natural or minimally processed foods and fewer processed or ultra-processed foods.[6]

People with Chronic Stable Heart Failure May Have Low Levels of Some Micronutrients Such As Copper

In an observational study published in 2017 in the *Journal of Cardiovascular Nursing,* researchers from the United Kingdom wanted to learn more about the association between the medical problem known as chronic stable heart failure and levels of micronutrients, such as copper, in the body. (Micronutrients are substances that are needed only in small amounts for normal body function.) As a result, the researchers decided to assess the dietary micronutrient intake and micronutrient status of 79 patients with heart failure. These patients had a mean age of 64.5 years, and 19 percent were women. Food frequency questionnaires were completed, and blood concentrations of several micronutrients, including copper, were measured with fasting blood samples. More than 20 percent of the subjects reported inadequate intakes of copper. Why is this important? According to the researchers "Poor nutritional status is associated with mortality in patients with heart failure." While it is not immediately evident why the subjects were consuming fewer micronutrients, the researchers offered several explanations, including decreased hunger sensation, psychological issues, nausea, and shortness of breath.[7]

There May Be an Association between Copper and Alzheimer's Disease

In a study published in 2013 in the journal *Proceedings of the National Academy of Sciences,* researchers from Rochester, New York, investigated the association between copper and Alzheimer's disease in mice and human brain cells. Over a three-month period of time, normal mice took in trace amounts of copper in their drinking water. The amounts of copper were similar to what people would consume in a diet. The researchers found that the copper entered the blood system and accumulated in the vessels that feed blood to the brain. Over time, there were toxic effects. The copper inhibited the removal of amyloid beta from the brain and stimulated the buildup of amyloid beta. Thus, plaques, which are seen in the brains of people with Alzheimer's disease, were allowed to form. Copper also promoted the inflammation of brain tissue. But copper is essential to the functioning of the body. Therefore, it is important that researchers find a balance between the consumption of too little or too much copper.[8]

Herbal Infusions May Be a Source of Copper

In a study published in 2012 in the *International Journal of Food Sciences and Nutrition*, researchers from Poland examined the copper and other mineral content of five herbs: chamomile, mint, St. John's wort, sage, and nettle. Content analyses were conducted for dried herb samples and prepared infusions. The researchers found the highest amount of copper in the dry and infused chamomile. Still, the researchers cautioned that the mineral content of herbs is related to several factors, such as their place of origin, the cultivation conditions, and the degree of environmental pollution. The results may be variable. The researchers noted that consuming an average of one herbal tea a day should not make an "important" difference in human nutrition.[9] The fact that many people consume larger amounts of herbal teas was not addressed.

NOTES

1. The George Mateljan Foundation. "Copper." December 28, 2017. http://whfoods.com/genpage-php?tname=nutrient&dbid=53.

2. Li, Si-ou, Jia-liang Wang, Geir Bjørklund, et al. "Serum Copper and Zinc Levels in Individuals with Autism Spectrum Disorders." *NeuroReport* 25 (2014): 1216–1220.

3. Xue, Yong, Eva Lee, Ke Ning, et al. "Prevalence of Picky Eating Behaviour in Chinese School-Age Children and Associations with Anthropometric Parameters and Intelligence Quotient: A Cross-Sectional Study." *Appetite* 91 (August 2015): 248–255.

4. Duncan, Andrew, Calum Yacoubian, Neil Watson, and Ian Morrison. "The Risk of Copper Deficiency in Patients Prescribed Zinc Supplements." *Journal of Clinical Pathology* 68, no. 9 (September 2015): 723–725.

5. Mahdavi-Roshan, Marjan, Mehrangiz Ebrahimi, and Aliasgar Ebrahimi. "Copper, Magnesium, Zinc and Calcium Status in Osteopenic and Osteoporotic Post-Menopausal Women." *Clinical Cases in Mineral and Bone Metabolism* 12, no. 1 (2015): 18–21.

6. Louzada, Maria Laura da Costa, Ana Paula Bortoletto Martins, Daniela Silva Canella, et al. "Impact of Ultra-Processed Foods on Micronutrient Content in the Brazilian Diet." *Revista de Saúde Pública* 49 (2015): 45.

7. McKeag, Nicolas A., Michelle C. McKinley, Mark T. Harbinson, et al. "Dietary Micronutrient Intake and Micronutrient Status in Patients with Chronic Stable Heart Failure: An Observational Study." *Journal of Cardiovascular Nursing* 32, no. 2 (March–April 2017): 148–155.

8. Singh, Itender, Abhay P. Sagare, Mireia Coma, et al. "Low Levels of Copper Disrupt Brain Amyloid-β Homeostasis by Altering Its Production and Clearance." *Proceedings of the National Academy of Sciences* 110, no. 36 (September 3, 2013): 14771–14776.

9. Suliburska, Joanna and Karolina Kaczmarek. "Herbal Infusions as a Source of Calcium, Magnesium, Iron, Zinc and Copper in Human Nutrition." *International Journal of Food Sciences and Nutrition* 63, no. 2 (March 2012): 194–198.

REFERENCES AND FURTHER READINGS

Duncan, Andrew, Calum Yacoubian, Neil Watson, and Ian Morrison. "The Risk of Copper Deficiency in Patients Prescribed Zinc Supplements." *Journal of Clinical Pathology* 68, no. 9 (September 2015): 723–725.

The George Mateljan Foundation. "Copper." December 28, 2017. http://whfoods.com/genpage.php?tname=nutrient&dbid=53.

Li, Si-ou, Jia-liang Wang, Geir Bjørklund, et al. "Serum Copper and Zinc Levels in Individuals with Autism Spectrum Disorders." *NeuroReport* 25 (2014): 1216–1220.

Louzada, Maria Laura da Costa, Ana Paula Bortoletto Martins, Daniela Silva Canella, et al. "Impact of Ultra-Processed Foods on Micronutrient Content in the Brazilian Diet." *Revista de Saúde Pública* 49 (2015): 45.

Mahdavi-Roshan, Marjan, Mehrangiz Ebrahimi, and Aliasgar Ebrahimi. "Copper, Magnesium, Zinc and Calcium Status in Osteopenic and Osteoporotic Post-Menopausal Women." *Clinical Cases in Mineral and Bone Metabolism* 12, no. 1 (2015): 18–21.

McKeag, Nicolas A., Michelle C. McKinley, Mark T. Harbinson, et al. "Dietary Micronutrient Intake and Micronutrient Status in Patients with Chronic Stable Heart Failure: An Observational Study." *Journal of Cardiovascular Nursing* 32, no. 2 (March–April 2017): 148–155.

Singh, Itender, Abhay P. Sagare, Mireia Coma, et al. "Low Levels of Copper Disrupt Brain Amyloid-β Homeostasis by Altering Its Production and Clearance." *Proceedings of the National Academy of Sciences* 110, no. 36 (September 3, 2013): 14771–14776.

Suliburska, Joanna and Karolina Kaczmarek. "Herbal Infusions as a Source of Calcium, Magnesium, Iron, Zinc and Copper in Human Nutrition." *International Journal of Food Sciences and Nutrition* 63, no. 2 (March 2012): 194–198.

Xue, Yong, Eva Lee, Ke Ning, et al. "Prevalence of Picky Eating Behaviour in Chinese School-Age Children and Associations with Anthropometric Parameters and Intelligence Quotients: A Cross-Sectional Study." *Appetite* 91 (August 2015): 248–255.

Fluoride

Fluorides, which are usually referred to as fluoride, are minerals containing fluorine, one of the most reactive elements found on the periodic table. Unlike some minerals that are harder to obtain, fluorides are commonly found in the earth's crust and water supply. The most common fluorides are sodium fluoride and calcium fluoride, which are naturally found in water and in some foods. Other fluorides, such as hexafluorosilicic acid and sodium hexafluorosilicate, are added to city water supplies to aid in the prevention of tooth decay. Sodium fluoride, stannous fluoride, and sodium monofluorophosphate are fluorine compounds that may be in toothpaste.

Fluoride is best known for helping to prevent tooth decay and cavities and promoting strong teeth and enamel. Adding fluoride to city and town water supplies is a practice that began in the United States in the 1940s. It is believed that adults and children who live in communities with fluoridated water experience 40 to 60 percent reductions in tooth decay. Although they tend to market themselves as if they come from the most pristine of sources, bottled water may be obtained from the tap or another fluoride-containing water source. As a result, bottled waters may contain fluoride.

Still, not everyone agrees that even small amounts of fluoride should be added to the water. In fact, many people cite studies that have found an association between fluoride and a number of different medical problems and concerns. The American Dental Association disagrees. "More than 70 years of scientific research has consistently shown that an optimal level of fluoride in community water is safe and effective in preventing tooth decay by at least 25% in both children and adults."[1]

FOOD SOURCES AND SUPPLEMENTS

The best source of fluoride is fluoridated water. In general, well water contains little or no fluoride. Food cooked in fluoridated water also has fluoride. Tea and gelatin are food sources of fluoride. People who know that their water supply is not fluoridated may want to discuss fluoride supplementation with their medical provider. Fluoride supplementation is available as a liquid, tablet, and chewable tablet. Normally, it is taken once a day by mouth. Fluoride may be taken by itself or combined with a food, such as cereal, or a liquid, such as juice. Fluoride supplements should not be taken at the same time as dairy products. A wait of at least one hour between fluoride and dairy is advised. Missed doses should be taken as soon as possible. However, if it is almost time for the next dose, the missed dose should be skipped. Double doses should be avoided. Supplemental fluoride may cause a number of side effects, including stained teeth, increases in saliva, a salty or soapy taste in the mouth, stomach pain, gastrointestinal upset, vomiting, diarrhea, rash, tremors, weakness, and/or seizures.

Even if a mother drinks fluoridated water, breast milk contains little fluoride. Babies who are breastfed or drink formula prepared with water that is not fluoridated may require supplementation at around six months of age. Babies who are fed formula prepared with fluoridated water probably obtain sufficient amounts of fluoride. It is best to discuss these concerns with a medical provider.

INTAKE RECOMMENDATIONS

In order to meet adequate intake requirements, the National Institutes of Health recommends that adult males take in 4 mg per day and adult females, including those who are pregnant or lactating, take in 3 mg per day. Teens between the ages of 14 and 18 years should take in 3 mg per day, and children between the ages of 9 and 13 years should take in 2 mg per day. Children between the ages of four and eight years should take in 1 mg per day, while children between the ages of one and three years should take in 0.7 mg per day. Infants between the ages of 7 and 12 months should take in 0.5 mg per day, while infants between the ages of birth and 6 months should take in 0.1 mg per day.[2]

For males and females eight years of age and older, the Tolerable Upper Intake level is 10 mg per day. For children between the ages of 4 and 8 years, the level is 2.2 mg per day; for children 1 to 3 years, that level is 1.3 mg per day; for children 7 to 12 months that level is 0.9 mg per day; and for children under the age of 6 months, that level is 0.7 mg per day.[3]

DEFICIENCY AND EXCESS

A deficiency of fluoride may result in more cavities and weak bones and teeth. It is almost impossible to obtain an excess of fluoride from the diet. When consumed in excess supplementation, fluoride is toxic. Large doses may result in nausea, abdominal pain, and vomiting.

Though it is rarely seen, infants who take in too much fluoride before their teeth have broken through the gums may have changes in the enamel, such as faint white lines or streaks. The following recommendations may help to ensure that infants and young children do not take in too much fluoride. When preparing formula, it is important to check the type of water that is advised. Fluoride supplements should not be used without the recommendation of a trusted medical provider. Children under the age of two years should not use a toothpaste that contains fluoride. Until they are six years old, children should not use a mouthwash containing fluoride.

KEY RESEARCH FINDINGS

Fluoride Appears to Be Useful for People at Increased Risk for Caries (Cavities)

In a retrospective, longitudinal analysis published in 2014 in the *Journal of the American Dental Association*, researchers from various Veterans' Administration dental clinics in the United States tested the use of fluoride applications on veterans at increased risk for caries—those who have two or more fillings during a one-year period of time. During fiscal year 2009, the first year of the trial, the goal was to provide fluoride treatments to at least 60 percent of high-risk patients.

By fiscal year 2012, the dental providers were providing the treatment to 81 percent. That meant that 8 out of every 10 clinics gave fluoride treatments to at least 90 percent of high-risk patients. And the fluoride treatments translated into a significant reduction in the need for new fillings. In fact, the high-risk dental patients experienced a 10-point drop in the rate of new fillings. The researchers noted that their fluoride treatment program demonstrated how positive changes may be made in a "large system of care."[4]

Fluoride Cessation May Increase the Number of Caries in the Primary Teeth of Children

In a study published in 2016 in the journal *Community Dentistry and Oral Epidemiology*, researchers from Alberta, Canada, investigated the short-term impact of fluoride cessation on children's cavities. The data were obtained from population-based samples of grade 2 school children in two similar cities in the province of Alberta, Canada. Pre-cessation data were collected during the 2004–2005 school year, and post-cessation data were collected during the 2013–2014 school year. One of the cities, Calgary, stopped fluoridating its water in May 2011; the other city, Edmonton, continued to add fluoride to its water supply. The researchers focused on smooth tooth surfaces, where fluoride is more likely to make a difference. The researchers found an increase in decay in primary teeth in both cities, but the magnitude of the increase was much more in Calgary than Edmonton. Among the primary teeth, there was "consistent indication of an adverse short-term effect of cessation." On the other hand, in both cities, there were decreases in caries in permanent teeth. The researchers suggested that the "absence of an increase in permanent teeth may have reflected the short time frame since cessation in our study." And, as a result, they advised continued monitoring and additional future data collection.[5]

Community Water Fluoridation Appears to Be Associated with Adult Tooth Loss

In a study published in 2010 in the *American Journal of Public Health*, researchers from New York City investigated the association between community water fluoridation and adult tooth loss. They used data from the 1995 to 1999 Behavioral Risk Factor Surveillance System, an annual survey of more than 350,000 adults, which they combined with data from the 1992 Water Fluoridation Census. Almost 60 percent of the subjects had no tooth loss, and less than 2 percent had lost all their teeth. While the researchers found no association between current community water fluoridation levels and tooth loss, they did find a significant association between the community water fluoridation levels at the time of the respondent's birth and tooth loss as an adult. Thus, fluoridation appears to be less important once permanent teeth have formed, and it seems to have a lasting effect.

The researchers noted that because they focused only on tooth loss, their results may not demonstrate all of the benefits people derive from water fluoridation. "This study suggests that the benefits of CWF [community water fluoridation] may be larger than previously believed."[6]

There May Be an Association between Fluoride Levels in Drinking Water and Hypothyroidism

In an observational, cross-sectional study published in 2015 in the *Journal of Epidemiology and Community Health*, researchers from the United Kingdom wanted to determine if there is an association between the levels of fluoride in the water supply and the incidence of hypothyroidism or abnormally low activity of the thyroid gland. The researchers obtained data on the fluoridation of the water supply and rates of hypothyroidism from 7,935 medical practices in England. They learned that communities with higher levels of fluoride in the drinking water had higher rates of hypothyroidism. Moreover, communities with higher levels of fluoride in the drinking water had significantly higher rates of hypothyroidism than communities with lower rates of fluoride in the drinking water. This study did not account for nondrinking water sources of fluoride. The researchers commented that their findings suggest a "substantial cause for public health concern." The researchers added that their data included only patients diagnosed with hypothyroidism. Many more people may have subclinical hypothyroidism or may not be diagnosed. The researchers said that their findings raise questions about the safety of fluoridation "and consideration should be given to reducing all sources of fluoride in the environment."[7]

Tea Drinkers May Consume Too Much Fluoride

In a study published in 2016 in the *International Journal of Environmental Research and Public Health*, researchers from Ireland, Oklahoma (United States), Canada, and New Zealand noted that Ireland has the highest consumption of black tea in the entire world. In addition, Ireland requires the fluoridation of drinking water. Are the Irish consuming too much fluoride? The researchers purchased 54 brands of commercially available black tea bags, and the infusions made with tap water were tested for levels of fluoride. The researchers found that all of the black tea infusions had amounts of fluoride that exceeded that legal limit. As a result, the researchers concluded that the population of Ireland is at "a significant risk for excessive intake of fluoride from tea consumption." Moreover, "a significant percentage of the general population is at risk of chronic fluoride intoxication," and the high intake of fluoride "may also be contributing to other disease states." The researchers recommended the establishment of maximum limits for the amount of fluoride permitted in teas and the end of the fluoridation of drinking water supplies.[8]

There May Be an Association between Excess Consumption of Fluoride and Hypertension (Elevated Blood Pressure)

In a study published in 2013 in the journal *Science of the Total Environment*, researchers from China wanted to learn if the excess consumption of fluoride was associated with hypertension (elevated blood pressure). The cohort consisted of 487 men and women between the ages of 40 and 75, who lived in eight villages in Zhaozhou County in the Heilongjiang Province of China. All of the participants, who had similar incomes and dietary habits, were divided into four groups according to the concentrations of fluoride in their water—normal, mild, moderate, and high levels of fluoride. The prevalence of hypertension in each group was, respectively, 20.16 percent, 24.54 percent, 32.30 percent, and 49.23 percent. As the concentrations of fluoride rose, so did the rates of people with elevated blood pressure. The researchers commented that their findings "might have policy implications for a country such as China that will lead to a recommendation to put more effort into improving the water and engaging in defluoridation projects to alleviate the toxicity of long-term effects of fluoride exposure to local residents and their offspring."[9]

Exposure to Elevated Levels of Fluoride in Water May Impair Childhood Cognitive Development

In a pilot study published in 2015 in the journal *Neurotoxicology and Teratology*, researchers from Boston, China, and Denmark examined the association between fluoride and childhood cognitive development. The cohort consisted of 51 first-grade children, between the ages of six and eight years, who lived in southern Sichuan China. There were slightly more females than males. Apart from seasonal changes, over the years, the drinking water fluoride concentrations remained stable, and the residents, who had limited mobility, tended to have a single source for their drinking water needs. Assessments were conducted on the fluoride intake and cognitive functioning of the children. The researchers found an association between fluoride in the drinking water and "developmental neurotoxicity."

These same researchers conducted a systematic review and meta-analysis of 27 cross-sectional studies of children exposed to fluoride in drinking water. Most of these studies were conducted in China. The researchers found that the children who had higher exposure to fluoride had lower IQ scores. The difference was around seven points. The researchers wrote that their "review highlighted a need to further characterize the dose-response association including improving assessment and control of potential confounders."[10]

High Levels of Fluoride May Also Impair Cognitive Health of the Elderly

In a study published in 2016 in the journal *Biological Trace Element Research*, researchers from China wanted to learn more about the effect of the excess consumption of fluoride on the cognitive abilities of the elderly. The cohort consisted of 511 subjects, who ranged in age from 60 to 86 years. The subjects were divided into four groups: normal cognition, mild, moderate, and severe cognition impairment. Most of the participants had mild or moderate cognitive impairment. Only about one-fifth of the subjects were in the normal group. As may have been predicted, the researchers found that cognitive impairment was most often found in people over the age of 80 years. The researchers found that certain low doses of fluoride may have a potential protective effect on cognition. At the same time, "high fluoride exposure is a potential risk factor for cognitive impairment in [an] elderly population."[11]

NOTES

1. American Dental Association. "Fluoride in Water." January 2, 2018. http://www.ada.org/en/public-programs/advocating-for-the-public/fluoride-and-fluoridation.

2. National Library of Medicine, National Institutes of Health. "Fluoride." January 2, 2018. https://www.ncbi.nlm.nig.gov/books/NBK109832/.

3. National Library of Medicine, National Institutes of Health. "Fluoride." January 2, 2018. https://www.ncbi.nlm.nih.gov/books/NBK109832/.

4. Gibson, Gretchen, M. Marianne Jurasic, Carolyn J. Wehler, et al. "Longitudinal Outcomes of Using a Fluoride Performance Measure for Adults at High Risk of Experiencing Caries." *Journal of the American Dental Association* 145, no. 5 (May 2014): 443–451.

5. McLaren, L., S. Patterson, S. Thawer, et al. "Measuring the Short-Term Impact of Fluoridation Cessation on Dental Caries in Grade 2 Children Using Tooth Surface Indices." *Community Dentistry and Oral Epidemiology* 44, no. 3 (June 2016): 274–282.

6. Neidell, Matthew, Karin Herzog, and Sherry Glied. "The Association between Community Water Fluoridation and Adult Tooth Loss." *American Journal of Public Health* 100, no. 10 (October 2010): 1980–1985.

7. Peckham, S., D. Lowery, and S. Spencer. "Are Fluoride Levels in Drinking Water Associated with Hypothyroidism Prevalence in England? A Large Observational Study of GP Practice Data and Fluoride Levels in Drinking Water." *Journal of Epidemiology and Community Health* 69, no. 7 (July 2015): 619–624.

8. Waugh, D. T., W. Potter, H. Limeback, and M. Godfrey. "Risk Assessment of Fluoride Intake from Tea in the Republic of Ireland and Its Implications for Public Health and Water Fluoridation." *International Journal of Environmental Research and Public Health* 13, no. 3 (2016): 259+.

9. Sun, Liyan, Yanhui Gao, Hui Liu, et al. "An Assessment of the Relationship between Excess Fluoride Intake from Drinking Water and Essential Hypertension in Adults Residing in Fluoride Endemic Areas." *Science of the Total Environment* 443 (2013): 864–869.

10. Choi, Anna L., Ying Zhang, Guifan Sun, et al. "Association of Lifetime Exposure to Fluoride and Cognitive Functions in Chinese Children: A Pilot Study." *Neurotoxicology and Teratology* 47 (2015): 96–101.

11. Li, M., Y. Gao, J. Cui, et al. "Cognitive Impairment and Risk Factors in Elderly People Living in Fluorosis Areas in China." *Biological Trace Element Research* 172, no. 1 (July 2016): 53–60.

REFERENCES AND FURTHER READINGS

American Dental Association. "Fluoride in Water." January 2, 2018. http://www.ada.org/en/public-programs/advocating-for-the-public/fluoride-and-fluoridation.

Choi, Anna L., Ying Zhang, Guifan Sun, et al. "Association of Lifetime Exposure to Fluoride and Cognitive Functions in Chinese Children: A Pilot Study." *Neurotoxicology and Teratology* 47 (2015): 96–101.

Gibson, Gretchen, M. Marianne Jurasic, Carolyn J. Wehler, et al. "Longitudinal Outcomes of Using a Fluoride Performance Measure for Adults at High Risk of Experiencing Caries." *Journal of the American Dental Association* 145, no. 5 (May 2014): 443–451.

Li, M., Y. Gao, J. Cui, et al. "Cognitive Impairment and Risk Factors in Elderly People Living in Fluorosis Areas in China." *Biological Trace Element Research* 172, no. 1 (July 2016): 53–60.

McLaren, L., S. Patterson, S. Thawer, et al. "Measuring the Short-Term Impact of Fluoridation Cessation on Dental Caries in Grade 2 Children Using Tooth Surface Indices." *Community Dentistry and Oral Epidemiology* 44, no. 3 (June 2016): 274–282.

National Library of Medicine, National Institutes of Health. "Fluoride." January 2, 2018. https://www.ncbi.nlm.nih.gov/books/NBK109832/.

Neidell, Matthew, Karin Herzog, and Sherry Glied. "The Association between Community Water Fluoridation and Adult Tooth Loss." *American Journal of Public Health* 100, no. 10 (October 2010): 1980–1985.

Peckham, S., D. Lowery, and S. Spencer. "Are Fluoride Levels in Drinking Water Associated with Hypothyroidism Prevalence in England? A Large Observational Study of GP Practice Data and Fluoride Levels in Drinking Water." *Journal of Epidemiology and Community Health* 69, no. 7 (July 2015): 619–624.

Sun, Liyan, Yanhui Gao, Hui Liu, et al. "An Assessment of the Relationship between Excess Fluoride Intake from Drinking Water and Essential Hypertension in Adults Residing in Fluoride Endemic Areas." *Science of the Total Environment* 443 (2013): 864–869.

Waugh, D. T., W. Potter, H. Limeback, and M. Godfrey. "Risk Assessment of Fluoride Intake from Tea in the Republic of Ireland and Its Implications for Public Health and Water Fluoridation." *International Journal of Environmental Research and Public Health* 13, no. 3 (2016): 259+.

Iodine

Found in many foods and in iodized salt, iodine is a mineral that the body requires to make thyroid hormones. Thyroid hormones control the metabolism of the body as well as other functions such as bone and brain development during pregnancy and infancy. Since the body is unable to make iodine, people must obtain it from their diet and, sometimes, supplementation.

Historically, iodine deficiency was fairly common in northern parts of the United States. However, the introduction of iodized salt almost a century ago virtually eliminated severe iodine deficiency. Still, in many other parts of the world, large numbers of people are unable to obtain sufficient amounts of dietary iodine and may be iodine deficient. In fact, the American Thyroid Association has noted that about 40 percent of the world's population is at risk for iodine deficiency.[1]

Although iodine is found naturally in soil and seawater, the actual amount of iodine varies from location to location. Since the amount of iodine in a particular product may not be listed on nutrition labels, it may be difficult to determine the actual iodine in a specific food. Likewise, when cooking iodine-rich foods in water, a large amount of the iodine may seep into the water. This is fine if the water will be consumed, as in a soup, but this is an unfortunate waste of a valuable mineral when the water is discarded.

FOOD SOURCES AND SUPPLEMENTS

Sea vegetables, such as the various forms of edible seaweed, are the best sources of iodine. Brown sea vegetables have more iodine than red sea vegetables. But there are other excellent sources such as scallops and cod. Very good sources of iodine include yogurt, shrimp, cow's milk, eggs, and strawberries. Sardines, salmon, and tuna are good sources.[2] Iodine is readily available as a dietary supplement, generally as potassium iodide or sodium iodide. Multivitamins often contain iodine, and kelp and some other types of seaweed may be purchased as a supplement.

INTAKE RECOMMENDATIONS

The Food and Nutrition Board has established the following Recommended Dietary Allowances for iodine. Lactating women should consume 290 mcg per day, while pregnant women should consume 220 mcg per day. Males and females aged 14 years and older should take in 150 mcg, while children between the ages of 9 and 13 years should take in 120 mcg. Children between the ages of 1 and 8 years should take in 90 mcg; children between the ages of 7 and 12 months should take in 130 mcg; and children between birth and 6 months should take in 110 mcg. There are also tolerable upper intake levels for iodine. Adults 19 years and older should consume no more than 1,000 mcg per day, while teens between the ages of 14 and 18 years should consume no more than 900 mcg. For children between the ages of 9 and 13 years, the upper limit is 600 mcg; for children between the ages of 4 and 8 years, the limit is 300 mcg; and children between the ages of 1 and 3 years should take in no more than 200 mcg per day. No upper limits have been established for infants. People who are taking supplemental iodine under the supervision of a medical provider should ignore these limits.[3]

DEFICIENCY AND EXCESS

While most residents of the United States are believed to obtain a sufficient amount of iodine from their diets, certain people are at increased risk for deficiencies. These include people who avoid using iodized salt, women who are pregnant, people who do not eat any animal products, and people who live in regions with iodine-deficient soil. People who are iodine deficient may be unable to make adequate amounts of thyroid hormones. As a result, they may have trouble thinking clearly and completing necessary tasks. An iodine deficiency during pregnancy may harm the growing fetus, causing stunted growth, mental retardation, lower-than-average intelligence quotient (IQ), and delayed sexual development. Frequently, the first sign of an iodine deficiency is a goiter or an enlarged thyroid gland. ("Goiter" comes from the Latin word *guttur*, which means throat.) Deficiency is more common in women than men.

Excess amounts of iodine are also harmful. Excessive iodine is associated with goiter, thyroid gland inflammation, thyroid cancer, burning of the throat and mouth, stomach burning and pain, fever, nausea, vomiting, diarrhea, weak pulse, and coma.[4]

KEY RESEARCH FINDINGS

Pasteurization May Lower the Amount of Iodine in Milk

In a study published in 2015 in the *International Journal of Endocrinology & Metabolism*, researchers from Iran investigated the effects that pasteurization and sterilization have on concentrations of iodine in milk. The cohort consisted of 30 Holstein dairy cows. They were fed a diet that contained 10 mg potassium iodide per kilogram of dry diet matter. Milk samples were taken on several different days and sterilized with ultrahigh temperature technology. The results were compared to another study in which milk was pasteurized. The researchers determined that feeding iodine supplement to the cows significantly increased the iodine content of the milk. The sterilization process also increased the iodine content. On the other hand, pasteurization decreased the amount of iodine. The researchers concluded that "supplemented sterilized milk could be a good alternative vehicle for dietary iodine in the prevention of iodine deficiency."[5]

Maternal Iodine Supplementation May Impact the Neuro-Intellectual Outcomes of Children

In a pilot, prospective, observational study published in 2016 in the journal *Thyroid*, researchers from Messina, Italy, examined the IQ of children born to mothers with different levels of iodine supplementation. The initial cohort consisted of four groups, each including 15 mother–child pairs from northeastern Sicily, who were matched according to their use of iodized salt and thyroid medication before and during pregnancy. The women in the first group used iodized salt; the women in the second group did not use iodized salt; the women in the third group used iodized salt and took thyroid medication; the women in the fourth group did not use iodized salt but took thyroid medication. The children were between the ages of 6 and 12 years. The researchers found an association between the iodine status of the mothers and the intellectual abilities of the children. The mothers who used iodized salt had children with higher intelligence scores. In addition, the researchers learned that more than 40 percent of the children had defective cognitive outcomes, especially verbal problems, and the vast majority were born to mothers not using iodized salt. "These results support the growing body of evidence that prenatal, mild-to-moderate iodine deficiency adversely affects cognitive development later in life, with a seemingly greater impact on verbal abilities."[6]

In a longitudinal study published in 2013 in the *Journal of Clinical Endocrinology & Metabolism*, researchers from Australia examined the association between mild iodine deficiency during pregnancy and longer-term educational outcomes of the offspring. The researchers examined the standardized test scores of 228 children whose mothers attended The Royal Hobart Hospital prenatal clinics in Tasmania, Australia, between 1999 and 2001. The children were born between March 2000 and December 2001, during a period of mild iodine deficiency in the population. In October 2001, the conditions changed; bread manufacturers began using iodized salt. Still, the greater part of their gestation occurred in a deficient environment. And the period of iodine deficiency appeared to have lasting effects. When the children were tested as nine-year-olds, they were found to score lower on standardized literacy tests. This was particularly evident in spelling. On the other hand, mild iodine deficiency was not associated with lower scores in math tests. The researchers commented that "even mild iodine deficiency during pregnancy can have long-term adverse impacts on fetal neurocognition that are not ameliorated by iodine sufficiency during childhood."[7]

High Intake of Iodine during Pregnancy May Result in Hypothyroidism in Newborns

In a report published in 2012 in the *Journal of Pediatrics*, researchers from Portland, Oregon, and Boston, Massachusetts, described three infants who developed congenital hypothyroidism or thyroid hormone deficiency because their mothers consumed supplements with excess amounts of iodine during pregnancy or breastfeeding. The three infants had blood iodine levels that were 10 times higher than those of healthy control infants. The researchers noted that iodine easily crosses the placenta, and it is essential for thyroid function and neurocognitive development. However, excessive amounts of iodine may decrease the amount of thyroid hormone production. All three of the infants were found to have elevated iodine content in their blood and urine. The researchers noted that their findings highlighted a potential problem associated with "nutritional supplements containing iodine in amounts far higher than the recommended daily allowance during pregnancy."[8]

Iodine Supplementation May Be Useful for Thyroid Disorders and May Lower Cholesterol Levels in Overweight Women

In a randomized, controlled study published in 2015 in the *Journal of Nutrition*, researchers from Zurich, Switzerland, and Marrakesh, Morocco, wanted to learn more about the effect iodine supplementation has on thyrotropin (also known as the thyroid stimulating hormone) and levels of serum cholesterol. Iodine is required for the production of thyroid hormones. A deficiency of iodine may lead to elevated levels of thyrotropin, which, in turn, is a predictor of higher levels of cholesterol. The cohort consisted of 163 overweight or obese Moroccan women, between the ages of 20 and 50 years, who were iodine deficient. For six months, the women took a daily 200 mcg iodine supplement or a placebo. The researchers found that the subjects with elevated baseline cholesterol levels who took iodine experienced an 11 percent reduction in total cholesterol. At a six-month follow-up, the levels of thyrotropin were 33 percent lower in the treatment group than the placebo group. But the most dramatic results were in levels of cholesterol. Only 21.5 percent of the subjects in the iodine supplementation group continued to have elevated levels of cholesterol. That was in contrast to 34.8 percent of the placebo group. The researchers commented that iodine supplementation in people who are deficient may decrease thyroid disorders and help to reduce cardiovascular disease.[9]

Physicians May Not Be Well-Versed in the Iodine Requirements of Pregnant Women

In a study published in 2015 in the *Journal of Endocrinological Investigation*, researchers from Turkey wanted to learn more about the knowledge, attitudes, and behaviors of physicians concerning thyroid disorders and iodine requirements during pregnancy. The cohort consisted of 322 physicians (endocrinologists, family physicians, and obstetricians) from seven geographical regions in Turkey. All of the physicians completed a questionnaire. While the physicians varied in their knowledge about thyroid disorders, the researchers determined that 67.1 percent of the physicians thought that iodine supplementation during pregnancy was not necessary. According to these researchers, physicians in all of the regions "have a lack of knowledge about treating and monitoring hypothyroidism and iodine supplementation in pregnancy." And, as a result, too many pregnant women are consuming insufficient amounts of iodine "despite the nationwide progress in resolving iodine deficiency."[10]

Fortifying Bread with Iodized Salt Improves the Iodine Status of School Children

In a study published in 2016 in the journal *Nutrients*, researchers from New Zealand noted that iodine deficiency emerged in the 1990s as a country-wide medical problem. As a result, since 2009, New Zealand has required the mandatory fortification of bread with iodized salt. Is this fortification having an impact on the iodine status of the children of New Zealand? From March to May 2015, the researchers conducted a cross-sectional survey of children between the ages of 8 and 10 years in the cities of Auckland and Christchurch. The final sample size was 415, and there were slightly more females than males. Urine and blood samples were taken from the children, and the children completed questionnaires on their intake of iodine from all sources. The researchers learned that the situation had improved since the initiation of the mandatory fortification of bread with iodized salt; children were consuming sufficient amounts of iodine—about twice the amount they consumed before fortification. Most of the iodine was obtained from breads and bread-based foods. Children of Asian ethnicity had the highest intake of iodine. This may be because they consume more seaweed, fish, and other seafood. "In conclusion, the results of this study confirmed that the iodine status in New Zealand school children is now adequate."[11]

Maternal Iodine Insufficiency Has the Potential to Trigger an Adverse Pregnancy Outcome

In a longitudinal study published in 2016 in the journal *Maternal & Child Nutrition*, researchers from Thailand assessed the iodine status of pregnant women during each trimester and compared the pregnancy outcomes between groups with iodine insufficiency and iodine sufficiency. There were 384 women in the first trimester, 325 women in the second trimester, and 221 women in the third trimester. The researchers measured levels of iodine in the urine. Almost half of all the samples indicated iodine insufficiency; only 2 percent of the samples had excessive levels of iodine. The researchers determined that rates of preterm birth and low birth weight were significantly higher in women with insufficient levels of iodine. In fact, the researchers found that "the prevalence of iodine insufficiency was higher than expected." Moreover, "it seemed unethical not to supplement iodine during pregnancy."[12]

NOTES

1. American Thyroid Association. "Iodoine." December 28, 2017. www.thyroid.org/?s=iodine.

2. The George Mateljan Foundation. "Iodine." December 28, 2017. http://whfoods.com/genpage.php?tname=nutrient&dbid=69.

3. Office of Dietary Supplements, National Institutes of Health. "Iodine." December 28, 2017.https://ods.od.nih.gov/factsheets/Iodine-Consumer/.

4. American Thyroid Association.

5. Nazeri, P., M. A. Norouzian, P. Mirmiran, et al. "Heating Process in Pasteurization and Not in Sterilization Decreases the Iodine Concentration of Milk." *International Journal of Endocrinology & Metabolism* 13, no. 4 (October 2015): e27995.

6. Moleti, Mariacarla, Francesco Trimarchi, Gaetano Tortorella, et al. "Effects of Maternal Iodine Nutrition and Thyroid Status on Cognitive Development in Offspring: A Pilot Study." *Thyroid* 26, no. 2 (February 2016): 296–305.

7. Hynes, Kristen L., Petr Otahal, Ian Hay, and John R. Burgess. "Mild Iodine Deficiency during Pregnancy Is Associated with Reduced Educational Outcomes in the Offspring: 9-Year Follow-Up of the Gestational Iodine Cohort." *Journal of Clinical Endocrinology & Metabolism* 98 (2013): 1954–1962.

8. Connelly, Kara J., Bruce A. Boston, Elizabeth N. Pearce, et al. "Congenital Hypothyroidism Caused by Excess Prenatal Maternal Iodine Ingestion." *Journal of Pediatrics* 161 (2012): 760–762.

9. Herter-Aeberli, I., M. Cherkaoui, N. El Ansari, et al. "Iodine Supplementation Decreases Hypercholesterolemia in Iodine-Deficient, Overweight Women: A Randomized Controlled Trial." *Journal of Nutrition* 145, no. 9 (September 2015): 2067–2075.

10. Kut, A., H. Kalli, C. Anil, et al. "Knowledge, Attitudes and Behaviors of Physicians towards Thyroid Disorders and Iodine Requirements in Pregnancy." *Journal of Endocrinological Investigation* 38, no. 10 (October 2015): 1057–1064.

11. Jones, Emma, Rachael McLean, Briar Davies, et al. "Adequate Iodine Status in New Zealand School Children Post-Fortification of Bread with Iodised Salt." *Nutrients* 8, no. 5 (2016): 298.

12. Charoenratana, C., P. Leelapat, K. Traisrisilp, and T. Tongsong. "Maternal Iodine Insufficiency and Adverse Pregnancy Outcomes." *Maternal & Child Nutrition* 12, no. 4 (October 2016): 680–687.

REFERENCES AND FURTHER READINGS

American Thyroid Association. "Iodoine." December 28, 2017. www.thyroid.org/?s=iodine.

Charoenratana, C., P. Leelapat, K. Traisrisilp, and T. Tongsong. "Maternal Iodine Insufficiency and Adverse Pregnancy Outcomes." *Maternal & Child Nutrition* 12, no. 4 (October 2016): 680–687.

Connelly, Kara J., Bruce A. Boston, Elizabeth N. Pearce, et al. "Congenital Hypothyroidism Caused by Excess Prenatal Maternal Iodine Ingestion." *Journal of Pediatrics* 161 (2012): 760–762.

The George Mateljan Foundation. "Iodine." December 28, 2017. http://whfoods.com/genpage.php?tname=nutrient&dbid=69.

Herter-Aeberli, I., M. Cherkaoui, N. El Ansari, et al. "Iodine Supplementation Decreases Hypercholesterolemia in Iodine-Deficient, Overweight Women: A Randomized Controlled Trial." *Journal of Nutrition* 145, no. 9 (September 2015): 2067–2075.

Hynes, Kristen L., Petr Otahal, Ian Hay, and John R. Burgess. "Mild Iodine Deficiency during Pregnancy Is Associated with Reduced Educational Outcomes in the Offspring: 9-Year Follow-Up of the Gestational Iodine Cohort." *Journal of Clinical Endocrinology & Metabolism* 98 (2013): 1954–1962.

Jones, Emma, Rachael McLean, Briar Davies, et al. "Adequate Iodine Status in New Zealand School Children Post-Fortification of Bread with Iodised Salt." *Nutrients* 8, no. 5 (2016): 298.

Kut, A., H. Kalli, C. Anil, et al. "Knowledge, Attitudes and Behaviors of Physicians towards Thyroid Disorders and Iodine Requirements in Pregnancy." *Journal of Endocrinological Investigation* 38, no. 10 (October 2015): 1057–1064.

Moleti, Mariacarla, Francesco Trimarchi, Gaetano Tortorella, et al. "Effects of Maternal Iodine Nutrition and Thyroid Status on Cognitive Development of Offspring: A Pilot Study." *Thyroid* 26, no. 2 (February 2016): 296–305.

Nazeri, P., M. A. Norouzian, P. Mirmiran, et al. "Heating Process in Pasteurization and Not in Sterilization Decreases the Iodine Concentration of Milk." *International Journal of Endocrinology & Metabolism* 13, no. 4 (October 2015): e27995.

Office of Dietary Supplements, National Institutes of Health. "Iodine." December 28, 2017. https://ods.od.nih.gov/factsheets/Iodine-Consumer/.

Iron

Iron is a mineral that the body needs for a number of different functions related to growth and development. For example, the body uses iron to make hemoglobin, a protein in red blood cells that carries oxygen from the lungs to all parts of the body, and myoglobin, a protein that provides oxygen to muscles. To maintain life, all of the cells in the body must have a constant supply of oxygen. The body also needs iron to make some hormones and connective tissue.

At any given time, an adult male has about 2 g of iron in his blood cells; women have about 1.6 g. If the daily intake of iron falls below what the body requires, the body will use stored iron. But then the body does not have all the iron that it requires.

Iron in food comes in two forms: heme iron and nonheme iron. Heme is primarily found in animal foods such as meat. The body absorbs more iron from heme foods. Nonheme iron is from plant sources.

FOOD SOURCES AND SUPPLEMENTS

Although people often associate iron with meat, iron is actually found in many different foods. Excellent sources of iron include spinach, Swiss chard, parsley, and turmeric. Very good sources of iron include bok choy, beef, clams, mussels, asparagus, leeks, and romaine lettuce. Good sources of iron include soybeans, lentils, sesame seeds, garbanzo beans, olives, navy beans, green peas, Brussels sprouts, beets, kale, broccoli, cabbage, and green beans. Iron is often added to multivitamins, but it is also available in supplements that contain only iron, often in the form of ferrous sulfate, ferrous gluconate, ferric citrate, or ferric sulfate. Any supplement that has iron should not be given to children. Accidental overdose of iron-containing products is a leading cause of death among children under the age of six years.

INTAKE RECOMMENDATIONS

The following are the Dietary Reference Intake (DRI) standards for iron. These DRI standards include adequate intake (AI) levels for infants up to six months and Recommended Dietary Allowances for all other categories. Males and females 51 years old and older should take in 8 mg per day. Males between the ages of 19 and 50 years should take in 8 mg per day, while females between the ages of 19 and 50 years should take in 18 mg per day. Males between the ages of 14 and 18 should take in 11 mg per day, while females between the ages of 14 and 18 years should take in 15 mg per day. Males and females between the ages of 9 and 13 years should take in 8 mg per day, while children between the ages of 4 and 8 years should take in 10 mg per day. Children between the ages of 1 and 3 years should take in 7 mg per day, while infants between the ages of 7 and 12 months should take in 11 mg. The AI for infants between birth and six months is .27 mg. Pregnant teens and women should take in 27 mg per day; breastfeeding teens should take in 10 mg per day, and breastfeeding women should take in 9 mg per day. There are also tolerable upper intake levels for iron. Teens 14 years and older and adults should take in no more than 45 mg per day, while children from birth to 13 years should take in no more than 40 mg per day.[1]

DEFICIENCY AND EXCESS

Most people who live in the United States probably obtain a sufficient amount of iron from their diets. But certain people are at increased risk for deficiency. These include female teens and women who have heavy periods; pregnant teens and women; infants who are premature or have a low birth weight; frequent blood donors; and people who have cancer, gastrointestinal disorders that impair absorption, and/or heart failure. People who consistently eat poorer diets are also at increased risk.

Short-term iron deficiency does not cause any obvious medical problems. The body will obtain the iron it requires from iron stored in the muscles, liver, spleen, and bone marrow. When the levels of iron stored in the body are depleted, the body will demonstrate symptoms of iron-deficiency anemia. Red blood cells will decrease in size and contain less hemoglobin. That will cause less oxygen to travel from the lungs to the body. Symptoms of iron deficiency include fatigue, gastrointestinal upset, difficulty with concentration, problems with controlling body temperature, and an inability to fight off germs and infections. Infants and children with iron deficiency are at increased risk for learning difficulties.

On the other hand, the excess intake of iron, especially iron supplementation on an empty stomach, has the potential to cause other problems such as gastrointestinal upset, constipation, nausea, abdominal pain, vomiting, and fainting. High doses of iron may inhibit the absorption of zinc. Extremely high doses of iron have been associated with organ failure, coma, convulsions, and death.

In addition, there is an inherited medical problem known as hemochromatosis in which toxic levels of iron build up in the body. Without treatment, this condition may trigger other problems such as liver cirrhosis, liver cancer, and heart disease.

KEY RESEARCH FINDINGS

In Developed Countries, Higher Consumption of Animal Flesh Foods Appears to Be Associated with Better Iron Status

In a systematic review published in 2016 in the journal *Nutrients*, researchers from Australia noted that animal flesh foods provide "the richest and most bioavailable source" of dietary iron. They wanted to determine if a higher consumption of animal flesh foods is associated with better iron status. The researchers located 8 experimental and 41 observational studies on the topic that included a total of 111,846 participants. While less than 10 percent of the participants were males, the participants ranged in age from 18 to 93 years. The studies varied widely. Of the seven high-quality studies that they examined, five found a positive association between animal flesh intake and iron status. Still, it was unclear how much and how often animal flesh needed to be consumed in order to maintain a healthy iron status. The researchers stressed the need for more research on this topic.[2]

Iron Supplementation May Be Useful for Women with Heavy Menstrual Bleeding

In a study published in 2014 in the journal *Acta Obstetricia et Gynecologica Scandinavica*, researchers from Finland wanted to learn more about how iron supplementation would impact the quality of life of women with heavy menstrual bleeding. The cohort consisted of 236 women, between the ages of 35 and 49 years, who were referred to hospital-based medical providers because of their heavy menstrual bleeding. At baseline, 63 women were anemic and 140 were severely iron deficient. Only 8 percent of the women had taken iron supplementation. The women were randomly assigned to receive a hysterectomy or a levonorgestrel-releasing intrauterine system (an intrauterine device that prevents pregnancy). Hemoglobin concentrations were measured at baseline, at 12 months, and after 5 years. Ferritin (a blood cell protein that contains iron) concentrations and menstrual blood loss were measured before treatments, and after 6 and 12 months and 5 years. The researchers learned that after one year, hemoglobin was still low among anemic women, and it took five years to correct ferritin levels. As a result of their findings, the researchers recommended the earlier treatment of anemia and iron deficiency with iron supplementation. "Clinicians should actively screen for anemia in women with HMB [heavy menstrual bleeding] and emphasize early iron substitution as an integral part of treatment."[3]

Probiotics May Improve Iron Absorption

In a study published in 2015 in the *British Journal of Nutrition*, researchers from Sweden wanted to learn if probiotics could increase the absorption of iron. The cohort consisted of 22 young healthy Swedish women who were of reproductive age. Over four consecutive days, 11 women consumed a fruit juice containing 5 mg of iron and 11 women drank an iron-fortified fruit juice with probiotics. Two separate trials were performed. The researchers learned that the addition of probiotics increased the absorption of iron by approximately 50 percent. And they noted that "there might be practical applications of such lactobacilli products in populations with high prevalence of iron deficiency."[4]

Frequent Blood Donors May Benefit from Iron Supplementation

In a randomized, controlled trial published in 2015 in the journal *JAMA*, researchers from Canada and multiple locations in the United States noted that in the United States people who donate blood frequently are at increased risk for developing anemia. In fact, it has been determined that between 25 and 35 percent of regular blood donors become iron depleted. The researchers wanted to determine if iron supplementation would improve the time required for hemoglobin recovery and the replenishing of iron stores, thereby reducing the incidence of anemia. The cohort consisted of 215 participants who had not donated whole blood or red blood cells for four months. After donating a unit of whole blood (500 ml), they took either no iron supplementation or one daily tablet of ferrous gluconate (37.5 mg of elemental iron) for 24 weeks. The researchers found that the participants who received iron supplementation had improved rates of hemoglobin recovery and faster restoration of iron stores. "Among blood donors with normal hemoglobin levels, low-dose iron supplementation, compared to no supplementation, reduced time to 80 percent recovery of the postdonation decrease in hemoglobin concentration in donors with low ferritin (≤26 ng/mL) or higher ferritin (>26ng/mL)."[5]

Frequent Blood Donors May Wish to Extend the Time between Donations

In a study published in 2014 in the journal *Transfusion*, researchers from Denmark wanted to learn more about the association between frequent blood donors and iron deficiency. The data were obtained from the Danish Blood Donor Study, an ongoing epidemiologic cohort. For their study, the researchers included 14,737 blood donors. These included 7,922 men, 5,403 premenopausal women, and 1,412 postmenopausal women. About one-third of the premenopausal women took iron supplementation. The researchers found that 9 percent of the men who were frequent blood donors, defined as more than nine donations in the past three years, had iron deficiency. Premenopausal and postmenopausal women who were frequent blood donors had iron deficiency rates of 39 and 22 percent, respectively. The risk of iron deficiency was most often associated with sex, menopausal status, and donation frequency. Interestingly, "prolonging the time since last donation protected against development of iron deficiency." Dietary and supplemental iron intake appeared to have a much weaker effect. "In general, the blood donation frequency, the time since last donation, sex, and menopausal status were the most important predictors of current iron status, whereas physiologic, lifestyle or supplemental factors, and dietary factors were associated with iron stores but were less influential."[6]

Oral Iron Supplementation May Affect Cognition of Older Children and Adults

In a systematic review and meta-analysis published in 2010 in *Nutrition Journal*, researchers based in the United Kingdom wanted to learn if iron supplementation would impact the cognitive abilities of older children and adults. The researchers noted that previous observational studies have found that anemia and iron deficiency are associated with cognitive deficits. The cohort consisted of 14 randomized, controlled trials that included children six years and older, adolescents, and younger women. Only one study included women over 35 years old. The researchers were unable to locate randomized, controlled trials containing men, postmenopausal women, or the elderly. The researchers learned that irrespective of baseline iron status, iron supplementation improved attention and concentration. In groups that were anemic, supplementation improved intelligence, but the supplementation failed to improve the intelligence, memory, psychomotor skills, or scholastic achievement of nonanemic people. The researchers underscored the need for more studies on this topic. "Further well powered, blinded and independently funded studies of at least one year's duration in children, adolescents, adults and older people with varying levels of baseline iron status and using well validated tests of cognition are needed to confirm and extend these results."[7]

Iron Supplementation during Pregnancy May Impact an Infant's Birth Weight

In a double-blind, randomized, controlled trial published in 2015 in the *British Journal of Nutrition*, researchers from China and Atlanta, Georgia, wanted to learn more about the association between iron supplementation during pregnancy and the birth weight of newborns. The initial cohort consisted of 18,775 pregnant women from five counties in northern China. During a time period that began before 20 weeks of gestation and continued until delivery, the women took daily supplements that contained folic acid (control) or folic acid and iron, or multiple micronutrients including folic acid, iron, and 13 other vitamins and minerals. Mothers' hemoglobin levels were tested at enrollment and after birth; baby weights were also noted within the first hour of birth. The final cohort included 17,897 women. The researchers learned that the iron–folic acid combination and the multiple micronutrient supplements had no effect on the birth weight of the infants of women with normal or high baseline hemoglobin levels. On the other hand, in the women with very high baseline hemoglobin levels, the iron–folic acid combination and the multiple micronutrient supplements increased birth weight by 91.44 g and 107.63 g, respectively. The researchers concluded that "the effects of Fe[iron]-containing supplements on birth weight depended on baseline Hb [hemoglobin] concentrations."[8]

Overweight Women Tend to Have Lower Levels of Iron

In a study published in 2016 in the *European Journal of Clinical Nutrition*, researchers from Ann Arbor, Michigan, and Beijing, China, wanted to learn more about the effect of maternal obesity on the iron status of the mother and baby. The researchers examined longitudinal data from 1,613 participants in a pregnancy iron supplemental trial in rural China. The women, who had uncomplicated singleton pregnancies, were followed from the early second trimester of pregnancy until delivery. At enrollment, the researchers found a negative association between maternal BMI (body mass index) and iron status. Heavier women had lower levels of iron. On delivery, the researchers noted a negative association between maternal BMI and neonatal iron status. Heavier women had babies who had lower levels of iron, "suggesting that the placental transfer of iron may be inhibited among obese individuals." The researchers concluded that the prevalence of obesity and iron deficiency have profound public health consequences.[9]

Another study on the association between excess weight and iron deficiency was published in 2015 in the *American Journal of Clinical Nutrition*. In this study, researchers from Ann Arbor, Michigan, and China compared the amount of iron absorption from a wheat-based meal with ascorbic acid to a wheat-based meal without ascorbic acid in normal-weight women and in women who were overweight and obese. (Ascorbic acid is known to enhance the absorption of iron.) In total, the researchers recruited 62 women. Twenty-four women had a normal weight; 19 women were overweight; and 19 women were obese. The women ranged in age from 20 to 44 years. The researchers determined that iron absorption was lower in the overweight and obese women than in the normal-weight women, and the enhancing effect of ascorbic acid on the overweight and obese women was only one-half that of the normal-weight women. The researchers concluded that "the widespread increase in overweight and obesity may limit current dietary strategies to improve iron absorption in iron-deficit women."[10]

Iron Supplementation Appears to Be Useful for Postpartum Depression

In a randomized, double-blind, placebo-controlled study published in 2017 in the *European Journal of Nutrition*, researchers from Tehran, Iran, wanted to determine if iron supplementation would be useful for nonanemic mothers with postpartum depression. The cohort consisted of 70 mothers with postpartum depression. One week after the delivery of healthy infants, 35 mothers were assigned to receive a daily iron supplementation and 35 were assigned to take a placebo. After six weeks, the researchers learned that the early iron supplementation appeared to result in significant rates of improvement for postpartum depression. As a result of their findings, the researchers advised that iron evaluations should be conducted on all mothers with postpartum depression. "Daily iron supplementation should be considered for the early improvement in PPD [postpartum depression] and iron stores."[11]

NOTES

1. Office of Dietary Supplements, National Institutes of Health. "Iron." December 28, 2017. https://ods.od.nih.gov/factsheets/Iron-Consumer/.

2. Jackson, Jacklyn, Rebecca Williams, Mark McEvoy, et al. "Is Higher Consumption of Animal Flesh Foods Associated with Better Iron Status among Adults in Developed Countries? A Systematic Review." *Nutrients* 8, no. 2 (2016): 89+.

3. Peuranpää, Pirkko, Satu Heliövaara-Peippo, Ian Fraser, et al. "Effects of Anemia and Iron Deficiency on Quality of Life in Women with Heavy Menstrual Bleeding." *Acta Obstetricia et Gynecologica Scandinavica* 93, no. 7 (July 2014): 654–660.

4. Hoppe, Michael, Gunilla Önning, Anna Berggren, and Lena Hulthén. "Probiotic Strain *Lactobacillus Plantarum* 299v Increases Iron Absorption from an Iron-Supplemented Fruit Drink: A Double-Isotope Cross-Over Single-Blind Study in Women of Reproductive Age." *British Journal of Nutrition* 114 (2015): 1195–1202.

5. Kiss, Joseph E., Donald Brambilla, Simone A. Glynn, et al. "Oral Iron Supplementation after Blood Donation: A Randomized Clinical Trial." *JAMA* 313, no. 6 (2015): 575–583.

6. Rigas, Andreas Stribolt, Cecilie Juul Sørensen, Ole Birger Pedersen, et al. "Predictors of Iron Levels in 14,737 Danish Blood Donors: Results from the Danish Blood Donor Study." *Transfusion* 54 (March 2014): 789–796.

7. Falkingham, Martin, Asmaa Abdelhamid, Peter Curtis, et al. "The Effects of Oral Iron Supplementation on Cognition in Older Children and Adults: A Systematic Review and Meta-Analysis." *Nutrition Journal* 9 (2010): 4+.

8. Wang, Linlin, Zuguo Mei, Hongtian Li, et al. "Modifying Effects of Maternal Hb Concentration on Infant Birth Weight in Women Receiving Prenatal Iron-Containing Supplements: A Randomised Controlled Trial." *British Journal of Nutrition* 115 (2016): 644–649.

9. Jones, A. D., G. Zhao, Y. P. Jiang, et al. "Maternal Obesity during Pregnancy Is Negatively Associated with Maternal and Neonatal Iron Status." *European Journal of Clinical Nutrition* 70, no. 8 (August 2016): 918–924.

10. Cepeda-Lopez, A. C., A. Melse-Boonstra, M. B. Zimmermann, and I. Herter-Aeberli. "In Overweight and Obese Women, Dietary Iron Absorption Is Reduced and the Enhancement of Iron Absorption by Ascorbic Acid Is One-Half That in Normal-Weight Women." *American Journal of Clinical Nutrition* 102 (2015): 1389–1397.

11. Sheikh, Mahdi, Sedigheh Hantoushzadeh, Mamak Shariat, et al. "The Efficacy of Early Iron Supplementation on Postpartum Depression, A Randomized Double-Blind Placebo-Controlled Trial." *European Journal of Nutrition* 56, no. 2 (March 2017): 901–908.

REFERENCES AND FURTHER READINGS

Cepeda-Lopez, A. C., A. Melse-Boonstra, M. B. Zimmermann, and I. Herter-Aeberli. "In Overweight and Obese Women, Dietary Iron Absorption Is Reduced and the Enhancement of Iron Absorption by Ascorbic Acid Is One-Half That in Normal-Weight Women." *American Journal of Clinical Nutrition* 102 (2015): 1389–1397.

Falkingham, Martin, Asmaa Abdelhamid, Peter Curtis, et al. "The Effects of Oral Iron Supplementation on Cognition in Older Children and Adults: A Systematic Review and Meta-Analysis." *Nutrition Journal* 9 (2010): 4+.

Hoppe, Michael, Gunilla Önning, Anna Berggren, and Lena Hulthén. "Probiotic Strain *Lactobacillus plantarum* 299v Increases Iron Absorption from an Iron-Supplemented Fruit Drink: A Double-Isotope Cross-Over Single-Blind Study in Women of Reproductive Age." *British Journal of Nutrition* 114 (2015): 1195–1202.

Jackson, Jacklyn, Rebecca Williams, Mark McEvoy, et al. "Is Higher Consumption of Animal Flesh Foods Associated with Better Iron Status among Adults in Developed Countries? A Systematic Review." *Nutrients* 8, no. 2 (2016): 89+.

Jones, A. D., G. Zhao, Y. P. Jiang, et al. "Maternal Obesity during Pregnancy Is Negatively Associated with Maternal and Neonatal Iron Status." *European Journal of Clinical Nutrition* 70, no. 8 (August 2016): 918–924.

Kiss, Joseph E., Donald Brambilla, Simone A. Glynn, et al. "Oral Iron Supplementation after Blood Donation: A Randomized Clinical Trial." *JAMA* 313, no. 6 (2015): 575–583.

Office of Dietary Supplements, National Institutes of Health. "Iron." December 28, 2017. https://ods.od.nih.gov/factsheets/Iron-Consumer/.

Peuranpää, Pirkko, Satu Heliövaara-Peippo, Ian Fraser, et al. "Effects of Anemia and Iron Deficiency on Quality of Life in Women with Heavy Menstrual Bleeding." *Acta Obstetricia et Gynecologica Scandinavica* 93, no. 7 (July 2014): 654–660.

Rigas, Andreas Stribolt, Cecilie Juul Sørensen, Ole Birger Pedersen, et al. "Predictors of Iron Levels in 14,737 Danish Blood Donors: Results from the Danish Blood Donor Study." *Transfusion* 54 (March 2014): 789–796.

Sheikh, Mahdi, Sedigheh Hantoushzadeh, Mamak Shariat, et al. "The Efficacy of Early Iron Supplementation on Postpartum Depression, A Randomized Double-Blind Placebo-Controlled Trial." *European Journal of Nutrition* 56, no. 2 (March 2017): 901–908.

Wang, Linlin, Zuguo Mei, Hongtian Li, et al. "Modifying Effects of Maternal Hb Concentration on Infant Birth Weight in Women Receiving Prenatal Iron-Containing Supplements: A Randomised Controlled Trial." *British Journal of Nutrition* 115 (2016): 644–649.

Magnesium

The mineral magnesium, which is found in a wide variety of foods, plays a crucial role in human metabolism. In fact, it is known that magnesium is required for at least 300 chemical reactions in the human body. Probably the most important task performed by magnesium is the production of energy. To do this, magnesium is involved in numerous chemical reactions. In addition, magnesium is needed to maintain nervous system balance. Studies have even shown that supplemental magnesium may alleviate at least some degree of depression.

About 50 to 60 percent of the body's magnesium is stored in the bones. As a result, magnesium serves a vital role in bone metabolism. Therefore, even a small magnesium deficiency may result in a significant amount of bone loss. In laboratory studies, researchers have triggered bone loss when they feed animals low magnesium diets. It is assumed that this also occurs in people.

Many people contend that magnesium is useful for a wide variety of medical concerns such as cardiovascular problems, high blood pressure, high levels of bad cholesterol, metabolic syndrome, and plaque-clogged arteries. Magnesium is also said to be effective for treating attention deficit hyperactivity disorder, anxiety, chronic fatigue syndrome, Lyme disease, mania, leg cramps at night and during pregnancy, kidney stones, migraine headaches, restless leg syndrome, asthma, and multiple sclerosis, and for preventing hearing loss and cancer.[1]

FOOD SOURCES AND SUPPLEMENTS

Only a few foods, such as spinach, Swiss chard, and beet greens, are excellent sources of magnesium. Pumpkin seeds, summer squash, and turnip greens have very good amounts of magnesium. But many foods have good amounts. These include soybeans, sesame seeds, black beans, quinoa, cashews, buckwheat, brown rice, barley, tofu, millet, almonds, wheat, tuna scallops, kale, green beans, raspberries, beets, broccoli, tomatoes, cantaloupe, asparagus, and strawberries. Other sources of magnesium include dairy products, meats, chocolate, and coffee. Water that contains high levels of minerals has magnesium. Magnesium is often included in multivitamins. But magnesium supplementation may be sold as a single ingredient or combined with calcium in a supplement that supports bone health. The most absorbable forms of magnesium are magnesium aspartate, magnesium citrate, magnesium lactate, and magnesium chloride. Magnesium is frequently an ingredient in antacids used for acid indigestion, and magnesium may be contained in strong laxatives used for constipation and to prepare the bowel for diagnostic or surgical procedures.

INTAKE RECOMMENDATIONS

The Recommended Dietary Allowance (RDA) for magnesium varies according to age and sex. The recommendation for infants from birth to 12 months is an adequate intake recommendation. Pregnant women should take in 350 to 360 mg per day, while pregnant teens should take in 400 mg per day. Breastfeeding women should take in 310 to 320 mg per day, while breastfeeding teens should take in 360 mg per day. Adult men should take in 400 to 420 mg per day, while adult women should take in 310 to 320 mg per day. Male teens between the ages of 14 and 18 years should take in 410 mg per day, while female teens between the ages of 14 and 18 should take in 360 mg per day. Children between the ages of 9 and 13 years should take in 240 mg per day, while children between the ages of 4 and 8 years should take in 130 mg per day. Children between the ages of one and three years should take in 80 mg per day. The adequate intake for children from 7 to 12 months is 75 mg per day, and for children from birth to 6 months, it is 30 mg per day. There is no upper limit for the dietary intake of magnesium.[2]

DEFICIENCY AND EXCESS

In the United States, magnesium deficiency is believed to be somewhat common. It has been estimated that an average American takes in only about 75 percent of his or her magnesium requirements. While almost everyone should improve their intake of magnesium, some people are at increased risk for magnesium deficiency. People with high blood sugar levels and who are obese have an increased risk for magnesium deficiency. Magnesium deficiency increases with age, especially among those with heart failure and chronic obstructive pulmonary disease, and African Americans have higher rates of deficiency than Caucasians. People with chronic gastrointestinal problems, such as Crohn's disease, are also at risk for deficiency. Certain medications, including diuretics, reduce magnesium levels. Lower levels of magnesium are associated with poorer bone health, fatigue, depression, and increases in inflammation. It is almost impossible to take in too much magnesium from eating foods. Excess magnesium supplementation has a tendency to result in loose stools.

KEY RESEARCH FINDINGS

Magnesium Supplementation May Improve Blood Pressure

In a study published in 2012 in the *European Journal of Clinical Nutrition*, researchers from the United Kingdom wanted to learn more about the association between magnesium supplementation and blood pressure. As a result, they conducted a meta-analysis that included 22 trials and 23 sets of data, with a total of 1,173 people with both normal and elevated levels of blood pressure. The trials included follow-up periods of between 3 and 24 weeks and doses of supplemental magnesium that ranged from 120 to 973 mg per day—with a mean dose of 410 mg per day. The researchers determined that magnesium supplementation lowered blood pressure, with a greater reduction in systolic blood pressure. Higher doses of magnesium were more effective than lower doses. While the reduction was small, it was "clinically significant."[3]

Magnesium Is an Important Part of Childhood Bone Growth

In a study published in 2014 in the *Journal of Bone and Mineral Research*, researchers from Houston, Texas, wanted to learn more about the role that magnesium plays in the growth of children's bones. The initial cohort consisted of children who were between the ages of 4 and 8.9 years. In order to determine the consumption of magnesium and calcium, information on the children's eating habits was collected. Magnesium absorption studies were completed on 50 children. The researchers found an association between the consumption and absorption of magnesium and the amount of bone in the children. It appeared that magnesium intake was more important than magnesium absorption efficiency. The researchers concluded that "Mg [magnesium] intake may be important in optimizing bone mineral development in children."[4]

Dietary Intake of Magnesium and Calcium May Reduce the Risk of Metabolic Syndrome

In a study published in 2015 in the *British Journal of Nutrition*, researchers from Cleveland, Ohio, wanted to learn more about the association between intake of magnesium and calcium and metabolic syndrome. (Metabolic syndrome is a clustering of metabolic traits, including abdominal obesity, glucose intolerance, hypertension, and elevated levels of cholesterol.) The researchers used National Health and Nutrition Examination Survey (NHANES) data from 2001 to 2010 that included 9,148 adults (4,549 men and 4,599 women), with an average age of 50 years. The overall prevalence of metabolic syndrome was 39.1 percent. The researchers found an inverse association between intake of magnesium and calcium and risk of metabolic syndrome. The subjects with the highest intake of magnesium and calcium had the lowest risk of metabolic syndrome. The mean total daily intake of magnesium was 282.7 and 309.4 mg per day for individuals with and without metabolic syndrome, respectively. The women who met the RDA for both magnesium and calcium saw the greatest decrease in risk of metabolic syndrome. While the same association was not observed in the men, when the men increased their magnesium intake to over 386 mg and their calcium intake to over 1,224 mg per day, their odds of metabolic syndrome were lowered. The researchers commented that a strength of their study "is the use of a large, nationally represented sample of adults in the USA."[5]

Low Magnesium Levels Are Associated with Metabolic Syndrome

In a study published in 2016 in the journal *Biological Trace Element Research*, researchers from Korea noted that there is conflicting evidence about the association between magnesium deficiency and metabolic syndrome. In order to bring clarity to the varying results, they conducted a meta-analysis that included 13 relevant studies with 5,496 participants (2,358 cases and 3,138 controls). The participants ranged in age from 41 to 72 years and came from 10 different countries. The researchers determined that there was a "large difference" in magnesium levels between participants with metabolic syndrome and the healthy controls. And they concluded that despite a high level of heterogeneity, there was "an inverse association between magnesium levels and metabolic syndrome."[6]

In Mice, Magnesium Deficiency during Pregnancy Impairs Placental Size and Function

In a study published in 2016 in the journal *Placenta*, researchers from New York City, Manhasset, New York, and Hempstead, New York, investigated the effect of magnesium deficiency on placental size and function. Pregnant Webster Swiss mice were fed either 100 percent or 10 percent of the recommended amount of magnesium. The researchers determined that even this "moderate" level of magnesium deficiency significantly impaired the size and functioning of the placentas. In addition, the magnesium deficiency significantly reduced the nutrient update and increased oxidative stress. The researchers noted that studies are being conducted to determine "whether timely maternal Mg [magnesium] supplementation can reverse these effects in mice." And they added that their findings "highlight the adverse effects of maternal Mg deficiency on fetal weight and placental function."[7]

Magnesium May Be Useful for Migraines

In a meta-analysis published in 2016 in the journal *Pain Physician*, researchers from Taiwan wrote that migraine attacks have been associated with magnesium deficiency. That is why they wanted to learn more about the usefulness of intravenous magnesium for acute migraine attacks and the ability of oral magnesium supplements to prevent migraines. The meta-analysis included a total of 21 randomized, controlled trials written in English or Chinese. Eleven studies were on the effects of intravenous magnesium on acute migraines (948 participants) and 10 studies on the ability of oral magnesium to prevent migraines (789 participants). The researchers learned that both types of magnesium "produced substantial effects on migraine." Intravenous magnesium was beneficial 15 to 45 minutes after the initial infusion, 120 minutes after the infusion, and 24 hours after the infusion. And oral magnesium supplements were particularly effective in preventing migraine attacks. The researchers commented that their "findings support the beneficial effects of intravenous and oral magnesium on acute migraine attacks and the prophylaxis of migraine, respectively."[8]

Low Serum Magnesium May Be Associated with Incident Kidney Disease

In a study published in 2015 in the journal *Kidney International,* researchers from Baltimore, Maryland, Madison, Wisconsin, Chapel Hill, North Carolina, and Jackson, Mississippi, wanted to learn if there is an association between levels of serum magnesium and incident kidney disease in the general population. The researchers used data collected for the Atherosclerosis Risk in Communities study, which had 13,226 participants between the ages of 45 and 65 years. During a follow-up of 21 years, there were 1,965 cases of incident chronic kidney disease and 208 cases of end-stage renal disease. The researchers determined that low levels of serum magnesium were significantly associated with incident chronic kidney disease and end-stage renal disease. In fact, subjects in the lowest serum magnesium category were about 1.6 times more likely to develop incident chronic kidney disease and 2.4 times more likely to develop end-stage renal disease. "In a large sample of middle-aged adults, low total serum magnesium was independently associated with incident CKD [chronic kidney disease] and ESRD [end-stage renal disease]."[9]

Magnesium Supplementation May Improve Physical Performance in Elderly Women

In a randomized, controlled study published in 2014 in the *American Journal of Clinical Nutrition,* researchers based in Italy wanted to learn more about the association between magnesium supplementation and physical performance of the elderly. The cohort consisted of 139 healthy, physically active women with a mean age of 71.5 years. Sixty-two women were assigned to take 12 weeks of magnesium supplementation; seventy-seven women had no intervention. The final analysis included 53 women on magnesium supplementation and 71 women who had no intervention. At baseline, both groups of women had similar performance scores. By the end of the trial, the women in the intervention group had significantly better performance scores. The researchers commented that their findings "suggest a role for magnesium supplementation preventing or delaying the age-related decline in physical performance." Magnesium supplementation may be most useful for elderly people who are magnesium deficient.[10]

There May Be an Association between Magnesium Intake and Depression

In a study published in 2015 in the *Journal of the American Board of Family Medicine,* researchers from Burlington, Vermont, wanted to learn more about the association between magnesium dietary intake and depression. The researchers used data from the cross-sectional, population-based NHANES from 2007 to 2010, which included 8,894 U.S. adults with a mean age of 46.1 years. The data showed the total magnesium intake in milligrams per day from both diets and supplements. The researchers found a statistically significant relationship between low intake of magnesium and depression in subjects younger than 65 years. "After adjusting for all potential confounders, the strength of the association of low magnesium intake with depression was attenuated but remained statistically significant."[11]

Low Magnesium Intake May Be Associated with "Externalizing" Behaviors in Adolescents

In a study published in 2015 in the journal *Public Health Nutrition*, researchers from Australia examined the association between low dietary intake of magnesium and "externalizing behavior problems" such as aggressive/delinquent behaviors and attention difficulties and "internalizing behavior problems" such as somatic complaints, anxiety, and depression in adolescents. The initial cohort consisted of 684 adolescents. Mental health assessments were conducted when they were 14 and 17 years. The researchers found a significant inverse association between magnesium and externalizing behavior problems; this association did not exist for internalizing behavior problems. The researchers noted that since magnesium intake may be increased by eating certain foods and taking supplementation, their findings have "important public health implications." Promoting the consumption of magnesium-rich foods and supplementation "may be a useful strategy to prevent mental health and behavioural problems in adolescents."[12]

The Risk of Diabetes May Be Associated with the Intake of Dietary Magnesium

In a study published in 2017 in the *European Journal of Nutrition*, researchers from Japan noted that past research on the association between magnesium intake and risk of diabetes has yielded inconsistent results. As a result, the researchers decided to investigate the association using the Takayama study, a Japanese population-based cohort that included 13,525 male and female residents of Takayama City. Magnesium intake was determined from a food frequency questionnaire administered at baseline. During a follow-up of 10 years, 438 subjects reported being diagnosed with diabetes. The researchers determined that women with the highest intake of magnesium had the lowest risk; the women in the high quartile of magnesium intake had a 50 percent lower risk of developing diabetes than the women in the low quartile. This type of association was not observed in men. "These results suggest that diets with a high intake of magnesium may decrease the risk of diabetes in women."[13]

NOTES

1. The George Mateljan Foundation. "Magnesium." December 28, 2017. http://whfoods.com/genpage.php?tname=nutrient&dbid=75.

2. Office of Dietary Supplements, National Institutes of Health. "Magnesium." December 28, 2017. https://ods.od.nih.gov/factsheets/Magnesium-Consumer/.

3. Kass, L., J. Weekes, and L. Carpenter. "Effect of Magnesium Supplementation on Blood Pressure: A Meta-Analysis." *European Journal of Clinical Nutrition* 66 (2012): 411–418.

4. Abrams, Steven A., Zhensheng Chen, and Keli M. Hawthorne. "Magnesium Metabolism in 4-Year-Old to 8-Year-Old Children." *Journal of Bone and Mineral Research* 29, no. 1 (January 2014): 118–122.

5. Moore-Schiltz, Laura, Jeffrey M. Albert, Mendel E. Singer, et al. "Dietary Intake of Calcium and Magnesium and the Metabolic Syndrome in the National Health and Nutrition Examination (NHANES) 2001–2010 Data." *British Journal of Nutrition* 114 (2015): 924–935.

6. La, Sang A., June Young Lee, Do Hoon Kim, et al. "Low Magnesium Levels in Adults with Metabolic Syndrome: A Meta-Analysis." *Biological Trace Element Research* 170 (2016): 33–42.

7. Rosner, J. Y., M. Gupta, M. McGill, et al. "Magnesium Deficiency during Pregnancy in Mice Impairs Placental Size and Function." *Placenta* 39 (2016): 87–93.

8. Chiu, H. Y., T. H. Yeh, Y. C. Huang, and P. Y. Chen. "Effects of Intravenous and Oral Magnesium on Reducing Migraine: A Meta-Analysis of Randomized Controlled Trials." *Pain Physician* 19, no. 1 (January 2016): E97–E112.

9. Tin, Adrienne, Morgan E. Grams, Nisa M. Maruthur, et al. "Results from the Atherosclerosis Risk in Communities Study Suggest That Low Serum Magnesium Is Associated with Incident Kidney Disease." *Kidney International* 87 (2015): 820–827.

10. Veronese, Nicola, Linda Berton, Sara Carraro, et al. "Effect of Oral Magnesium Supplementation on Physical Performance in Healthy Elderly Women Involved in a Weekly Exercise Program: A Randomized Controlled Trial." *American Journal of Clinical Nutrition* 100 (2014): 974–981.

11. Tarleton, Emily K. and Benjamin Littenberg. "Magnesium Intake and Depression in Adults." *Journal of the American Board of Family Medicine* 28, no. 2 (March–April 2015): 249–256.

12. Black, Lucinda J., Karina L. Allen, Peter Jacoby, et al. "Low Dietary Intake of Magnesium Is Associated with Increased Externalising Behaviours in Adolescents." *Public Health Nutrition* 18, no. 10 (July 2015): 1824–1830.

13. Konishi, Kie, Keiko Wada, Takashi Tamura, et al. "Dietary Magnesium Intake and the Risk of Diabetes in the Japanese Community: Results from the Takayama Study." *European Journal of Nutrition* 56, no. 2 (March 2017): 767–774.

REFERENCES AND FURTHER READINGS

Abrams, Steven A., Zhensheng Chen, and Keli M. Hawthorne. "Magnesium Metabolism in 4-Year-Old to 8-Year-Old Children." *Journal of Bone and Mineral Research* 29, no. 1 (January 2014): 118–122.

Black, Lucinda J., Karina L. Allen, Peter Jacoby, et al. "Low Dietary Intake of Magnesium Is Associated with Increased Externalising Behaviours in Adolescents." *Public Health Nutrition* 18, no. 10 (July 2015): 1824–1830.

Chiu, H. Y., T. H. Yeh, Y. C. Huang, and P. Y. Chen. "Effects of Intravenous and Oral Magnesium on Reducing Migraine: A Meta-Analysis of Randomized Controlled Trials." *Pain Physician* 19, no. 1 (January 2016): E97–E112.

The George Mateljan Foundation. "Magnesium." December 28, 2017. http://whfoods.com/genpage.php?tname=nutrient&dbid=75.

Kass, L., J. Weekes, and L. Carpenter. "Effect of Magnesium Supplementation on Blood Pressure: A Meta-Analysis." *European Journal of Clinical Nutrition* 66 (2012): 411–418.

Konishi, Kie, Keiko Wada, Takashi Tamura, et al. "Dietary Magnesium Intake and the Risk of Diabetes in the Japanese Community: Results from the Takayama Study." *European Journal of Nutrition* 56, no. 2 (March 2017): 767–774.

La, Sang A., June Young Lee, Do Hoon Kim, et al. "Low Magnesium Levels in Adults with Metabolic Syndrome: A Meta-Analysis." *Biological Trace Element Research* 170 (2016): 33–42.

Moore-Schiltz, Laura, Jeffrey M. Albert, Mendel E. Singer, et al. "Dietary Intake of Calcium and Magnesium and the Metabolic Syndrome in the National Health and Nutrition Examination (NHANES) 2001–2010 Data." *British Journal of Nutrition* 114 (2015): 924–935.

Office of Dietary Supplements, National Institutes of Health. "Magnesium." December 28, 2017. https://ods.od.nih.gov/factsheets/Magnesium-Consumer/.

Rosner, J. Y., M. Gupta, M. McGill, et al. "Magnesium Deficiency during Pregnancy in Mice Impairs Placental Size and Function." *Placenta* 39 (2016): 87–93.

Tarleton, Emily K. and Benjamin Littenberg. "Magnesium Intake and Depression in Adults." *Journal of the American Board of Family Medicine* 28, no. 2 (March–April 2015): 249–256.

Tin, Adrienne, Morgan E. Grams, Nisa M. Maruthur, et al. "Results from the Atherosclerosis Risk in Communities Study Suggest That Low Serum Magnesium Is Associated with Incident Kidney Disease." *Kidney International* 87 (2015): 820–827.

Veronese, Nicola, Linda Berton, Sara Carraro, et al. "Effect of Oral Magnesium Supplementation on Physical Performance in Healthy Elderly Women Involved in a Weekly Exercise Program: A Randomized Controlled Trial." *American Journal of Clinical Nutrition* 100 (2014): 974–981.

Manganese

Though many people have never heard of manganese (Mn), it is a trace mineral that the body requires in tiny amounts to maintain proper health and function. Manganese helps the body build connective tissue, bones, blood clotting factors, and sex hormones. Fortunately, manganese is found in a wide variety of plant-based foods. Adults are able to store very small amounts of manganese in their bodies—about 15 to 20 mg—primarily in bones, the liver, kidneys, and the pancreas.

Manganese functions as an antioxidant in skin cells and other types of cells, and it assists in protecting skin against oxygen-related damage and from ultraviolet light. In so doing, manganese may play a role in anti-aging and preventing or delaying the development of a number of health conditions, such as heart disease and cancer. Manganese is also required for a process known as gluconeogenesis, which is the conversion of substances like amino acids and organic acids into glucose. Some of the enzymes in this process require manganese. Moreover, manganese is thought to play a role in fat and carbohydrate metabolism, blood sugar control, calcium absorption, and normal brain and nerve function. And it is believed to be useful for arthritis, premenstrual syndrome, diabetes, and epilepsy.

FOOD SOURCES AND SUPPLEMENTS

There are many foods that contain excellent amounts of manganese. These include oats, brown rice, garbanzo beans, spinach, pineapple, raspberries, beet greens, kale, turnip greens, summer squash, sea vegetables, garlic, and bok choy. Large numbers of foods contain very good amounts of manganese. These include pumpkin seeds, soybeans, tofu, barley, quinoa, wheat, walnuts, sweet potatoes, lentils, green peas, buckwheat, beets, almonds, blueberries, winter squash, cranberries, broccoli, asparagus, tomatoes, cauliflower, crimini mushrooms, and cabbage. Lots of foods have good amounts of manganese. These include pinto beans, black beans, kidney beans, peanuts, sunflower seeds, cashews, potatoes, bananas, onions, carrots, shiitake mushrooms, corn, eggplants, bell peppers, kiwifruit, and cucumbers.[1] Manganese may also be obtained through supplementation. It is sold by itself, or it may be combined with other trace minerals. Manganese is often included in multivitamin supplements.

INTAKE RECOMMENDATIONS

The following are the Dietary Reference Intake standards for manganese. These standards are adequate intake levels. Pregnant women should take in 2 mg per day, while lactating women should take in 2.6 mg per day. Males 19 years and older should take in 2.3 mg per day, while females 19 years and older should take in 1.8 mg per day. Male teens between the ages of 14 and 18 years should take in 2.2 mg per day, while female teens between the ages of 14 and 18 years should take in 1.6 mg per day. Male children between the ages of 9 and 13 years should take in 1.9 mg per day, while female children between the ages of 9 and 13 should take in 1.6 mg per day. Children between the ages of four and eight years should take in 1.5 mg per day, while children between the ages of one and three years should take in 1.2 mg per day. Infants between the ages of 7 and 12 months should take in 0.6 mg per day, while infants from birth to 6 months should take in 0.003 mg per day. Manganese has a tolerable upper intake level of 11 mg per day.[2]

DEFICIENCY AND EXCESS

Animal studies have determined that very low intakes of manganese are associated with poor bone formation. It is not known if low levels of manganese contribute to bone loss. People who take in insufficient amounts of manganese may have skin problems, such as rashes. Low levels of manganese intake have also been associated with infertility, bone malformation, weakness, and seizures. On the other hand, too much dietary manganese may result in high levels of the mineral in body tissues, which have the potential to cause neurological problems.

Elevated levels of manganese have been associated with poor cognitive performance and learning disabilities in school children. People may also be exposed to excessive amounts of manganese through air and water supplies. For example, it is known that welders and steel workers have higher-than-desirable exposure to manganese. It is not uncommon for steel workers to have nervous system problems.

KEY RESEARCH FINDINGS

There May Be an Association between Manganese Intake and Children's Attention, Cognition, Behavior, and Academic Performance

In a cross-sectional study published in 2013 in the journal *Experimental Research*, researchers from Korea wanted to learn if a high or low exposure to manganese was associated with academic and attention problems among school children. The cohort consisted of 1,089 children between the ages of 8 and 11 years, who lived in five representative areas in South Korea. The researchers selected two or three schools from each region. After the children had a variety of tests, the researchers divided the data into three different levels of manganese—a high-manganese group, a middle-manganese group, and a low-manganese group. The researchers determined that higher intake of manganese was associated with lower scores in thinking, reading, calculation, and intelligence quotient and increased risk of errors. On the other hand, a lower intake of manganese was associated with lower scores on a color naming test. Why are these results so important? The researchers commented that the school children were at an age of rapid brain development that includes the maturation of the frontal brain, which deals with attention and concentration. "The findings of this cross-sectional study suggest that excess exposure or deficiency of Mn can cause harmful effects in children."[3]

There Seems to Be an Association between Levels of Manganese in the Hair and Symptoms of Attention Deficit Hyperactivity Disorder

In a study published in 2015 in the journal *Psychiatry Investigation*, researchers from Korea investigated the association between levels of manganese in the hair and symptoms of attention deficit hyperactivity disorder. The cohort consisted of 40 children with attention deficit hyperactivity disorder and 43 control children without this disorder. The children, who had an average age of 9.72 years, mostly lived in the urban area of Seoul, Korea. Evaluations were conducted to assess the severity of the attention deficit hyperactivity disorder, and hair samples were taken to determine the levels of manganese. The researchers found a significant association between manganese levels and the presence of attention deficit hyperactivity disorder. In fact, both high levels and deficient levels of manganese were associated with attention deficit hyperactivity disorder. The researchers commented that "further research is needed to understand the causal relationship between Mn exposure and children's health, and to enable an improved risk assessment."[4]

There May Be an Association between Low Levels of Manganese and Preeclampsia in Pregnant Women

In a case-controlled study published in 2013 in the journal *Biological Trace Element Research*, researchers from Bangladesh evaluated the association between the serum concentrations of four trace elements, including manganese, and the rates of preeclampsia in Bangladesh women. (Preeclampsia is a disorder in which a pregnant woman experiences high blood pressure; it has the potential to damage other organs, often the kidneys.) Reducing the rates of preeclampsia is important. According to the researchers, preeclampsia occurs in about 2 to 8 percent of all pregnancies, and "it is one of the leading causes of maternal mortality and preterm delivery in the world." Preeclampsia threatens the life of both the mother and the growing fetus. The cohort consisted of 50 preeclamptic pregnant women and 58 pregnant women with normal blood pressure. Data were collected during routine obstetric visits from June 2012 to February 2013. When the researchers compared the levels of manganese in the women, they determined that the women with preeclampsia had significantly lower levels. Interestingly, the levels of the other trace elements—zinc, copper, and iron—were also lower. The researchers noted that "decreased concentration of trace element may play a major role in the development of preeclampsia."[5]

Serum Manganese Levels Appear to Be Associated with Type 2 Diabetes

In a case-controlled study published in 2016 in the journal *Environmental Health Perspectives*, researchers from China and Boston wanted to learn more about the association between levels of manganese in the blood and the incidence of newly diagnosed type 2 diabetes. The cohort consisted of 3,228 participants from China; 1,614 were newly diagnosed with type 2 diabetes and 1,614 were normal controls. When compared to the controls, the subjects with type 2 diabetes had higher body mass index and total cholesterol values and a greater prevalence of family history of diabetes and hypertension. The researchers found a U-shaped association between levels of serum manganese and incidence of newly diagnosed type 2 diabetes. Both low and high levels of manganese were associated with higher rates of newly diagnosed type 2 diabetes. The researchers commented that "further studies with large samples, especially prospective studies, are warranted to confirm the association between manganese levels and T2D [type 2 diabetes]."[6]

Manganese Levels Appear to Be Associated with Diabetes and Renal Dysfunction

In a cross-sectional study published in 2014 in the journal BMC Endocrine Disorders, researchers from Korea investigated the association between levels of manganese in the blood and diabetes and renal dysfunction. Data were obtained from the Korean National Health and Nutrition Examination Survey (KNAHNES). The cohort included 3,996 participants who were at least 20 years old. All of the participants had been evaluated for the presence of five chronic disease: diabetes, renal dysfunction, hypertension, ischemic heart disease, and stroke. The researchers found significantly lower levels of manganese in the diabetes and renal dysfunction groups. Thus, the participants with lower levels of serum manganese were at increased risk for diabetes and renal dysfunction. There was no significant association between manganese and the other groups. According to the researchers, their findings suggested that serum manganese deficiency "might be involved in the pathophysiological processes of diabetes and renal dysfunction."[7]

Blood Levels of Manganese May Influence Blood Pressure

The previously noted KNAHNES data were also used for a study published in 2011 in the journal Environmental Research. In this study, researchers from Korea examined the association between levels of serum manganese and blood pressure readings. The cohort included 1,991 adults 20 years of age or older. The researchers learned that the geometric mean level of manganese was significantly higher in the women than the men. And the geometric mean level of blood manganese of the subjects with normal blood pressure was significantly lower than the subjects with prehypertension or hypertension (high blood pressure). The researchers concluded that blood manganese levels were "associated with an increased risk of hypertension in data representative of the Korean adult population." This finding "may have important implications for health policy and disease prevention."[8]

Manganese Deficiency May Be Related to Breast Cancer

In a study published in 2015 in the International Journal of Clinical and Experimental Medicine, researchers from China wrote that there have been conflicting reports on the association between manganese levels and breast cancer. To learn more, they conducted a meta-analysis that included 11 case-controlled studies published in English and Chinese with 1,302 subjects. The studies, which were published between 2000 and 2013, each included between 50 and 285 subjects. They were conducted in China, Turkey, and Korea. When compared to the healthy controls, the subjects with breast cancer from China and Korea had lower levels of manganese in their blood or hair. Why was this association not evident in the Turkish women? The researchers suggest that the answer may be obtained from additional research. "This finding needs further confirmation by trans-regional multicenter, long-term observation in a cohort design to obtain better understanding of causal relationships between Mn levels and breast cancer."[9]

Manganese in Drinking Water May Negatively Impact the Neurobehavioral Functioning of School-Age Children

In a cross-sectional study published in 2014 in the journal *Environmental Health Perspectives*, researchers from Boston and several locations in Canada wanted to examine the association between the intake of manganese in drinking water and several aspects of neurobehavioral functioning—memory, attention, motor function, and parent- and teacher-reported hyperactive behavior. The cohort consisted of 375 children, between the ages of 6 and 13 years, from eight municipalities located in southern Quebec, Canada. The researchers measured the amounts of manganese in the home water supplies and in the hair of the children. During home visits, researchers administered food frequency questionnaires. Other tests and scales were used to assess neurobehavioral functioning. The researchers learned that the children with the higher intake of manganese had poorer memory, attention, and motor function. The manganese did not appear to have any impact on hyperactive behavior. The researchers concluded that "exposure to manganese in water was associated with poorer neurobehavioral performance in children, even at low levels commonly encountered in North American."[10]

Chronic Manganese Exposure May Impair Attention and Working Memory of Nonhuman Primates

In a study published in 2015 in the journal *NeuroToxicology*, researchers from Philadelphia, Pennsylvania, and New York City wanted to learn more about cognitive problems associated with chronic manganese exposure. Specifically, the researchers focused on the effect of chronic manganese exposure on attention, working memory, and executive function in nine monkeys who were between five and six years old when the study began. The monkeys were all trained to do various cognitive tasks. During a period of 12 months, six of the monkeys were exposed to manganese and three served as controls. The researchers observed that deficits began a few months after manganese exposure. After several months, the exposed monkeys had essentially no problems with the easiest tasks but significant impairments with the more difficult tasks. In contrast, the control monkeys demonstrated either no change or improvements in performance. The researchers commented that their findings "add to the literature on the detrimental effects of chronic Mn exposure on cognition."[11]

There Appears to Be Some Association between Dietary Intake of Manganese and Metabolic Syndrome

In a study published in 2016 in the *British Journal of Nutrition*, researchers from different locations in China noted that animal studies have found associations between intake of manganese and some aspects of metabolic syndrome. Only a few such studies have been conducted on Chinese adults. In order to complete their own trial, the researchers used data obtained from the Fifth Chinese National Nutrition and Health Survey (2010–2012), which provided relevant information on 2,111 adults. The participants completed questionnaires, dietary assessments, and physical examinations. Rice was determined to be the major food source of manganese. Twenty-eight percent of the subjects (n = 590) had metabolic syndrome. In men, a higher intake of manganese was associated with a lower risk of metabolic syndrome. However, in women, a high intake of manganese was associated with an increased risk of metabolic syndrome. A high intake of manganese was associated with an increased risk of low HDL ("good") cholesterol among both men and women. The researchers commented that "the inverse association between Mn intake and the MetS [metabolic syndrome] in women might be due to the increased risk for low HDL-cholesterol."[12]

There May Be an Association between a Pregnant Woman's Levels of Urinary Manganese and Her Newborn's Birth Weight

In a study published in 2016 in the journal *BMC Public Health*, researchers from China and several locations in the United States wanted to learn more about the role that different levels of maternal urinary manganese has on the birth weight of newborns. Between 2012 and 2014, researchers in China collected maternal urine samples from 816 women before they delivered their babies. Following delivery of these babies, the researchers analyzed data on 204 low-birth-weight newborns and 612 matched controls. When compared to the control mothers, the researchers determined that the mothers of the low-birth-weight infants had significantly higher levels of urinary manganese. The mothers of low-birth-weight infants also tended to have low levels of manganese, though this relationship was not significant. The researchers commented that manganese "may contribute to adverse birth outcomes at both low and high exposure levels." In addition, "this observation suggests that Mn during pregnancy may be important for fetal growth."[13]

NOTES

1. The George Mateljan Foundation. "Manganese." December 28, 2017. http://whfoods.com/genpage.php?tname=nutrient&dbid=77.
2. University of Maryland Medical Center. "Manganese." December 28, 2017. http://umm.edu/health/medical/altmed/supplement/manganese.
3. Bhang, Soo-Young, Soo-Churl Cho, Jae-Won Kim, et al. "Relationship between Blood Manganese Levels and Children's Attention, Cognition, Behavior, and Academic Performance—A Nationwide Cross-Sectional Study." *Environmental Research* 126 (2013): 9–16.
4. Shin, Dong-Won, Eun-Ji Kim, Se-Won Lim, et al. "Association of Hair Manganese Level with Symptoms in Attention-Deficit/Hyperactivity Disorder." *Psychiatry Investigation* 12, no. 1 (January 2015): 66–72.
5. Sarwar, M.S., S. Ahmed, M.S. Ullah, et al. "Comparative Study of Serum Zinc, Copper, Manganese, and Iron in Preeclamptic Pregnant Women." *Biological Trace Element Research* 154 (2013): 14–20.
6. Shan, Z., S. Chen, T. Sun, et al. "U-Shaped Association between Plasma Manganese Levels and Type 2 Diabetes." *Environmental Health Perspectives* 124, no. 12 (December 2016): 1876–1881.
7. Koh, Eun Sil, Sung Jun Kim, Hye Eun Yoon, et al. "Association of Blood Manganese Level with Diabetes and Renal Dysfunction: A Cross-Sectional Study of the Korean General Population." *BMC Endocrine Disorders* 14 (2014): 24.
8. Lee, Byung-Kook and Yangho Kim. "Relationship between Blood Manganese and Blood Pressure in the Korean General Population according to KNHANES 2008." *Environmental Research* 111 (2011): 797–803.
9. Shen, Fei, Wen-Song Cai, Jiang-Lin Li, et al. "The Association between Deficient Manganese Levels and Breast Cancer: A Meta-Analysis." *International Journal of Clinical and Experimental Medicine* 8, no. 3 (March 15, 2015): 3671–3680.
10. Oulhote, Youssef, Donna Mergler, Benoit Barbeau, et al. "Neurobehavioral Function in School-Age Children Exposed to Manganese in Drinking Water." *Environmental Health Perspectives* 122, no. 12 (December 2014): 1343–1350.
11. Schneider, J.S., C. Williams, M. Ault, and T.R. Guilarte. "Effects of Chronic Manganese Exposure on Attention and Working Memory in Non-Human Primates." *NeuroToxicology* 48 (2015): 217–222.
12. Zhou, Biao, Xuefen Su, Danting Su, et al. "Dietary Intake of Manganese and the Risk of the Metabolic Syndrome in a Chinese Population." *British Journal of Nutrition* 116, no. 5 (2016): 853–863.
13. Xia, Wei, Yanqiu Zhou, Tongzhang Zheng, et al. "Maternal Urinary Manganese and Risk of Low Birth Weight: A Case-Control Study." *BMC Public Health* 16 (2016): 142+.

REFERENCES AND FURTHER READINGS

Bhang, Soo-Young, Soo-Churl Cho, Jae-Won Kim, et al. "Relationship between Blood Manganese Levels and Children's Attention, Cognition, Behavior, and Academic Performance—A Nationwide Cross-Sectional Study." *Environmental Research* 126 (2013): 9–16.
The George Mateljan Foundation. "Manganese." December 28, 2017. http://whfoods.com/genpage.php?tname=nutrient&dbid=77.

Koh, Eun Sil, Sung Jun Kim, Hye Eun Yoon, et al. "Association of Blood Manganese Level with Diabetes and Renal Dysfunction: A Cross-Sectional Study of the Korean General Population." *BMC Endocrine Disorders* 14 (2014): 24.

Lee, Byung-Kook and Yangho Kim. "Relationship between Blood Manganese and Blood Pressure in the Korean General Population according to KNHANES 2008." *Environmental Research* 111 (2011): 797–803.

Oulhote, Youssef, Donna Mergler, Benoit Barbeau, et al. "Neurobiological Function in School-Age Children Exposed to Manganese in Drinking Water." *Environmental Health Perspectives* 122, no. 12 (December 2014): 1343–1350.

Sarwar, M. S., S. Ahmed, M. S. Ullah, et al. "Comparative Study of Serum Zinc, Copper, Manganese, and Iron in Preeclamptic Pregnant Women." *Biological Trace Element Research* 154 (2013): 14–20.

Schneider, J. S., C. Williams, M. Ault, and T. R. Guilarte. "Effects of Chronic Manganese Exposure on Attention and Working Memory in Non-Human Primates." *NeuroToxicology* 48 (2015): 217–222.

Shan, Z., S. Chen, T. Sun, et al. "U-Shaped Association between Plasma Manganese Levels and Type 2 Diabetes." *Environmental Health Perspectives* 124, no. 12 (December 2016): 1876–1881.

Shen, Fei, Wen-Song Cai, Jiang-Lin Li, et al. "The Association between Deficient Manganese Levels and Breast Cancer: A Meta-Analysis." *International Journal of Clinical and Experimental Medicine* 8, no. 3 (March 15, 2015): 3671–3680.

Shin, Dong-Won, Eun-Ji Kim, Se-Won Lim, et al. "Association of Hair Manganese Level with Symptoms of Attention-Deficit/Hyperactivity Disorder." *Psychiatry Investigation* 12, no. 1 (January 2015): 66–72.

University of Maryland Medical Center. "Manganese." December 28, 2017. http://umm.edu/health/medical/altmed/supplement/manganese.

Xia, Wei, Yanqiu Zhou, Tongzhang Zheng, et al. "Maternal Urinary Manganese and Risk of Low Birth Weight: A Case-Control Study." *BMC Public Health* 16 (2016): 142+.

Zhou, Biao, Xuefen Su, Danting Su, et al. "Dietary Intake of Manganese and the Risk of the Metabolic Syndrome in a Chinese Population." *British Journal of Nutrition* 116, no. 5 (2016): 853–863.

Molybdenum

Though not as well known as many other minerals, molybdenum is a key trace mineral that plays a role in numerous different body systems. Molybdenum is needed for at least seven body enzymes to function. For example, molybdenum is required for the enzyme sulfite oxidase to work in many of the organ systems of the body, especially the liver and brain. And molybdenum is a cofactor for an enzyme called xanthine oxidase, which helps convert hypoxanthine and xanthine into uric acid. While too much uric acid is associated with the painful condition known as gout, the body requires healthy amounts of uric acid.

In addition, because molybdenum is a cofactor of the enzyme aldehyde dehydrogenase, it probably plays a role in nervous system metabolism, specifically metabolism of the nervous system messaging molecules such as serotonin and melatonin. Molybdenum is also needed to form unique proteins called amidoxine-reducing component proteins.[1] Without molybdenum, the body cannot break down certain amino acids.

FOOD SOURCES AND SUPPLEMENTS

Excellent sources of molybdenum include lentils, dried peas, lima beans, kidney beans, soybeans, black beans, pinto beans, garbanzo beans, oats, tomatoes, romaine lettuce, cucumbers, and celery. Very good sources of molybdenum include barley, eggs, carrots, bell peppers, and fennel. Good sources of molybdenum include yogurt, peanuts, sesame seeds, walnuts, green peas, almonds, and cod.[2] Though it may be a little difficult to find in retail stores, molybdenum is sold online as a single-ingredient supplement. It is available in a variety of forms, including capsules, tablets, and liquid. Molybdenum may be combined with other trace minerals and may be included in daily multivitamin formulas.

INTAKE RECOMMENDATIONS

The Food and Nutrition Board of the National Academy of Sciences established Dietary Reference Intakes for molybdenum. The recommendations for infants under one year are adequate intake levels. Pregnant and lactating women should take in 50 mg per day. Men and women 19 years and older should take in 45 mcg per day, while teens between the ages of 14 and 18 years should take in 43 mcg per day. Children between the ages of 9 and 13 years should take in 34 mcg per day, while children between the ages of 4 and 8 years should take in 22 mcg per day. Children between the ages of one and three years should take in 17 mcg per day. Infants between the ages of 6 and 12 months should take in 3 mcg per day, while infants from birth to 6 months should take in 2 mcg per day.

There are also upper intake levels for molybdenum. Pregnant or lactating women over 19 years should not take in more than 2,000 mcg per day, while pregnant or lactating women under 19 years should not take in more than 1,700 mcg per day. Men and women who are 19 years or older should take in no more than 2,000 mcg per day, while teens between the ages of 14 and 18 should take in no more than 1,700 mcg per day. Children between the ages of 9 and 13 years should take in no more than 1,000 mcg per day, while children between the ages of 4 and 8 should take in no more than 600 mcg per day. Children between the ages of one and three years should take in no more than 300 mcg per day. There is no established limit for infants under 12 months.[3]

DEFICIENCY AND EXCESS

In the United States, it is believed that people have a very low risk of molybdenum deficiency. The typical American diet contains far more molybdenum than the body needs. At the same time, there appears to be a low risk of dietary toxicity. But these topics have not been sufficiently studied.

KEY RESEARCH FINDINGS

There May Be an Association between Low Levels of Molybdenum and Esophageal Cancer

In a study published in 2012 in the *Global Journal of Health Science*, researchers from India and South Africa examined the association between molybdenum, zinc, and esophageal cancer. Their cohort consisted of two different ethnic populations. One group was from Eastern Cape, South Africa, where there are high rates of esophageal cancer. The other group was from West Bengal, India, where there are low rates of the illness. Each ethnic group was divided into two groups of 30 people—one group consisted of esophageal cancer patients and the other group had volunteers who were controls. Hair samples were taken from all of the participants, and food grains from both regions were analyzed. The researchers found a strong correlation between reduced levels of molybdenum in the hair and the development of esophageal cancer in South Africa. The food grains from South Africa also had lower levels of molybdenum. And they concluded that the low levels of molybdenum may be an explanation for the higher rates of esophageal cancer.[4]

There Appears to Be a Low Risk of Excessive or Inadequate Consumption of Molybdenum

In a study published in 2014 in the journal *Food Additives & Contaminants*, researchers from Cameroon (central Africa), Maryland (United States), Italy, and France examined the dietary exposure of 14 toxic and essential trace elements, including molybdenum. Food consumption data were obtained from the Second Cameroon Household Budget Survey. In addition, there were 1,773 individual food samples that were pooled into 64 analytical samples. The researchers determined that the risk of the excess or inadequate consumption of molybdenum was low. Among the surveyed population, molybdenum "can be considered not to pose a public health problem."[5]

Levels of Molybdenum in U.S. and Canadian Infant Formulas May Be Higher Than Desired

In a study published in 2011 in the journal *Biological Trace Element Research*, researchers from Canada wanted to learn more about the amounts of molybdenum in infant formulas sold in the United States and Canada. A total of 81 infant formulas were purchased in Canada and multiple locations in the United

States. The levels of molybdenum in the formulas were compared to the amount of molybdenum in powdered milk and human milk. The researchers learned that full-term, premature, and soy-based formulas had significantly higher mean molybdenum content than human milk and "special" formulas. Meanwhile, the molybdenum content and quality of the raw materials were consistent among the manufacturers of the products studied. And there were no significant differences in molybdenum content between the same formulas purchased at different locations. The researchers concluded that there is a need for more study of the higher amounts of molybdenum in the formulas, especially with premature babies. "The high intake may pose health risks."[6]

People on Parenteral and Enteral Nutrition May or May Not Require Supplemental Molybdenum

In a study published in 2014 in the *Asia Pacific Journal of Clinical Nutrition*, researchers from Australia and New Zealand reviewed the available research on the need for supplemental trace elements during parenteral and enteral nutrition. (Parenteral nutrition involves the intravenous feeding of the body; enteral nutrition usually involves feeding the body via a feeding tube, but it may consist of other types of gastrointestinal supplementation.) The researchers reviewed several trace elements, including molybdenum. The researchers found that there were few studies on the topic. "A paucity of available literature and limitations with currently available methods of monitoring trace element status are acknowledged." Still, they noted that people on shorter-term treatment probably do not require supplemental molybdenum. People on longer-term treatment may require low-dose supplementation.[7]

Exercise Appears to Raise Levels of Serum Molybdenum

In a study published in 2014 in *Global Journal of Health Science*, researchers from Turkey investigated the effect of maximal exercise on several serum trace elements, including molybdenum. The cohort consisted of 28 "well-trained" and "elite" wrestlers. Blood samples were taken before exercise, immediately after exercise, and one hour after the exercise was completed. The researchers determined that exercise significantly raised blood levels of molybdenum immediately after training. One hour later, there was a nonsignificant decrease of serum molybdenum.[8]

Pasteurization of Breast Milk Does Not Affect the Levels of Molybdenum

In a study published in 2016 in the *Journal of Perinatology*, researchers from Australia explained that children who are born prematurely often need to be fed pasteurized donor milk from other breastfeeding mothers. Does this milk retain the same nutrient content of non-pasteurized breast milk? It has not always been clear. The researchers obtained breast milk from 16 mothers, and the samples were divided into pre- and post-pasteurization groups. All of the samples were tested for eight essential trace elements, including molybdenum. The researchers found no significant nutrient differences in the concentrations of molybdenum in the pre- and post-pasteurizing samples. And they concluded that "pasteurization does not appear to affect concentrations of most trace elements."[9]

NOTES

1. The George Mateljan Foundation. "Molybdenum." December 28, 2017. http://whfoods.com/genpage.php?tname=nutrient&dbid=128.
2. Ibid.
3. Linus Pauling Institute, Oregon State University. http://oregonstate.edu/.
4. Ray, S. S., D. Das, T. Ghosh, and A. K. Ghosh. "The Levels of Zinc and Molybdenum in Hair and Food Grain in Areas of High and Low Incidence of Esophageal Cancer: A Comparative Study." *Global Journal of Health Science* 4, no. 4 (2012): 168–175.
5. Gimou, M. M., R. Pouillot, U. R. Charrondiere, et al. "Dietary Exposure and Health Risk Assessment for 14 Toxic and Essential Trace Elements in Yaoundé: The Cameroonian Total Diet Study." *Food Additives & Contaminants: Part A* 31, no. 6 (2014): 1064–1080.
6. Abramovich, Milana, Angela Miller, Haifeng Yang, and James K. Friel. "Molybdenum Content of Canadian and US Infant Formulas." *Biological Trace Element Research* 143, no. 2 (November 2011): 844–853.
7. Osland, Emma J., Azmat Ali, Elisabeth Isenring, et al. "Australasian Society for Parental and Enteral Nutrition Guidelines for Supplementation of Trace Elements during Parenteral Nutrition." *Asia Pacific Journal of Clinical Nutrition* 23, no. 4 (November 2014): 545–554.
8. Otağ, Aynur, Muhsin Hazar, İlhan Otağ, et al. "Responses of Trace Elements to Aerobic Maximal Exercise in Elite Sportsmen." *Global Journal of Health Science* 6, no. 3 (2014): 90–96.
9. Mohd-Taufek, N., D. Cartwright, M. Davies, et al. "The Effect of Pasteurization on Trace Elements in Donor Breast Milk." *Journal of Perinatology* 36, no. 10 (October 2016): 897–900.

REFERENCES AND FURTHER READINGS

Abramovich, Milana, Angela Miller, Haifeng Yang, and James K. Friel. "Molybdenum Content of Canadian and US Infant Formulas." *Biological Trace Element Research* 143, no. 2 (November 2011): 844–853.
The George Mateljan Foundation. "Molybdenum." December 28, 2017. http://whfoods.com/genpage.php?tname=nutrient&dbid=128.
Gimou, M. M., R. Pouillot, U. R. Charrondiere, et al. "Dietary Exposure and Health Risk Assessment for 14 Toxic and Essential Trace Elements in Yaoundé: The Cameroonian Total Diet Study." *Food Additives & Contaminants: Part A* 31, no. 6 (2014): 1064–1080.
Linus Pauling Institute, Oregon State University. http://lpi.oregonstate.edu/.

Mohd-Taufek, N., D. Cartwright, M. Davies, et al. "The Effect of Pasteurization on Trace Elements in Donor Breast Milk." *Journal of Perinatology* 36, no. 10 (October 2016): 897–900.

Osland, Emma J., Azmat Ali, Elisabeth Isenring, et al. "Australasian Society for Parenteral and Enteral Nutrition Guidelines for Supplementation of trace Elements during Parenteral Nutrition." *Asia Pacific Journal of Clinical Nutrition* 23, no. 4 (November 2014): 545–554.

Otağ, Aynur, Muhsin Hazar, İlhan Otağ, et al. "Responses of Trace Elements to Aerobic Maximal Exercise in Elite Sportsmen." *Global Journal of Health Science* 6, no. 3 (2014): 90–96.

Ray, S. S., D. Das, T. Ghosh, and A. K. Ghosh. "The Levels of Zinc and Molybdenum in Hair and Food Grain in Areas of High and Low Incidence of Esophageal Cancer: A Comparative Study." *Global Journal of Health Science* 4, no. 4 (2012): 168–175.

Phosphorus

Next to calcium, phosphorus is the most abundant mineral in the body. Calcium and phosphorus work together to keep bones and teeth strong. About 85 percent of the body's phosphorus is stored in the bones and teeth. Smaller amounts of phosphorus may be found in all the cells and tissues throughout the body; it helps maintain, repair, and grow cells and tissues and in the production of the genetic building blocks DNA and RNA. The body needs phosphorus to use and store energy, and the kidneys use phosphorus to filter waste. Phosphorus is required to maintain a normal heartbeat and correct nerve signaling. Adequate amounts of phosphorus reduce the muscle pain that may follow a strenuous workout. In addition to all these functions, phosphorus plays a role in balancing the body's levels of vitamin D, iodine, magnesium, and zinc.

Nutritional experts recommend consuming about the same amounts of dietary calcium and phosphorus. This may be problematic. A typical Western diet normally has two to four times more phosphorus than calcium. Meat, poultry, and many carbonated beverages contain higher amounts of phosphorus. When the body has more phosphorus than calcium, it tends to use calcium stored in bones, which may result in weakened bones and teeth problems.

FOOD SOURCES AND SUPPLEMENTS

Only a small number of foods are excellent sources of phosphorus. These include scallops, cod, and crimini mushrooms. Many foods have very good amounts of phosphorous. These include tuna, turkey, chicken, beef, pumpkin seeds, lentils, yogurt, tofu, oats, green peas, broccoli, cow's milk, spinach, asparagus, Brussels sprouts, summer squash, bok choy, tomatoes, and cauliflower. There are also large numbers of foods with good amounts of phosphorus. These include garbanzo, navy, pinto, kidney, and black beans; cashews; sunflower seeds; sesame seeds; rye; millet; barley; brown rice; peanuts; potatoes; buckwheat; onions; beets; cucumbers; sea vegetables; strawberries; and corn.[1] Most balanced diets should contain sufficient amounts of phosphorus.

While it is possible to purchase phosphorus as a single supplement, it is more often combined with other bone-supporting nutrients, such as calcium and magnesium. In the United States there is concern that people take in too much phosphorus. Phosphorus also has the potential to interact with some prescription and nonprescription medications. Unless recommended by a medical provider, it is generally advised to avoid phosphorus supplementation.

INTAKE RECOMMENDATIONS

The Food and Nutrition Board at the Institute of Medicine has developed Dietary Reference Intakes for phosphorus for adults and children and adequate intake levels for infants. Males and females 19 years and older should take in 700 mg per day, while children and teens between the ages of 9 and 18 years should take in 1,250 mg per day. Children between the ages of four and eight years should take in 500 mg per day, while children between the ages of one and three years should take in 460 mg per day. Infants between the ages of six months and one year should take in 275 mg per day, while infants between birth and six months should take in 100 mg per day.

There are also tolerable upper intake levels for phosphorus. Lactating women should take in no more than 4,000 mg per day, while pregnant women should take in no more than 3,500 mg per day. People 70 years or older should take in no more than 3,000 mg per day, while people between the ages of 9 and 70 years should take in no more than 4,000 mg per day. Children between the ages of one and eight years should take in no more than 3,000 mg per day, while there is no upper limit for infants.[2]

DEFICIENCY AND EXCESS

True phosphorus deficiency is believed to be rare in the United States. Most people take in too much rather than too little phosphorus. Still, there are people who are deficient in this nutrient. People with diabetes, alcoholism, or a gastrointestinal malabsorption problem are at increased risk for deficiency, as are those who are severely malnourished. Certain medications, such as some antacids and diuretics, may cause phosphorus levels to drop. Angiotensin-converting enzyme (ACE) inhibitors and medications to lower blood pressure may also reduce phosphorus levels. Alcohol may leach phosphorus from the bones. Symptoms of phosphorus deficiency include loss of appetite, anxiety, bone pain, stiff joints, weakening of bones, fatigue, irregular breathing, irritability, numbness, weakness, and weight change.[3]

Excess amounts of phosphorus in the body are most often caused by kidney disease or consuming too much phosphorus. Processed foods, such as lunch meats, sausages, baking mixes, and frozen patties, nuggets, and strips tend to contain high amounts of phosphorus. Adding phosphorus to these foods enables them to be stored for longer periods of time. Excess phosphorus may be toxic. It may cause a number of symptoms such as diarrhea and the hardening (calcification) of organs and soft tissue. It may increase the risk of cardiovascular disease. Excess phosphorus may interfere with the body's ability to use iron, calcium, magnesium, and zinc. Though the practice is strongly discouraged, athletes who take phosphorus supplementation before competitions or heavy workouts, must increase their intake of calcium.

KEY RESEARCH FINDINGS

Higher Intakes of Phosphorus May Trigger Kidney Problems in Subjects with Normal Renal Function

In a retrospective study published in 2013 in *The American Journal of Medicine*, researchers from three locations in California wanted to learn more about the association between higher levels of phosphorus intake and kidney (renal) function. From January 1, 1998, to December 31, 2008, the researchers identified 94,989 ethnically diverse subjects who were members of Kaiser Permanente Southern California. They had a mean age of 50 years. While 61 percent of the subjects were white, 14 percent were black and 25 percent were Hispanic. During the 11 years of the study, end-stage renal disease occurred in 130 subjects (0.1%). The subjects who consumed higher amounts of phosphorus were at increased risk for this serious medical problem. Interestingly, "this relationship was present despite the fact that phosphorus levels for the most part were within normal reference ranges."[4]

Higher Serum Phosphorus Levels Appear to Be Associated with Increases in Cardiovascular and All Causes of Mortality

In a meta-analysis published in 2016 in the journal *Clinica Chimica Acta*, researchers from China examined the association between elevated serum phosphorous levels and cardiovascular and all-cause mortality. The researchers identified six prospective studies that included 120,269 subjects and 7,002 total death events. After analyzing the data, the researchers found that the highest levels of serum phosphorus had a strong association with cardiovascular and all-cause mortality. In the general population, the subjects who had the highest concentrations of serum phosphorus had "excessive risk" of cardiovascular and all-cause mortality. Moreover, the effect of serum phosphorus on all-cause mortality appeared to be "pronounced" in men but not in women. The researchers underscored the need for more studies to confirm their findings.[5]

Another study on the same association was published in 2016 in the *American Journal of Kidney Diseases*. In this study, Korean researchers collected clinical and biochemical data from adults who were undergoing routine health checkups at three tertiary hospitals that shared similar health-care protocols. When subjects had multiple hospital visits, the researchers used the data only from the first visit. Subjects with possible chronic kidney disease were excluded. The final cohort consisted of 92,756 subjects between the ages of 40 and 79 years. The researchers found that the women tended to have higher phosphorus levels than the men. Men with higher levels of phosphorus were younger and less likely to have high blood pressure; the women with higher levels of phosphorus were older and more likely to have diabetes and high blood pressure. During a median follow-up of 75 months, 1,646 subjects died. In the overall population, higher serum phosphorus levels were an independent predictor for all-cause mortality in people with normal kidney function. The researchers commented that "further investigations are warranted to identify the contributing mechanisms of the sex- and age-specific association between serum phosphorus levels and mortality in the general population."[6]

There Appears to Be an Association between Higher Levels of Serum Phosphorus and Coronary Atherosclerosis in Young Adults

In a study published in 2009 in the *Journal of the American Society of Nephrology*, researchers from Minnesota and the United Kingdom explained that phosphorus levels are associated with atherosclerosis in both animals and humans with advanced chronic kidney disease. They wanted to learn if there was also an association when the subjects had normal kidney function. The cohort consisted of 3,015 healthy young adults in the prospective Coronary Artery Risk Development in Young Adults study. The subjects had a mean age of 25.2 years. As part of their baseline evaluations, measurements were taken of serum phosphate levels. Fifteen years later, researchers found minimal coronary artery calcification in 3.2 percent of the participants, mild calcification in 4.8 percent of the participants, moderate calcification in 1.1 percent of the participants, and severe calcification in 0.5 percent of the participants. Higher phosphate levels were found to be associated with higher rates of coronary artery calcification. The researchers concluded that "higher serum phosphorus levels, even within the normal range, may be a risk factor for coronary artery atherosclerosis in healthy young adults."[7]

There Appears to Be an Association between Serum Phosphate and Risk of Cardiovascular Events in People with or without Chronic Kidney Disease

In a study published in 2013 in the online journal *PLoS ONE*, researchers from the United Kingdom examined the association between serum levels of phosphate (a salt that contains phosphorus) and cardiovascular events in people with or without chronic kidney disease. The researchers followed three groups from the adult cohort of Quality Improvement in Chronic Kidney Disease for a period of 2.5 years. One group, which consisted of 24,184, had normal kidney function. Another group, which consisted of 20,356, had stages 1 and 2 of chronic kidney disease; and another group, which consisted of 13,292, had stages 3 to 5 of chronic kidney disease. (In stage 1, kidney function is normal; by stage 5, kidney function is profoundly impaired.) During the follow-up period, 1,005 people suffered from one or more adverse cardiovascular events. Of these, 521 died. The researchers learned that serum phosphate levels were associated with cardiovascular events and mortality in people with or without chronic kidney disease. The researchers commented that their findings "add to the growing weight of evidence that phosphate is an independent predictor of cardiovascular disease, in both people with and without CKD [chronic kidney disease]."[8]

Many Beverages Contain Very High Levels of Phosphorus

In a letter to the editor that was published in 2015 in the *American Journal of Kidney Diseases*, healthcare professionals from Baltimore, Maryland, San Diego, California, and Danville, Pennsylvania, commented that most people do not realize that many popular beverages contain large amounts of phosphorus. Companies are not required to include information on phosphorus on food labels. As a result, consumers are unable to compare the phosphorus content of different food products. The professionals decided to conduct their own research on 46 beverage products purchased in central Pennsylvania between September and December 2013. These included sodas, lemonades, teas, and enhanced waters. Powdered beverages and water enhancers were prepared according to the package instructions. Measured phosphorus content was compared with reference values from the Nutrition Data System for Research (NDSR). All of the products tested contained some phosphorus; 78 percent had higher amounts of phosphorus than the NDSR reference values. The difference in phosphorus content between measured and reference values ranged from –8 to +261 mg per 8 fluid ounces. The values differed widely, even with the same brands in the same categories. For example, among the iced tea beverages, the amounts of phosphorus ranged from 3 to 105 mg per 8 fluid ounces. The health professionals concluded that the "current nutritional databases capture phosphorus content poorly in many popular beverages with phosphorus-based additives."[9]

High Intake of Phosphorus Aggravates High Blood Pressure and Cardiac Problems in Rats with Metabolic Syndrome

In a study published in 2014 in the journal *Cardiovascular Pathology*, researchers from Japan investigated some of the cardiac problems associated with a high phosphorus/zinc-free diet in rats bred to have high blood pressure (hypertension) and develop metabolic syndrome. The rats, which were six weeks old when the study began, were fed either a control diet or a high phosphorus/zinc-free diet for 18 weeks. The researchers determined that the high phosphorus/zinc-free diet induced high blood pressure and harmed cardiac functioning in the rats. Since processed foods contain high amounts of phosphorus and low amounts of zinc, the researchers noted that their "study sounds a warning on [the] consumption of high amounts of processed food."[10]

People with Fewer Financial Resources Tend to Have a Higher Intake of Phosphorus

In a cross-sectional analysis published in 2010 in the *Journal of the American Society of Nephrology*, researchers from several locations in the United States examined the association between race, socioeconomic status, and serum phosphate. The cohort consisted of 2,879 participants in the Chronic Renal Insufficiency Cohort Study. The researchers determined that the white and black participants who had the lowest income or were unemployed had higher serum phosphate concentrations than the white and black participants with the highest incomes or who were employed. Intake of serum phosphate appeared to be strongly associated with income levels. "Although small differences in serum phosphate concentrations were also noted by race, this relationship was modified by income." Thus, "low socioeconomic status is a novel risk factor for increased serum phosphate concentrations."[11]

NOTES

1. The George Mateljan Foundation. "Phosphorus." December 28, 2017. http://www.whfoods.com/genpage.php?pfriendly=1&tname=nutrient&dbid=127.
2. Ibid.
3. University of Maryland Medical Center. "Phosphorus." December 28, 2017. http://www.umm.edu/health/medical/altmed/supplement/phosphorus.
4. Sim, John J., Simran K. Bhandari, Ning Smith, et al. "Phosphorus and Risk of Renal Failure in Subjects with Normal Renal Function." *The American Journal of Medicine* 126 (2013): 311–318.
5. Bai, Wenwei, Jing Li, and Juan Liu. "Serum Phosphorus, Cardiovascular and All-Cause Mortality in the General Population: A Meta-Analysis." *Clinica Chimica Acta* 461 (2016): 76–82.
6. Yoo, Kyung Don, Soohee Kang, Yunhee Choi, et al. "Sex, Age, and the Association of Serum Phosphorus with All-Cause Mortality in Adults with Normal Kidney Function." *American Journal of Kidney Diseases* 67, no. 1 (2016): 79–88.
7. Foley, Robert N., Allan J. Collins, Charles A. Herzog, et al. "Serum Phosphorus Levels Associate with Coronary Atherosclerosis in Young Adults." *Journal of the American Society of Nephrology* 20 (2009): 397–404.
8. McGovern, Andrew Peter, Simon de Lusignan, Jeremy van Vlymen, et al. "Serum Phosphate as a Risk Factor for Cardiovascular Events in People with and without Chronic Kidney Disease: A Large Community Based Cohort Study." *PLoS ONE* 8, no. 9 (September 2013): e74996.

9. Moser, Melissa, Karen White, Bobbie Henry, et al. "Phosphorus Content of Popular Beverages." *American Journal of Kidney Diseases* 65, no. 6 (2015): 967–971.

10. Suzuki, Yuka, Shingo Mitsushima, Ai Kato, et al. "High-Phosphorus/Zinc-Free Diet Aggravates Hypertension and Cardiac Dysfunction in a Rat Model of the Metabolic Syndrome." *Cardiovascular Pathology* 23 (2014): 43–49.

11. Gutiérrez, Orlando M., Cheryl Anderson, Tamara Isakova, et al. "Low Socioeconomic Status Associates with Higher Serum Phosphate Irrespective of Race." *Journal of the American Society of Nephrology* 21 (2010): 1953–1960.

REFERENCES AND FURTHER READINGS

Bai, Wenwei, Jing Li, and Juan Liu. "Serum Phosphorus, Cardiovascular and All-Cause Mortality in the General Population: A Meta-Analysis." *Clinica Chimica Acta* 461 (2016): 76–82.

Foley, Robert N., Allan J. Collins, Charles A. Herzog, et al. "Serum Phosphorus Levels Associate with Coronary Atherosclerosis in Young Adults." *Journal of the American Society of Nephrology* 20 (2009): 397–404.

The George Mateljan Foundation. "Phosphorus." December 28, 2017. http://www.whfoods.com/genpage.php?pfriendly=1&tname=nutrient&dbid=127.

Gutiérrez, Orlando M., Cheryl Anderson, Tamara Isakova, et al. "Low Socioeconomic Status Associates with Higher Serum Phosphate Irrespective of Race." *Journal of the American Society of Nephrology* 21 (2010): 1953–1960.

McGovern, Andrew Peter, Simon de Lusignan, Jeremy van Vlymen, et al. "Serum Phosphate as a Risk Factor for Cardiovascular Events in People with and without Chronic Kidney Disease: A Large Community Based Cohort Study." *PLoS ONE* 8, no. 9 (September 2013): e74996.

Moser, Melissa, Karen White, Bobbie Henry, et al. "Phosphorus Content of Popular Beverages." *American Journal of Kidney Diseases* 65, no. 6 (2015): 967–971.

Sim, John J., Simran K. Bhandari, Ning Smith, et al. "Phosphorus and Risk of Renal Failure in Subjects with Normal Renal Function." *The American Journal of Medicine* 126 (2013): 311–318.

Suzuki, Yuka, Shingo Mitsushima, Ai Kato, et al. "High-Phosphorus/Zinc-Free Diet Aggravates Hypertension and Cardiac Dysfunction in a Rat Model of the Metabolic Syndrome." *Cardiovascular Pathology* 23 (2014): 43–49.

University of Maryland Medical Center. "Phosphorus." December 28, 2017. http://www.umm.edu/health/medical/altmed/supplement/phosphorus.

Yoo, Kyung Don, Soohee Kang, Yunhee Choi, et al. "Sex, Age, and the Association of Serum Phosphorus with All-Cause Mortality in Adults with Normal Kidney Function." *American Journal of Kidney Diseases* 67, no. 1 (2016): 79–88.

Potassium

Potassium is a mineral that is found in many foods, especially vegetables. It is most abundant in green leafy vegetables. But potassium is also found in meat, chicken, and fish, as well as many fruits.

Potassium is believed to improve the control of blood pressure. As a result, it is not uncommon for medical providers to suggest that their patients with high blood pressure increase their intake of dietary potassium. Keeping blood pressure under control helps protect kidney health. In addition, potassium prevents the leaching of calcium from the bones, which reduces the amount of calcium in the urine. This impedes the formation of painful stones in the kidneys.

Potassium helps build proteins, breaks down and uses carbohydrates, builds muscle, and maintains normal body growth. It helps to maintain the acid balance in the body and is necessary for the electrical activity of the heart.

FOOD SOURCES AND SUPPLEMENTS

A few foods have excellent amounts of potassium. These include beet greens, dried figs, Swiss chard, spinach, and bok choy. Many more foods have very good amounts of potassium. These include beets, Brussels sprouts, broccoli, cantaloupe, tomatoes, asparagus, cabbage, summer squash, crimini mushrooms, kale, turnip greens, celery, romaine lettuce, and bell peppers. And countless numbers of foods have good amounts of potassium. These include lima beans, sweet potatoes, soybeans, pinto beans, lentils, avocadoes, kidney beans, tuna, papaya, winter squash, salmon, bananas, green peas, scallops, strawberries, kiwifruit, cauliflower, eggplant, and watermelon.[1] Potassium is often added to multivitamins, but people who wish to take extra potassium may purchase it as a single- or fewer-ingredient supplement.

INTAKE RECOMMENDATIONS

The Food and Nutrition Board of the Institute of Medicine recommends the following dietary intake of potassium. Adults 19 years and older should take in 4.7 g per day, while women who are breast-feeding should take in 5.1 g per day. Teens between the ages of 14 and 18 years should take in 4.7 g per day, while children between the ages of 9 and 13 years should take in 4.5 g per day. Children between the ages of four and eight years should take in 3.8 g per day, while children between the ages of one and three should take in 3 g per day. Infants between the ages of 7 and 12 months should take in 0.7 g per day, while newborns up to 6 months should take in 0.4 g per day.[2] There is no tolerable upper limit for potassium.

DEFICIENCY AND EXCESS

In the United States, potassium deficiency is believed to be very common. This is thought to be the direct result of the heavy reliance on processed foods. But other factors increase the risk of a deficiency. Women and African Americans appear to be at increased risk for deficiency. People who undergo an activity that increases fluid loss—such as exercising or working outside in hot weather—may lose potassium. Moreover, potassium deficiency is seen in people who suffer from frequent vomiting and acute or chronic diarrhea, as well as those with ongoing gastrointestinal problems. Symptoms of low levels of blood potassium, a condition known as hypokalemia, are weak muscles, abnormal heart rhythms, and a rise in blood pressure.

"Hyperkalemia" is the name for excess amounts of potassium in the blood. It may trigger abnormal and dangerous heart rhythms. Hyperkalemia may be caused by poor kidney function, certain heart medications, such as angiotensin-converting enzyme inhibitors and angiotensin 2 receptor blockers, potassium-sparing diuretics, and severe infections.

KEY RESEARCH FINDINGS

Potassium Supplementation Appears to Lower Blood Pressure

In a randomized, placebo-controlled crossover study published in 2015 in the *Journal of Human Hypertension*, researchers from the Netherlands examined the effects of potassium and sodium supplementation on blood pressure and arterial stiffness in 37 untreated prehypertensive people. During the study, the subjects ate a "fully controlled diet" that was relatively low in potassium and sodium. The subjects were told to keep other lifestyle behaviors, such as physical activity, "constant." After a one-week "run-in" period, the subjects took capsules with supplemental potassium, supplemental sodium, or a placebo, each for four weeks. Thirty-six subjects completed the study. They had a mean pretreatment blood pressure of 145/81 mm Hg, and 69 percent had a systolic blood pressure at or above 140 mm Hg. When the participants were taking the potassium supplementation, they experienced significant reductions in blood pressure. The researchers concluded that "increasing potassium intake, on top of a relatively low-sodium diet, had a beneficial effect on BP [blood pressure]."[3]

In a meta-analysis published in 2015 in the *Journal of Hypertension*, researchers from Switzerland wanted to learn more about the ability of potassium to lower blood pressure in nonmedicated people with or without high blood pressure. In addition, the researchers examined the association between potassium intake, sodium-to-potassium ratio, and reductions in blood pressure. The cohort consisted of 15 randomized, controlled trials with a total of 917 patients. All of the studies, which were published between 1984 and 2010, were conducted for at least four weeks. The researchers learned that potassium supplementation reduced levels of systolic blood pressure, especially in people who were hypertensive. And they concluded that their findings "support the overall benefit of increased potassium intake by patients with elevated BP, specifically those who are not taking any antihypertensive treatment."[4]

There May Be an Association between the Sodium-to-Potassium Ratio and High Blood Pressure

In a study published in 2016 in the journal *Nutrients*, researchers from Korea explained that high blood pressure is a massive public health concern in Korea. "Hypertension causes some of the heaviest social burdens through medical insurance and personal suffering." More needs to be done to find ways to reduce blood pressure levels. As a result, the researchers investigated the impact that the sodium-to-potassium (Na:K) ratio has on blood pressure. The cohort consisted of data from the Korean National Health and Nutrition Examination Surveys from 2010 to 2014. There were 30,206 subjects between the ages of 20 and 79 years. Based on the sodium-to-potassium ratios, the cohort was divided into quartiles. The researchers learned that the groups with higher sodium-to-potassium ratios had higher rates of high blood pressure. People with higher sodium-to-potassium ratios consumed more cereal, salty vegetables, meats, and meat products than those with lower ratios. Researchers noted that "a good way" to achieve a lower ratio is to consume "sufficient fresh vegetables, fruits, and low fat dairy." The researchers concluded that "a lower sodium to potassium ratio diet than a usual diet is recommended to control high blood pressure in Korea."[5]

In a study published in 2013 in the online journal *PLoS ONE*, researchers from Atlanta, Georgia, and Ames, Iowa, used data collected in the United States to examine the importance of the sodium-to-potassium ratio. The cohort consisted of 10,563 participants, aged 20 years or older, in the 2005–2010 National Health and Nutrition Examination Survey (NHANES). Participants did not take medication for high blood pressure or consume a low-sodium diet. Data on dietary sodium and potassium were assessed using two 24-hour dietary recalls. The researchers determined that the mean sodium-to-potassium ratio was higher among the participants with high blood pressure. "These results support those from randomized controlled trials showing reduced sodium consumption and increased potassium consumption can help prevent hypertension, and hence, cardiovascular disease."[6]

Craniosacral Therapy for Chronic Low Back Pain May Increase Levels of Serum Potassium

In a study published in 2016 in *The Journal of Alternative and Complementary Medicine*, researchers from Spain examined the association between craniosacral therapy in patients with chronic low back pain and a number of different factors, including the amount of serum potassium in the body. The cohort consisted of 64 patients, between the ages of 18 and 65 years, with chronic low back pain, who were referred for physical therapy at a clinic at the University of Almeria in Spain. The patients were randomly assigned to receive 10 sessions of craniosacral therapy or 10 sessions of classic massage. "Craniosacral treatment focuses on the connective tissues of the skull and spine and on cerebrospinal fluid." Outcome measures were assessed before the first treatment session, after the 10-session intervention, and one month after the last treatment. The researchers found that the patients in both groups had statistically similar results in a number of factors, such as reduction in disability and pain intensity. However, the patients in the craniosacral groups had better improvements in several factors, including an increase in serum potassium. "Changes over time were significantly better in the craniosacral group than in the massage group for potassium."[7]

Potassium Supplementation Does Not Appear to Affect Heart Rate

In a meta-analysis published in 2016 in the journal *Nutrition, Metabolism & Cardiovascular Diseases*, researchers from the Netherlands wanted to learn if potassium supplementation had any effect on the heart rate of healthy adults. Having an elevated resting heart rate could place people at increased risk for cardiovascular problems. The researchers assembled a cohort that consisted of 22 trials with 1,056 subjects. Five of the trials were parallel and 17 were crossover. The subjects had a median potassium dose of 2.5 g per day and a median intervention of four weeks. The researchers determined that the supplementation "showed no overall effect" on the heart rates of the subjects. However, the researchers did not rule out "potential adverse effects" of long-term use of potassium supplementation and noted that the subject "warranted further investigation."[8]

Potassium-Rich Diets May Help Protect the Kidneys and Cardiovascular Systems of People with Diabetes

In an observational study published in 2015 in the *Clinical Journal of the American Society of Nephrology*, researchers from Japan explained that people with type 2 diabetes are at increased risk for a variety of health concerns, such as kidney and cardiovascular problems. In fact, it has been shown that people with type 2 diabetes have a significantly higher risk of developing end-stage renal disease and cardiovascular disease. Should people with type 2 diabetes consume more potassium? The cohort, which was formed between 1996 and 2003, consisted of 623 people who had type 2 diabetes and normal renal functioning. Follow-up continued until 2013; the median follow-up period was 11 years. The study measured amounts of potassium in the urine; people with higher amounts of potassium in their urine took in higher amounts of potassium. The researchers found that higher intakes of potassium were associated with lower risk of renal dysfunction and low risk of cardiovascular problems. And they concluded that "higher urinary potassium excretion was associated with the slower decline of renal function and the lower incidence of cardiovascular complications in type 2 diabetic patients with normal renal function."[9]

Adolescents May Wish to Increase Their Intake of Dietary Potassium

In a prospective study published in 2015 in *JAMA Pediatrics*, researchers from Boston and Colorado examined the effect of dietary potassium and sodium and the potassium-to-sodium ratio on adolescent blood pressure. The researchers obtained data from the National Heart, Lung, and Blood Institute's Growth and Health Study, which had statistics collected from Richmond, California, Cincinnati, Ohio, and Washington, DC. The initial cohort, which was obtained from March 1987 through February 1988, included data on 2,185 white and black females aged 9 and 10 years. Follow-up continued until February 1999. The researchers determined that the teens in the group with the highest daily consumption of potassium (2,400 mg per day or more) had lower blood pressure levels in their late adolescence. In contrast, there was no evidence that sodium had an effect on these teens. The potassium-to-sodium ratio was inversely associated only with systolic blood pressure. The researchers concluded that "the beneficial effects of dietary potassium-rich foods during childhood may help suppress the adolescent increase in blood pressure." In fact, "black and white adolescent girls who consumed more dietary potassium had lower BPs in later adolescence."[10]

Toddlers Benefit from Consuming Vegetables High in Potassium

In a study published in 2016 in the journal *Advances in Nutrition*, researchers from Virginia examined the average nutrient intakes and total vegetable and white potato consumption among children between the ages of one and three years. Data were obtained from the NHANES 2009–2012 and the Food Patterns Equivalents Database 2009–2012. The researchers calculated the mean intake of several nutrients, including potassium. While the average intakes of most nutrients among this age group met or exceeded recommendations, the toddlers consumed too little potassium. Most of their potassium was obtained from dairy and fruit. Their mean total vegetable intake was less than the recommended amount of one cup per day; their mean intake of potassium was "far below recommendations." According to the researchers, toddlers should be encouraged to eat more foods with higher amounts of potassium.[11]

Preschool Children Need to Take in More Potassium

In a study published in 2016 in the journal *Nutrients*, researchers from Australia wanted to learn more about the intake of potassium among preschool children. Were the children taking in enough potassium? What were the food sources for potassium and what was the sodium-to-potassium ratio? The cohort consisted of 251 Australian children with a mean age of 3.5 years. Nutritionists collected data during telephone-administered 24-hour dietary recalls. The researchers learned that 54 percent of the children did not meet the Australian recommended adequate intake for potassium (2,000 mg per day). Potassium consumption was mostly derived from milk, fruits, and vegetables. The sodium-to-potassium ratio exceeded the recommended level of 1. Foods with the highest ratio were processed meats, white bread and rolls, and sauces and condiments. The researchers commented that increases in consumption of vegetables may help improve levels of potassium intake and lower the sodium-to-potassium ratio. "An increase in vegetable consumption in pre-school children is recommended to increase dietary potassium and has the potential to decrease the Na:K ratio which is likely to have long-term health benefits."[12]

Insufficient Intake of Potassium in Young Women May Contribute to the Later Development of Osteoporosis

In a study published in 2016 in the journal *Roczniki Państwowego Zakładu Higieny*, researchers from Poland examined the association between intake of potassium and other nutrients in young women and the risk of the later development of osteoporosis. Osteoporosis or the serious loss of bone mass density is associated with a number of medical problems such as fractures and disability. The cohort consisted of 75 Polish women between the ages of 20 and 30 years. Data were collected from September to November 2014. After the women prepared three-day dietary records, the researchers analyzed the nutrient intakes of their diets, focusing on nutrients that support bone health such as potassium. They learned that the majority of women had an inadequate intake of potassium, and this may ultimately contribute to the development of osteoporosis. Moreover, "it may be associated not only to the increased osteoporosis risk, but also other diet-related diseases."[13]

Higher Dietary Intake of Potassium Appears to Reduce the Risk of Stroke

In a meta-analysis published in 2011 in the journal *Stroke*, researchers from Sweden examined the association between intake of potassium and risk of stroke. The cohort consisted of 10 independent prospective studies, published between 1987 and 2011, that contained a total of 8,695 cases of stroke and 268,276 participants. Half of the studies were conducted in the United States. The other studies took place in Europe, Japan, and Taiwan. The researchers found a statistically significant inverse association between potassium intake and the risk of stroke. For every 1,000 mg per day increase in potassium intake, the risk of total stroke decreased by 11 per cent. The reductions in stroke were most often seen in ischemic strokes or those caused by a blood clot that disrupts the blood supply to the brain.[14]

Adolescents Need to Increase Their Intake of Potassium

In a cross-sectional study published in 2016 in the journal *Food & Nutrition Research*, researchers from Portugal and Australia evaluated the amount of potassium and sodium excreted by 200 Portuguese adolescents as well as the food sources of these nutrients. On average, the teens were 14 years, and their body mass index was normal. The amounts of potassium and sodium were measured during one 24-hour urinary collection. Dietary sources of potassium and sodium, which were divided into 13 major food groups, were assessed for 24 hours. The main sources of potassium were milk, milk products, meats, and vegetables. The researchers determined that the teens consumed too little potassium. In fact, 96.1 percent did not meet recommendations for potassium intake. The researchers noted the need to develop "strategies to improve fruit and vegetable consumption." People who eat more fruits and vegetables take in more potassium.[15]

NOTES

1. The George Mateljan Foundation. "Potassium." December 29, 2017. http://whfoods.com/genpage.php?tname=nutrient&dbid=90.

2. Medlineplus. "Potassium." December 29, 2017. https://medlineplus.gov/potassium.html.

3. Gijsbers, L., J.I. Dower, M. Mensink, et al. "Effects of Sodium and Potassium Supplementation on Blood Pressure and Arterial Stiffness: A Fully Controlled Dietary Intervention Study." *Journal of Human Hypertension* 29 (2015): 592–598.

4. Binia, Aristea, Jonathan Jaeger, Youyou Hu, et al. "Daily Potassium Intake and Sodium-to-Potassium Ratio in the Reduction of Blood Pressure: A Meta-Analysis of Randomized Controlled Trials." *Journal of Hypertension* 33, no. 8 (August 2015): 1509–1520.

5. Park, Junhyung, Chang Keun Kwock, and Yoon Jung Yang. "The Effect of the Sodium to Potassium Ratio on Hypertension Prevalence: A Propensity Score Matching Approach." *Nutrients* 8, no. 8 (2016): 482+.

6. Zhang, Zefeng, Mary E. Cogswell, Cathleen Gillespie, et al. "Association between Usual Sodium and Potassium Intake and Blood Pressure and Hypertension among U.S. Adults: NHANES 2005–2010." *PLoS ONE* 8, no. 10 (October 2013): e75289.

7. Castro-Sánchez, A. M., I.C. Lara-Palomo, G. A. Matarán-Peñarrocha, et al. "Benefits of Craniosacral Therapy in Patients with Chronic Low Back Pain: A Randomized Controlled Trial." *The Journal of Alternative and Complementary Medicine* 22, no. 8 (2016): 650–657.

8. Gijsbers, L., F.J. Mölenberg, S.J. Bakker, and J.M. Geleijnse. "Potassium Supplementation and Heart Rate: A Meta-Analysis of Randomized Controlled Trials." *Nutrition, Metabolism & Cardiovascular Diseases* 26, no. 8 (August 2016): 674–682.

9. Araki, Shin-ichi, Masakazu Haneda, Daisuke Koya, et al. "Urinary Potassium Excretion and Renal and Cardiovascular Complications in Patients with Type 2 Diabetes and Normal Renal Function." *Clinical Journal of the American Society of Nephrology* 10 (2015): 2152–2158.

10. Buendia, Justin R., M. Loring Bradlee, Stephen R. Daniels, et al. "Longitudinal Effects of Dietary Sodium and Potassium on Blood Pressure in Adolescent Girls." *JAMA Pediatrics* 169, no. 6 (2015): 560–568.

11. Storey, Maureen L. and Patricia A. Anderson. "Nutrient Intakes and Vegetable and White Potato Consumption by Children Aged 1 to 3 Years." *Advances in Nutrition* 7, Supplement (2016): 241S–246S.

12. O'Halloran, S. A., C. A. Grimes, K. E. Lacy, et al. "Dietary Intake and Sources of Potassium and the Relationship to Dietary Sodium in a Sample of Australian Pre-School Children." *Nutrients* 8, no. 8 (2016): 496+.

13. Sidor, Patrycja, Dominika Gląbska, and Dariusz Włodarek. "Analysis of the Dietary Factors Contributing to the Future Osteoporosis Risk in Young Polish Women." *Roczniki Państwowego Zakładu Higieny* 67, no. 3 (2016): 279–285.

14. Larsson, Susanna C., Nicola Orsini, and Alicja Wolk. "Dietary Potassium Intake and Risk of Stroke: A Dose-Response Meta-Analysis of Prospective Studies." *Stroke* 42, no. 10 (October 2011): 2746–2750.

15. Gonçalves, C., S. Abreu, P. Padrão, et al. "Sodium and Potassium Urinary Excretion and Dietary Intake: A Cross-Sectional Analysis in Adolescents." *Food & Nutrition Research* 60 (2016): 29442+.

REFERENCES AND FURTHER READINGS

Araki, Shin-ichi, Masakazu Haneda, Daisuke Koya, et al. "Urinary Potassium Excretion and Renal and Cardiovascular Complications in Patients with Type 2 Diabetes and Normal Renal Function." *Clinical Journal of the American Society of Nephrology* 10 (2015): 2152–2158.

Binia, Aristea, Jonathan Jaeger, Youyou Hu, et al. "Daily Potassium Intake and Sodium-to-Potassium Ratio in the Reduction of Blood Pressure: A Meta-Analysis of Randomized Controlled Trials." *Journal of Hypertension* 33, no. 8 (August 2015): 1509–1520.

Buendia, Justin R., M. Loring Bradlee, Stephen R. Daniels, et al. "Longitudinal Effects of Dietary Sodium and Potassium on Blood Pressure in Adolescent Girls." *JAMA Pediatrics* 169, no. 6 (2015): 560–568.

Castro-Sánchez, A. M., I. C. Lara-Palomo, G. A. Matarán-Penarrocha, et al. "Benefits of Craniosacral Therapy in Patients with Chronic Low Back Pain: A Randomized Controlled Trial." *The Journal of Alternative and Complementary Medicine* 22, no. 8 (2016): 650–657.

The George Mateljan Foundation. "Potassium." December 29, 2017. http://whfoods.com/genpage.php?tname=nutrient&dbid=90.

Gijsbers, L., J. I. Dower, M. Mensink, et al. "Effects of Sodium and Potassium Supplementation on Blood Pressure and Arterial Stiffness: A Fully Controlled Dietary Intervention Study." *Journal of Human Hypertension* 29 (2015): 592–598.

Gijsbers, L., F. J. Möleberg, S. J. Bakker, and J. M. Geleijnse. "Potassium Supplementation and Heart Rate: A Meta-Analysis of Randomized Controlled Trials." *Nutrition, Metabolism & Cardiovascular Diseases* 26, no. 8 (August 2016): 674–682.

Gonçalves, C., S. Abreu, P. Padrão, et al. "Sodium and Potassium Urinary Excretion and Dietary Intake: A Cross-Sectional Analysis in Adolescents." *Food & Nutrition Research* 60 (2016): 29442+.

Larsson, Susanna C., Nicola Orsini, and Alicja Wolk. "Dietary Potassium Intake and Risk of Stroke: A Dose-Response Meta-Analysis of Prospective Studies." *Stroke* 42, no. 10 (October 2011): 2746–2750.

Medlineplus. "Potassium." December 29, 2017. https://medlineplus.gov/potassium.html.

O'Halloran, S. A., C. A. Grimes, K. E. Lacy, et al. "Dietary Intake and Sources of Potassium and the Relationship to Dietary Sodium in a Sample of Australian Pre-School Children." *Nutrients* 8, no. 8 (2016): 496+.

Park, Junhyung, Chang Keun Kwock, and Yoon Jung Yang. "The Effect of the Sodium to Potassium Ratio on Hypertension Prevalence: A Propensity Score Matching Approach." *Nutrients* 8, no. 8 (2016): 482+.

Sidor, Patrycja, Dominika Gląbska, and Dariusz Włodarek. "Analysis of the Dietary Factors Contributing to the Future Osteoporosis Risk in Young Polish Women." *Roczniki Państwowego Zakładu Higieny* 67, no. 3 (2016): 279–285.

Storey, Maureen L. and Patricia A. Anderson. "Nutrient Intakes and Vegetable and White Potato Consumption by Children Aged 1 to 3 Years." *Advances in Nutrition* 7, Supplement (2016): 241S–246S.

Zhang, Zefeng, Mary E. Cogswell, Cathleen Gillespie, et al. "Association between Usual Sodium and Potassium Intake and Blood Pressure and Hypertension among U.S. Adults: NHANES 2005–2010." *PLoS ONE* 8, no. 10 (October 2013): e75289.

Selenium

Selenium (Se) is a trace element that is found naturally in many foods. Only a very small amount is needed in the daily diet. The actual selenium content of plant foods relates to the selenium content of the soil in which they were grown. It is known that the amount of selenium in the soil may vary widely. Soil in the Midwestern and Western sections of the United States tends to have more selenium than soil in the South and Northeast.

In the human body, selenium functions as an antioxidant, especially when combined with vitamin E. It helps fight free radicals, particles that damage cell membranes and DNA, and may well contribute to the development of conditions such as cardiovascular disease and cancer. Selenium plays a role in the functioning of the thyroid gland; a selenium-containing enzyme transforms a less-active thyroid hormone T4 into a more-active T3. In addition, selenium and iodine work together to maintain a strong thyroid gland. And selenium supports the immune system. It is known that people who have the autoimmune disorder rheumatoid arthritis have low levels of selenium, as do people with certain types of cancer. It is still uncertain if selenium is the cause or the effect of these medical problems.[1]

FOOD SOURCES AND SUPPLEMENTS

Excellent sources of selenium include tuna, shrimp, sardines, salmon, cod, asparagus, and crimini and shiitake mushrooms. Very good sources of selenium include chicken, lamb, scallops, beef, barley, tofu, and eggs. Good sources of selenium include brown rice, sunflower seeds, sesame seeds, cow's milk, flaxseeds, cabbage, spinach, garlic, broccoli, and Swiss chard.[2] Selenium may be included in a multivitamin, and it may be sold as a single ingredient or combined with other ingredients, often as a thyroid support product.

INTAKE RECOMMENDATIONS

The Food and Nutrition Board of the Institute of Medicine recommends the following dietary intake of selenium. The Recommended Dietary Allowances are listed in micrograms. Women who are pregnant should take in 60 mcg per day, while women who are breast-feeding should take in 70 mcg per day. Beginning at age 14, males and females should take in 55 mcg per day. Children between the ages of 9 and 13 years should take in 40 mcg per day, while children between the ages of 4 and 8 years should take in 30 mcg per day. Children between the ages of one and three years should take in 20 mcg per day. The recommendations for infants are adequate intakes. Infants between the ages of 7 and 12 months should take in 20 mcg per day, while children between birth and six months should take in 15 mcg per day.[3] The tolerable upper limit levels for selenium is 400 mcg per day.

DEFICIENCY AND EXCESS

It is believed that most Americans consume adequate amounts of selenium. As a result, selenium deficiency is thought to be rare. Still, certain people are at increased risk for selenium deficiency. These include people undergoing kidney dialysis and people living with HIV. People who have weight loss surgeries or who have malabsorption problems are also at increased risk. Symptoms of selenium deficiency include hair loss, skin and fingernail discoloration, low immunity, constant tiredness and fatigue, brain fog and difficulty concentrating, reproductive problems, and hypothyroidism (low levels of thyroid hormone).

While it is difficult to obtain excess selenium from food, people who take selenium supplementation may take in high amounts. Symptoms of excess selenium include nausea, diarrhea, skin rashes, mottled teeth, irritability, and nervous system problems.

KEY RESEARCH FINDINGS

There May Be an Association between Low Levels of Selenium and Liver Cancer

In a study published in 2016 in the *American Journal of Clinical Nutrition*, researchers from locations throughout the world, who were led by a researcher from Ireland, examined the association between levels of selenium and incidence of liver cancer. Data were derived from the European Prospective Investigation into

Cancer and Nutrition study (EPIC), which included about 520,000 men and women between the ages of 25 and 70 years from 10 European countries. The subjects were tracked from 1992 to 2000. They completed questionnaires, and laboratory testing evaluated the blood samples for selenium and selenoprotein P (SePP), the major circulating selenium transfer protein. The researchers calculated the incidence of three different types of liver cancer—hepatocellular carcinoma (HCC), gallbladder and biliary tract cancers (GBTC), and intrahepatic bile duct cancer (IHBC). The researchers found that subjects with two types of liver cancer, HCC and GBTC, had significantly lower amounts of circulating selenium and SePP concentrations. This association was not seen with HBC. Higher-circulating selenium was associated with a significantly lower HCC risk, but not with the risk of GBTC or IHCC. Higher SePP concentrations were associated with lowered IHCC risk. The researchers concluded that selenium may play a role in the development of some cases of liver cancer. "There are several lines of evidence to support a strong preventative effect of higher selenium concentrations against hepatobiliary cancers."[4]

Selenium May Provide Protection against a Pre-cervical Cancer Condition as Well as Metabolic Benefits

In a randomized, double-blind, placebo-controlled trial published in 2015 in the *British Journal of Nutrition*, researchers from Iran examined the association between the long-term consumption of selenium and the development of a precancerous cervical condition known as cervical intraepithelial neoplasia (CIN). With CIN, there are changes in the squamous cells of the cervix. Left untreated, CIN may develop into cervical cancer. The initial cohort consisted of 58 women, between the ages of 18 and 55 years, who were diagnosed with low-grade CIN. For six months, the women took either a selenium supplement or a placebo. Fifty subjects completed the trial. The researchers determined that the women taking the selenium supplement experienced a regression in their CIN. In addition, they had significant reductions in fasting plasma glucose levels, serum insulin levels, and serum triglyceride levels, and increases in HDL or "good" cholesterol levels. According to the researchers, "the effects of Se administration in patients with CIN have not been evaluated so far."[5]

Selenium Supplementation May Reduce the Incidence of Preeclampsia in Pregnant Women

In a randomized, double-blind, placebo-controlled study published in 2010 in the *Taiwanese Journal of Obstetrics and Gynecology*, researchers from Iran and the United Kingdom wanted to determine if selenium supplementation could help prevent preeclampsia in high-risk pregnant women. (Preeclampsia is a pregnancy complication characterized by high blood pressure and damage to another organ system, often the kidneys.) The initial cohort consisted of 166 primigravid women, who were in the first trimester of pregnancy. Until delivery of their children, a period of about six months, half of the women took selenium supplementation and half took a placebo. The women who took selenium supplementation had significant increases in their mean serum selenium concentrations. Normally, without supplementation, serum selenium levels fall significantly during pregnancy, and this decrease is progressive. While three of the women in the control group became preeclamptic, none of the women taking selenium developed this medical problem. According to the researchers, further studies on the topic should include larger numbers of women. "Any definitive judgment about the efficacy of selenium supplementation in pregnancy for the purpose of preventing the development of preeclampsia will depend on the results of future trials with a larger number of participants."[6]

There May Be an Association between Breast Cancer and Levels of Serum Selenium

In a study published in 2012 in the journal *Breast Cancer Research and Treatment*, researchers from Sweden and Boston commented that some nutrition intervention trials have found that selenium supplementation reduced cancer mortality. Would selenium be useful against breast cancer? The researchers investigated the efficacy in 3,146 women diagnosed with invasive breast cancer in the population-based Swedish Mammography Cohort. The mean age at diagnosis was 65 years. Using food frequency questionnaires, the researchers determined selenium intakes before breast cancer diagnosis. During 28,172 person-years of follow-up from 1987 to 2009, there were 416 deaths from breast cancer and 964 total deaths. The researchers found that dietary selenium intake was inversely associated with death from breast cancer and overall mortality. The researchers commented that their findings "suggest that selenium intake before breast cancer diagnosis may improve breast-cancer specific survival and overall survival." The main sources of dietary selenium were fish, dairy products, meat, eggs, and hard bread. However, the researchers cautioned that their "findings may be limited to populations with low intakes of selenium."[7]

Higher Selenium Status May Be Associated with Lower Risk of Prostate Cancer

In a study published in 2016 in the *Journal of the National Cancer Institute*, researchers from multiple locations throughout the world evaluated the findings of 15 prospective studies on the association between selenium in the blood and toenails and the risk of prostate cancer. In total, the studies included 6,497 men with prostate cancer and 8,107 men without prostate cancer. Data were available for 4,527 case patients and 6,021 control subjects for blood selenium and 1,970 cases and 2,086 controls for nail selenium. The researchers found an inverse association between nail, but not blood, selenium concentrations and prostate cancer. Why were there differences? The researchers commented that "nails are a more reliable marker of long-term selenium exposure." High concentrations of both serum and nail selenium were associated with a reduced risk of aggressive prostate cancer. The researchers underscored the need for further research.[8]

But Another Study Found No Association between Selenium and Prostate Cancer

In a phase 3, randomized, double-blind, placebo-controlled clinical trial which was published in 2013 in the journal *The Prostate*, researchers from multiple locations in the United States as well as New Zealand investigated the association between selenium supplementation and prostate cancer incidence in high-risk men. The initial cohort consisted of 699 men under the age of 80 years; as a result of laboratory or clinical testing, all of the subjects were deemed at high risk for prostate cancer. The subjects were placed on either two different doses of selenium or a placebo, and they were followed every six months for up to five years. Two hundred and ninety-two subjects (41.8%) completed the trial. The researchers determined that neither dose of selenium appeared to have a significant effect on the incidence of prostate cancer. "Selenium supplementation appeared to have no effect on the incidence of prostate cancer in men at high risk."[9]

There Appears to Be a Positive Association between Dietary Selenium Intake and Diabetes

In a cross-sectional study published in 2015 in *Nutrition Journal*, researchers from China examined the association between dietary intake of selenium and the risk of diabetes. The cohort consisted of 5,423 subjects (2,882 males and 2,541 females), who were 40 years or older. They lived in Hunan Province of China. Demographic and other data were obtained by registered nurses during medical examinations. Among the subjects studied, the average intake of selenium was 43.51 mcg per day. The overall prevalence of diabetes was 9.7 percent. The researchers observed several significant differences between the subjects without diabetes and those with diabetes, including variations in the intake of selenium. Subjects with diabetes consumed more selenium. There was a significant positive association between dietary selenium intake and the prevalence of diabetes. As a result, people who consume more selenium may be at increased risk for diabetes. The researchers emphasized the need for more studies on the topic.[10]

In another study, published in 2016 in the journal *BMJ Open Diabetes Research & Care*, researchers from Taiwan investigated the association between selenium blood levels and the prevalence of diabetes. This hospital-based, case-controlled study included 847 male and female adults 40 years of age or older from Northern Taiwan. The average age of the subjects was 63.9 years, and 69.2 percent were male. Data were gathered from 2007 to 2014 at one medical center in Taipei. The subjects were divided into quartiles, according to the serum selenium levels. The researchers found that higher levels of serum selenium were correlated with increased risk for diabetes. When compared to the subjects in the lowest quartile of selenium intake, the subjects in the quartile with the highest intake of selenium had a 3.79-fold risk of diabetes. "Serum selenium levels were positively associated with prevalence of diabetes." This association was "independent of insulin resistance and central obesity."[11]

In Order to Function Properly, the Thyroid Gland Requires Adequate Amounts of Selenium

In an observational study published in 2015 in the *Journal of Clinical Endocrinology & Metabolism*, researchers from China and Berlin wanted to learn more about the association between proper thyroid functioning and selenium. It is known that, in the body, the thyroid gland has the highest selenium concentration per gram of tissue. The researchers examined the prevalence of thyroid disease in people residing in two similar counties in Shaanxi Province in China. The primary difference between the counties was the amount of selenium in the soil. One of the counties (Ziyang) was determined to have adequate amounts of selenium in the soil; the other county (Ningshan) had low amounts of selenium in the soil. The initial cohort consisted of 6,152 adults between the ages of 18 and 70 years, who lived in one of the counties. There were 3,038 subjects from the adequate selenium county and 3,114 subjects from the inadequate selenium county. The subjects completed food frequency questionnaires and had clinical examinations as well as thyroid ultrasound tests and fasting blood tests. The researchers learned that the risk of thyroid disease was 69 percent higher for those living in the low-selenium county than the adequate-selenium county. While 18 percent of the subjects in the adequate-selenium area had thyroid disease, more than 30 percent of the subjects in the low-selenium area had thyroid disease. The researchers concluded that "increased selenium intake may reduce the risk in areas of low selenium intake that exist not only in China but also in many other parts of the world."[12]

People Who Are Newly Diagnosed with Graves' Disease Frequently Have Low Levels of Selenium

In a population-based study published in 2013 in the journal *Clinical Endocrinology*, researchers from Denmark and Germany wanted to learn more about the association between selenium serum levels and Graves' disease (GD), an autoimmune disorder that leads to an overactive thyroid gland. The researchers investigated 97 patients with newly diagnosed GD as well as patients with other medical problems. They compared their results to 830 random controls. The researchers found that the patients with newly diagnosed GD had significantly lower levels of serum selenium. Their findings "support the postulated link between inadequate selenium supply and overt autoimmune thyroid disease, especially GD." The researchers underscored the need for more research. "More studies are needed to elucidate whether selenium supplement has a more general beneficial effect in GD."[13]

Selenium May Support Bone Mineral Density in Aging Men

In a study published in 2016 in the online journal *PLoS ONE*, researchers from the Netherlands and Germany wanted to learn more about the association between selenium status and bone mineral density. The cohort consisted of 387 healthy elderly men with a median age of 77 years. The researchers determined that the overall selenium status of the population was low normal, but only 0.5 percent of the subjects met the criteria for deficiency. The researchers found a positive association between selenium status and bone mineral density in healthy aging European men. "This is the first study to show in men that Se status, even within this low normal range is positively associated with BMD." According to the researchers, "even in a population with borderline sufficiency there is a significant association with bone mineral density."[14]

Levels of Serum Selenium May Affect Depressive Moods

In a study published in 2015 in *The Journal of Nutrition*, researchers from New Zealand wanted to learn more about the association between selenium and psychiatric issues, such as depressive symptoms and negative moods. The cohort consisted of 978 young adults (36.5% male) between the ages of 17 and 25 years. The subjects completed the Center for Epidemiological Studies-Depression scale and reported their positive and negative moods for 13 days. The researchers found a U-shaped association between selenium intake and depressive symptoms; the subjects with the lowest and highest intakes of selenium had significantly higher symptoms of depression. Lower levels of selenium were associated with more depression than higher levels. As a result, lower levels appeared to be more detrimental than higher levels. People with the lowest levels of depression took in between 82 and 85 mcg of selenium per day. The researchers commented that this is the first study "to show that selenium concentration is related to daily negative mood in a similar way to depressive symptoms." These findings "may have important implications for people who eat a diet either low or very high in selenium and for people who take selenium supplements."[15]

NOTES

1. Office of Dietary Supplements, National Institutes of Health. "Selenium." December 29, 2017. https://ods.od.nih.gov/factsheets/Selenium-Consumer/.
2. The George Mateljan Foundation. "Selenium." December 29, 2017. http://whfoods.com/genpage.php?tname=nutrient&dbid=95.
3. NIH Office of Dietary Supplements.
4. Hughes, David J., Talita Duarte-Salles, Sandra Hybsier, et al. "Prediagnostic Selenium Status and Hepatobiliary Cancer Risk in the European Prospective Investigation into Cancer and Nutrition Cohort." *American Journal of Clinical Nutrition* 104 (2016): 406–414.
5. Karamali, Maryam, Sepideh Nourgostar, Ashraf Zamani, et al. "The Favourable Effects of Long-Term Selenium Supplementation on Regression of Cervical Tissues and Metabolic Profiles of Patients with Cervical Intraepithelial Neoplasia: A Randomised, Double-Blind, Placebo-Controlled Trial." *British Journal of Nutrition* 114 (2015): 2039–2045.
6. Tara, Fatemeh, Gholamali Maamouri, Margaret P. Rayman, et al. "Selenium Supplementation and the Incidence of Preeclampsia in Pregnant Iranian Women: A Randomized, Double-Blind, Placebo-Controlled Pilot Trial." *Taiwanese Journal of Obstetrics and Gynecology* 49, no. 2 (2010): 181–187.
7. Harris, Holly R., Leif Bergkvist, and Alicja Wolk. "Selenium Intake and Breast Cancer Mortality in a Cohort of Swedish Women." *Breast Cancer Research and Treatment* 134 (2012): 1269–1277.
8. Allen, Naomi E., Ruth C. Travis, Paul N. Appleby, et al. "Selenium and Prostate Cancer: Analysis of Individual Participant Data from Fifteen Prospective Studies." *Journal of the National Cancer Institute* 108, no. 11 (2016): djw153.
9. Algotar, Amit M., M. Suzanne Stratton, Frederick R. Ahmann, et al. "Phase 3 Clinical Trial Investigating the Effect of Selenium Supplementation in Men at High-Risk for Prostate Cancer." *The Prostate* 73 (2013): 328–335.
10. Wei, Jie, Chao Zeng, Qian-yi Gong, et al. "The Association between Dietary Selenium Intake and Diabetes: A Cross-Sectional Study among Middle-Aged and Older Adults." *Nutrition Journal* 14 (2015): 18.
11. Lu, Chia-Wen, Hao-Hsiang Chang, Kuen-Cheh Yang, et al. "High Serum Selenium Levels Are Associated with Increased Risk for Diabetes Mellitus Independent of Central Obesity and Insulin Resistance." *BMJ Open Diabetes Research & Care* 4 (2016): e000253.
12. Wu, Qian, Margaret P. Rayman, Hongjun Lv, et al. "Low Population Selenium Status Is Associated with Increased Prevalence of Thyroid Disease." *Journal of Clinical Endocrinology & Metabolism* 100, no. 11 (November 2015): 4037–4047.
13. Pederson, Inge Bülow, Mils Knudsen, Allan Carlé, et al. "Serum Selenium Is Low in Newly Diagnosed Graves Disease: A Population-Based Study." *Clinical Endocrinology* 79 (2013): 584–590.
14. Beukhof, C. M., M. Medici, A. W. van den Beld, et al. "Selenium Status Is Positively Associated with Bone Mineral Density in Healthy Aging European Men." *PLoS ONE* 11, no. 4 (2016): e0152748.

15. Conner, Tamlin S., Aimee C. Richardson, and Jody C. Miller. "Optimal Serum Selenium Concentrations Are Associated with Lower Depressive Symptoms and Negative Mood among Young Adults." *The Journal of Nutrition* 145, no. 1 (January 1, 2015): 59–65.

REFERENCES AND FURTHER READINGS

Algotar, Amit M., M. Suzanne Stratton, Frederick R. Ahmann, et al. "Phase 3 Clinical Trial Investigating the Effect of Selenium Supplementation in Men at High-Risk for Prostate Cancer." *The Prostate* 73 (2013): 328–335.

Allen, Naomi E., Ruth C. Travis, Paul N. Appleby, et al. "Selenium and Prostate Cancer: Analysis of Individual Participant Data from Fifteen Prospective Studies." *Journal of the National Cancer Institute* 108, no. 11 (2016): djw153.

Beukhof, C. M., M. Medici, A. W. van den Beld, et al. "Selenium Status Is Positively Associated with Bone Mineral Density in Healthy Aging European Men." *PLoS ONE* 11, no. 4 (2016): e0152748.

Conner, Tamlin S., Aimee C. Richardson, and Jody C. Miller. "Optimal Serum Selenium Concentrations Are Associated with Lower Depressive Symptoms and Negative Mood among Young Adults." *The Journal of Nutrition* 145, no. 1 (January 1, 2015): 59–65.

The George Mateljan Foundation. "Selenium." December 29, 2017. http://whfoods.com/genpage.php?tname=nutrient&dbid=95.

Harris, Holly R., Leif Bergkvist, and Alicja Wolk. "Selenium Intake and Breast Cancer Mortality in a Cohort of Swedish Women." *Breast Cancer Research and Treatment* 134, no. 3 (2012): 1269–1277.

Hughes, David J., Talita Duarte-Salles, Sandra Hybsier, et al. "Prediagnostic Selenium Status and Hepatobiliary Cancer Risk in the European Prospective Investigation into Cancer and Nutrition Cohort." *American Journal of Clinical Nutrition* 104 (2016): 406–414.

Karamali, Maryam, Sepideh Nourgostar, Ashraf Zamani, et al. "The Favourable Effects of Long-Term Selenium Supplementation on Regression of Cervical Tissues and Metabolic Profiles of Patients with Cervical Intraepithelial Neoplasia: A Randomised, Double-Blind, Placebo-Controlled Trial." *British Journal of Nutrition* 114 (2015): 2039–2045.

Lu, Chia-Wen, Hao-Hsiang Chang, Kuen-Cheh Yang, et al. "High Serum Selenium Levels Are Associated with Increased Risk for Diabetes Mellitus Independent of Central Obesity and Insulin Resistance." *BMJ Open Diabetes Research & Care* 4 (2016): e000253.

Office of Dietary Supplements, National Institutes of Health. "Selenium." December 29, 2017. https://ods.od.nih.gov/factsheets/Selenium-Consumer/.

Pedersen, Inge Bülow, Nils Knudsen, Allan Carlé, et al. "Serum Selenium Is Low in Newly Diagnosed Graves Disease: A Population-Based Study." *Clinical Endocrinology* 79 (2013): 584–590.

Tara, Fatemeh, Gholamali Maamouri, Margaret P. Rayman, et al. "Selenium Supplementation and the Incidence of Preeclampsia in Pregnant Iranian Women: A Randomized, Double-Blind, Placebo-Controlled Pilot Trial." *Taiwanese Journal of Obstetrics and Gynecology* 49, no. 2 (2010): 181–187.

Wei, Jie, Chao Zeng, Qian-yi Gong, et al. "The Association between Dietary Selenium Intake and Diabetes: A Cross-Sectional Study among Middle-Aged and Older Adults." *Nutrition Journal* 14 (2015): 18+.

Wu, Qian, Margaret P. Rayman, Hongjun Lv, et al. "Low Population Selenium Status Is Associated with Increased Prevalence of Thyroid Disease." *Journal of Clinical Endocrinology & Metabolism* 100, no. 11 (November 2015): 4037–4047.

Sodium

Sodium is a mineral that occurs naturally in foods, such as celery, beets, and milk, or is added during manufacturing or processing. While sodium and salt tend to be used interchangeably, they are not the same. Everyday table salt is actually a combination of sodium and chloride. By weight, salt is about 40 percent sodium and 60 percent chloride.

Sodium is an important electrolyte. The human body requires sodium to support the functioning of nerves and muscles and to maintain the right balance of fluids. The kidneys control the amount of sodium in the body.

FOOD SOURCES AND SUPPLEMENTS

Sodium is most abundant in highly processed foods. Canned soups, lunch meats, and frozen dinners tend to have higher amounts of sodium. Other higher sources of sodium are bread products, pizza, sandwiches, and poultry. Sodium (in the form of salt) is also commonly added to dishes during cooking or at the table before eating. Some over-the-counter and prescription medications have sodium; people taking those drugs are probably unaware of this source. Although sodium can be purchased as a supplement, it should be taken only under the supervision of a health-care provider.

INTAKE RECOMMENDATIONS

The Food and Nutrition Board of the Institute of Medicine recommends that healthy people between the ages of 19 and 50 years should consume 1.5 g of sodium (1,500 mg) and 2.3 g of chloride each day or 3.8 g of salt. The tolerable upper intake level for salt is set at 5.8 g per day.

The American Heart Association recommends that people consume no more than one teaspoon of salt per day from all sources; one teaspoon of salt has about 2,300 mg of sodium. The association suggests that most adults would benefit from no more than 1,500 mg per day. But Americans tend to consume more than 3,400 mg per day of sodium. The American Heart Association asked 1,000 adults to estimate their sodium intake. One-third were unable to provide an estimate; another 54 percent thought they were taking in less than 2,000 mg sodium per day.[1]

DEFICIENCY AND EXCESS

The human body needs only a small amount of sodium—less than 500 mg per day. Therefore, a true deficiency rarely occurs.

On the other hand, as has been noted, excess sodium intake is common. When the kidneys are unable to eliminate all of the excess sodium, it builds up in the body and increases the amount of fluid inside blood vessels. This process elevates blood pressure. Hypertension, or elevated blood pressure, may trigger other cardiovascular concerns. For example, high blood pressure may increase the buildup of arterial plaque that blocks the blood flow through arteries. This may lead to a heart attack or stroke. About one-third of the U.S. adult population has hypertension. More than 40 percent of non-Hispanic black adults have high blood pressure; blacks also develop high blood pressure at younger ages than whites. Even people who don't have high blood pressure may benefit from eating lower amounts of sodium.[2]

KEY RESEARCH FINDINGS

In the United States, Children and Adolescents Are Not Following a Diet That Reduces the Risk of High Blood Pressure and Lowers the Risk of Cardiovascular Disease

In a study published in 2017 in the *Journal of the Academy of Nutrition and Dietetics*, researchers from Massachusetts explained that the Dietary Approaches to Stop Hypertension (DASH) diet is known to lower blood pressure and reduce the risk of cardiovascular disease in adults. (The DASH diet emphasizes fruits, vegetables, low-fat dairy, whole grains, and plant-based proteins and includes only small amounts of sodium.) But little is known about how the diet might benefit children and teens. As a result, the researchers obtained data on 9,793 children and teens between the ages of 8 and 18 years from the 2003–2012 National Health and Nutrition Examination Surveys. The researchers found that there was a low adherence to a DASH-like diet among the children and teens surveyed. Most of the children and teens met only one or two nutrient targets, and not a single participant met all nine of the nutrient targets. The researchers concluded that there was "poor accordance with a DASH-like nutrient pattern among US youth."[3]

High and Low Intakes of Sodium Are Associated with Increased Mortality and Higher Rates of Cardiovascular Disease

In a meta-analysis published in 2014 in the *American Journal of Hypertension*, researchers from Denmark investigated the incidence of all-cause mortality and cardiovascular disease events in populations exposed to low, low average, higher average, and high levels of sodium. The cohort consisted of 25 different studies; the vast majority of these studies were observational. The researchers noted their primary finding was that people who consumed both low and high amounts of sodium placed themselves at increased risk for all types of mortality and cardiovascular diseases. In fact, there was no difference in outcomes between the higher- and lower-sodium intake groups. The researchers concluded that their data were "consistent with the hypothesis that a U shape best describes the relationship of sodium to health care outcomes."[4]

Oral Sodium Supplementation Does Not Appear to Enhance or Hinder the Performance of Athletes

In a study published in 2015 in the *Journal of Sports Science & Medicine*, researchers from Saint Louis, Missouri, wanted to learn if supplementation with 1,800 mg of sodium would impact the performance of trained, endurance athletes. The cohort for the analysis consisted of 11 endurance athletes; they participated in two sessions of two hours of treadmill or cycling endurance exercise; during one session they were given a sodium capsule, and during a second session they were given a placebo. The number of days between the tests ranged from 7 to 26. The participants were instructed to adhere to a sodium-restricted diet and consume the same food and beverages for the 48 hours before each test. The researchers learned that high-sodium supplementation did not appear to improve or impair athletic performance. It did not have a significant effect on sweat rate, cardiovascular drift, heat stress, skin temperature, rating of perceived exertion, or time to exhaustion. The participants became dehydrated with or without sodium.

Although the researchers had hypothesized that the high-sodium supplementation would negatively impact the athletes, that did not prove to be true. Still, "in light of the possibility that high sodium intakes might have on other adverse effects, such as hypertension," the researchers recommended "that athletes interpret professional recommendations for sodium needs during exercise with caution."[5]

Sodium Phosphate Only Slightly Benefited Sprinting Athletes

In a study published in 2016 in the *Journal of Science and Medicine in Sport*, researchers from Australia wanted to determine if sodium and caffeine could benefit sprinting athletes. The researchers recruited 11 male athletes from various team sports—Australian football, basketball, hockey, and soccer. All of the athletes were around the age of 20 years; none had consumed any nutritional supplements for two months. Over a 14-week period, the subjects participated in experimental trials that tested the ability of sodium phosphate and caffeine, sodium phosphate and a placebo, caffeine and a placebo, and a placebo to have an effect on the speed of sprints. There were 17 days between each trial. Exercise testing was performed in an indoor gymnasium. The researchers found that the athletes taking sodium phosphate experienced only small improvements in the speed of their sprints, and this association was not significant. Yet the researchers commented that "there is some evidence" that sodium phosphate supplementation may improve repeated-sprint ability in male team-sports athletes. "These results are important to coaches and athletes who wish to improve repeated-sprint ability during a team-sport game."[6]

An Interaction between Dietary Sodium and Smoking May Increase the Risk of Rheumatoid Arthritis

In a study published in 2015 in the journal *Rheumatology*, researchers from Sweden examined the association between sodium consumption and rheumatoid arthritis. They used population-based prospective data from the Västerbotten Intervention Programme, which included 386 people who had described their dietary habits for a median of 7.7 years before the onset of symptoms of rheumatoid arthritis. There were also 1,886 matched controls. Initially, the researchers found no association between sodium intake and rheumatoid arthritis. However, when they included smoking in the analysis, a relationship emerged. Among smokers, who indicated that they smoked one or more cigarettes per day, higher sodium intake more than doubled the risk for rheumatoid arthritis. This association did not exist for nonsmokers. According to the researchers, their findings suggested "that high sodium consumption among smokers was associated with the risk of RA [and] may provide new insights into the impact of smoking on RA development."[7]

There Is an Association between High Sodium Intake and Mortality from Heart Disease, Stroke, and Type 2 Diabetes

In a study published in 2017 in *JAMA*, researchers from Boston, Massachusetts, Cambridge, England, and Bronx, New York, examined the association between the intake of 10 specific dietary factors, including sodium, and mortality from heart disease, stroke, and type 2 diabetes. The researchers used data from the National Health and Nutrition Examination Surveys 1999–2002 and 2009–2012 and the National Center for Health Statistics. The data indicated that in 2012 there were 702,308 cardiometabolic deaths in the United States. These included 506,100 from heart disease, 128,294 from stroke, and 67,914 from types 2 diabetes. Of these, the largest numbers of estimated cardiometabolic deaths—66,508 people—were related to the high consumption of sodium. Among unhealthful foods and nutrients, sodium should be "a key target." Governments need to find ways to implement policies that "educate the public and engage industry" to reduce the amount of salt in processed foods. Past efforts to reduce salt have been "effective, equitable, and highly cost-effective or even cost-saving."[8]

Reduced-Sodium Meals Appear to Be Readily Accepted by Uninformed Consumers

In a single-blind, randomized, controlled study published in 2015 in the *Journal of the Academy of Nutrition and Dietetics*, researchers from the Netherlands wanted to determine if people would readily accept eating food with less sodium. The cohort consisted of 74 people between the ages of 18 and 35 years. During a three-week period of time, all of the participants ate a lunchtime buffet. The

36 people in the intervention group ate food that contained 29 to 61 percent less sodium; the 38 participants in the control group ate food with the usual amount of sodium. While the participants were not aware of these changes, they generally liked the lower-sodium foods as much as the foods with regular amounts of sodium. The researchers learned that the subjects who ate the food with less sodium ate about the same amount of food. Urine tests determined that the subjects who ate less sodium had less sodium in their bodies. Moreover, the people who ate the lower-sodium lunches did not compensate by eating higher-sodium foods during the remainder of the day. "Offering reduced-sodium foods without explicitly informing consumers of the sodium reduction can contribute to reduced daily sodium intake."[9]

Dietary Sodium Intake Has Increased Among People with High Blood Pressure

In a study published in 2017 in the *Journal of Hypertension*, researchers from Newark, New Jersey, and New York City wanted to learn more about the sodium intake of people who have high blood pressure. Data were obtained from the National Health and Nutrition Examination Survey, 1999–2012, which included adults over the age of 20 years with self-reported high blood pressure. During the years of the survey, a total of 13,033 adults with hypertension were examined. Almost half were non-Hispanic white; 53 percent were men. The researchers determined that more than 83 percent of the participants were consuming more than 1,500 mg sodium per day. When compared to younger adults, adults over the age of 50 consumed less sodium. Men consumed more sodium than women. From 1999 to 2012, the mean sodium consumption of this cohort increased by 14.2 percent. The researchers commented that their findings demonstrated that "the vast majority of US adults diagnosed with hypertension consume sodium in far excess of dietary recommendations." There is a "need for improved population-based interventions, including more effective strategies and aggressive approaches to reduce the sodium consumption among hypertensive adults."[10]

There Are Group Variations to Sodium Intake, and the Vast Majority of Sodium in the Diet Comes from Food Prepared Outside the Home

In a study published in 2017 in the journal *Circulation*, researchers from several locations in the United States wanted to learn about sources of dietary sodium. The cohort consisted of 450 adults from three geographic locations—Birmingham, Alabama, Palo Alto, California, and Minneapolis–St. Paul, Minnesota. Each location had 150 adults. There were equal numbers of men and women who were black, Asian, Hispanic, and non-Hispanic white. Four 24-hour dietary recalls were collected from each participant, and each participant had a one-time visit to a clinic. The researcher determined that the mean total daily sodium intake was 3,501 mg per day, well above the previously noted recommended levels of 2,300 mg per day. Men consumed more sodium than women, and sodium intake was higher in blacks and Asians than Hispanics. College graduates consumed less sodium than those with high school or lower levels of education, and obese people consumed more sodium than normal-weight people. Sodium intake was higher in Alabama than California and Minnesota.

The researchers found that the sodium added to the food consumed outside the home was the leading source of sodium; in their cohort, 70.9 percent of the sodium was obtained from this outside food. The next highest contributor was sodium naturally found in food; that represented 14.2 percent. The third and fourth contributors were salt added during food preparation and salt from the salt shaker on the table. Other sources of sodium, such as nonprescription antacids, dietary supplements, and tap water, were minimal sources of sodium. The researchers concluded that there is a need "to reduce sodium intake in the United States through setting targets to reduce the sodium content of commercially processed and prepared foods."[11]

There Is an Association between Sodium Intake and Blood Pressure among Children and Teens in the United States

In a study published in 2012 in the journal *Pediatrics*, researchers based in Atlanta, Georgia, assessed the association between the intake of dietary sodium and blood pressure in children and adolescents in the United States. The cohort consisted of data from the National Health and Nutrition Examination Survey, 2003–2008; there were 6,235 children and adolescents between the ages of 8 and 18 years. Using 24-hour dietary recalls, estimates were made of the subjects' usual sodium intake. The researchers determined that the subjects consumed an average of 3,387 mg per day of sodium, and the average sodium intake increased with age. Consumption was higher among males and among those who were overweight/obese. Among the ethnic groups, non-Hispanic whites had the highest intake. These high levels of sodium intake were associated with elevated rates of systolic blood pressure and the risk of pre-high blood pressure and high blood pressure. The researchers underscored the need for "evidence-based interventions" to help children and teens reduce their intake of sodium.[12]

NOTES

1. American Heart Association. "Sodium and Salt." December 29, 2017. http://www.heart.org/HEARTORG/HealthyLiving/Healthy/eating/Nutrriton/Sodium-Salt-or-Sodium-Chloride_UCM_303290_Article.jsp#.WkbMCihOE_s.

2. Ibid.

3. Cohen, Juliana F. W., Megan E. Lehnerd, Robert F. Houser, and Eric B. Rimm. "Dietary Approaches to Stop Hypertension Diet, Weight Status, and Blood Pressure among Children and Adolescents: National Health and Nutrition Examination Surveys 2003–2012." *Journal of the Academy of Nutrition and Dietetics* 117, no. 9 (September 2017): 1437–1444.

4. Graudal, Niels, Gesche Jürgens, Bo Baslund, and Michael H. Alderman. "Compared with Usual Sodium Intake, Low- and Excessive-Sodium Diets Are Associated with Increased Mortality: A Meta-Analysis." *American Journal of Hypertension* 27, no. 9 (September 2014): 1129–1137.

5. Earhart, Elizabeth L., Edward P. Weiss, Rabia Rahman, and Patrick V. Kelly. "Effects of Oral Sodium Supplementation on Indices of Thermoregulation in Trained, Endurance Athletes." *Journal of Sports Science & Medicine* 14, no. 1 (2015): 172–178.

6. Kopec, Benjamin J., Brian T. Dawson, Christopher Buck, and Karen E. Wallman. "Effects of Sodium Phosphate and Caffeine Ingestion on Repeated-Sprint Ability in Male Athletes." *Journal of Science and Medicine in Sport* 19, no. 3 (March 2016): 272–276.

7. Sundström, Björn, Ingegerd Johansson, and Solbritt Rantapää-Dahlqvist. "Interaction between Dietary Sodium and Smoking Increases the Risk for Rheumatoid Arthritis: Results from a Nested Case-Control Study." *Rheumatology* 54 (2015): 487–493.

8. Micha, R., J. L. Peñalvo, F. Cudhea, et al. "Association between Dietary Factors and Mortality from Heart Disease, Stroke, and Type 2 Diabetes in the United States." *JAMA* 317, no. 9 (March 7, 2017): 912–924.

9. Janssen, Anke M., Stefanie Kremer, Willeke L. van Stipriaan, et al. "Reduced-Sodium Lunches Are Well-Accepted by Uninformed Consumers over a 3-Week Period and Result in Decreased Daily Dietary Sodium Intakes: A Randomized Controlled Trial." *Journal of the Academy of Nutrition and Dietetics* 115, no. 10 (October 2015): 1614–1625.

10. Dolmatova, Elena V., Kasra Moazzami, and Sameer Bansilal. "Dietary Sodium Intake among US Adults with Hypertension, 1999–2012." *Journal of Hypertension* 36, no. 2 (February 2018): 237–242.

11. Harnack, Lisa J., Mary E. Cogswell, James M. Shikany, et al. "Sources of Sodium in US Adults from 3 Geographic Regions." *Circulation* 135, no. 19 (May 9, 2017): 1775–1783.

12. Yang, Quanhe, Zefeng Zhang, Elena V. Kuklina, et al. "Sodium Intake and Blood Pressure among US Children and Adolescents." *Pediatrics* 130 (2012): 611–619.

REFERENCES AND FURTHER READINGS

American Heart Association. "Sodium and Salt." December 29, 2017. http://www.heart.org/HEARTORG/HealthyLiving/Healthy/eating/Nutrriton/Sodium-Salt-or-Sodium-Chloride_UCM_303290_Article.jsp#.WkbMCihOE_s.

Cohen, Juliana F. W., Megan E. Lehnerd, Robert F. Houser, and Eric B. Rimm. "Dietary Approaches to Stop Hypertension Diet, Weight Status, and Blood Pressure among Children and Adolescents: National Health and Nutrition Examination Surveys 2003–2012." *Journal of the Academy of Nutrition and Dietetics* 117, no. 9 (September 2017): 1437–1444.

Dolmatova, Elena V., Kasra Moazzami, and Sameer Bansilal. "Dietary Sodium Intake among US Adults with Hypertension, 1999–2012." *Journal of Hypertension* 36, no. 2 (February 2018): 237–242.

Earhart, Elizabeth L., Edward P. Weiss, Rabia Rahman, and Patrick V. Kelly. "Effects of Oral Sodium Supplementation on Indices of Thermoregulation in Trained, Endurance Athletes." *Journal of Sports Science & Medicine* 14, no. 1 (2015): 172–178.

Graudal, Niels, Gesche Jürgens, Bo Baslund, and Michael H. Alderman. "Compared with Usual Sodium Intake, Low- and Excessive-Sodium Diets Are Associated with Increased Mortality: A Meta-Analysis." *American Journal of Hypertension* 27, no. 9 (September 2014): 1129–1137.

Harnack, Lisa J., Mary E. Cogswell, James M. Shikany, et al. "Sources of Sodium in US Adults from 3 Geographic Regions." *Circulation* 135, no. 19 (May 9, 2017): 1775–1783.

Janssen, Anke M., Stefanie Kremer, Willeke L. van Stipriaan, et al. "Reduced-Sodium Lunches Are Well-Accepted by Uninformed Consumers over a 3-Week Period and Result in Decreased Daily Dietary Sodium Intakes: A Randomized Controlled Trial." *Journal of the Academy of Nutrition and Dietetics* 115, no. 10 (October 2010): 1614–1625.

Kopec, Benjamin J., Brian T. Dawson, Christopher Buck, and Karen E. Wallman. "Effects of Sodium Phosphate and Caffeine Ingestion on Repeated-Sprint Ability in Male Athletes." *Journal of Science and Medicine in Sport* 19, no. 3 (March 2016): 272–276.

Micha, R., J.L. Peñalvo, F. Cudhea, et al. "Association between Dietary Factors and Mortality from Heart Disease, Stroke, and Type 2 Diabetes in the United States." *JAMA* 317, no. 9 (March 7, 2017): 912–924.

Sundström, Björn, Ingegerd Johansson, and Solbritt Rantapää-Dahlqvist. "Interaction between Dietary Sodium and Smoking Increases the Risk for Rheumatoid Arthritis: Results from A Nested Case-Control Study." *Rheumatology* 54 (2015): 487–493.

Yang, Quanhe, Zefeng Zhang, Elena V. Kuklina, et al. "Sodium Intake and Blood Pressure Among US Children and Adolescents." *Pediatrics* 130 (2012): 611–619.

Vitamin A

Found in a wide variety of foods, vitamin A is a fat-soluble vitamin that is needed for normal vision, reproduction, and the proper development of a fetus. It supports the immune system as well as the heart, lungs, kidneys, and other organs. Vitamin A also plays a role in growth, bone formation, and wound healing.

There are actually two main types of vitamin A. The first, known as preformed vitamin A (retinoids), is found in meat, poultry, fish, and dairy products; the second, known as provitamin A (carotenoids), is contained in plant-based products such as fruits and vegetables. The most common type of provitamin A is beta-carotene.

FOOD SOURCES AND SUPPLEMENTS

Liver is by far the most potent food source of preformed vitamin A. There are many other excellent sources of vitamin A, including sweet potatoes, carrots, spinach, kale, mustard greens, collard greens, beet greens, turnip greens,

Swiss chard, winter squash, romaine lettuce, bok choy, cantaloupe, bell peppers, and parsley. Very good sources of vitamin A include broccoli, asparagus, sea vegetables, chili peppers, tomatoes, and basil. Good sources of vitamin A include papaya, shrimp, eggs, Brussels sprouts, grapefruit, cow's milk, green beans, watermelon, leeks, apricots, cilantro, and celery.[1] Vitamin A is generally found in multivitamins; it is also sold as a single-ingredient vitamin.

INTAKE RECOMMENDATIONS

The Office of Dietary Supplements of the National Institutes of Health cites the following recommendations for vitamin A. For people 14 years and older, recommendations range from 700 to 900 mcg of retinol activity equivalents (RAEs) per day. Recommended intakes for women who are breast-feeding range from 1,200 to 1,300 RAE per day, while lower values are recommended for infants and children younger than 14 years. However, product labels contain information on vitamin A in international units, not RAEs. And the process of converting RAEs to international units may be confusing. Most professionals agree that a varied diet should provide most residents of the United States with sufficient vitamin A. At the same time, the U.S. Food and Drug Administration has established a daily value (DV) of 5,000 IU of vitamin A for adults and children four years of age and older. (DVs are not recommended intakes; they don't vary by age and sex.)[2]

There are tolerable upper intake levels for preformed vitamin A. Pregnant or lactating women 19 years or older should take in not more than 3,000 mcg (10,000 IU) of preformed vitamin A per day, while pregnant or lactating women 18 years or younger should take in no more than 2,800 mcg (9,333 IU) per day. Adults 19 years and older should take in no more than 3,000 mcg (10,000 IU) of preformed vitamin A per day, while teenagers between the ages of 14 and 18 years should take in no more than 2,800 mcg (9,333 IU) per day. Children between the ages of 9 and 14 years should take in no more than 1,700 mcg (5,666 IU) of preformed vitamin A per day, while children between the ages of 4 and 8 years should take in no more than 900 mcg (3,000 IU) of preformed vitamin A per day. Children three years and younger should take in no more than 600 mcg (2,000 IU) per day.[3]

DEFICIENCY AND EXCESS

While vitamin A deficiency is common in developing countries, in the United States, the deficiency is believed to be rare. When young children and pregnant women take in too little vitamin A, they may develop an eye condition known as xerophthalmia, which is an inability to see in low light. If not treated, xerophthalmia may lead to blindness. Other medical conditions associated with vitamin A deficiency include dry eyes, diarrhea, and skin problems. People living with cystic fibrosis have an increased risk for vitamin A deficiency.

On the other hand, it is very important to avoid taking in too much vitamin A. Though it is almost impossible to consume too much vitamin A from food, supplemental vitamin A and/or vitamin A in certain medications may result in toxicity. Symptoms of excess vitamin A include dizziness, nausea, headaches, coma, and even death. Females who may be pregnant should not take high doses of vitamin A. Most cases of vitamin A toxicity occur from the continued intake of high amounts of supplemental vitamin A.

Consuming high amounts of beta-carotene or other forms of provitamin A may cause the skin to turn a yellow-orange color, most often in the palms of the hands and soles of the feet. This condition, which is known as carotenodermia, may be a nuisance and embarrassing, but it is harmless.

KEY RESEARCH FINDINGS

Vitamin A Supplementation May Be Useful for a Few Symptoms of Multiple Sclerosis

In a double-blind, placebo-controlled, randomized study published in 2016 in the *Iranian Journal of Allergy, Asthma and Immunology*, researchers from Iran wanted to learn if vitamin A supplementation was useful for the fatigue and depression associated with multiple sclerosis. (Multiple sclerosis is an autoimmune disorder of the central nervous system that is characterized by neurological disability.) The initial cohort consisted of 101 subjects with "relapsing-remitting" multiple sclerosis. All of the subjects, who ranged in age from 20 to 45 years, were treated at an outpatient clinic. The subjects in the treatment group took two different doses of vitamin A, each for six months. Four subjects from each of the two groups did not complete the study. Still, the results were notable. The patients taking vitamin A experienced significant improvements in fatigue and depression. "The present study demonstrated that vitamin A as an immune modulator can improve psychiatric signs in MS."[4]

Vitamin A Supplementation May or May Not Benefit New Mothers and Their Infants

In a systematic review published in 2015 in the journal *Revista Brasileira de Epidemiologia* (*Brazilian Journal of Epidemiology*), researchers from Brazil investigated the impact of vitamin A supplementation on adult pregnant women and women who have recently given birth. They were also interested in learning how the mothers' supplementation affected the newborns. The researchers located seven studies on the effects of vitamin A supplementation during the early newborn period that were published between January 2000 and January 2014, but they were unable to locate any relevant studies on the effects of vitamin A supplementation on pregnant women. The researchers found that the new mothers who were taking vitamin A supplementation had more vitamin A content in their colostrum than the controls. As a result, the newborns consumed more vitamin A. "Supplementation contributes to a better nutritional status of vitamin A for both the child and the puerperal woman and increased the offer of vitamin A for the newborn through the breast milk."[5]

In another systematic review published in 2016 in *Cochrane Database of Systematic Reviews,* researchers from Brazil, Germany, and Australia examined 14 trials that investigated the use of vitamin A supplementation for postpartum women. The trials, which included 25,758 women and infant pairs, focused on maternal and infant health. The studies compared women who took vitamin A supplementation to women who did not or compared a higher dose of vitamin A supplementation to a lower dose. In all the trials, a considerable proportion of the infants were at least partially breastfed until six months. The researchers found that the vitamin A supplementation increased the amount of this nutrient in the mother's breast milk. However, it did not appear to make a difference in the health or well-being of the mothers or babies. At the same time, no adverse effects were observed. "There was no evidence of benefit from different doses of vitamin A supplementation for postpartum women on maternal and infant mortality and morbidity, compared with other doses or placebo."[6]

Prenatal Vitamin A Supplementation May Be Associated with Adverse Childhood Behavior

In a prospective study published in 2016 in the journal *Pediatrics International,* researchers from Japan wanted to learn more about the association between intake of vitamin A supplementation during pregnancy and problematic childhood behaviors. Their cohort consisted of 1,271 pairs of Japanese pregnant women and their newborns; they were followed until the children were three years old. During their third trimester of pregnancy, the women completed a self-administered questionnaire. Another questionnaire was sent to the women one month after delivery. A few years later, to evaluate the behavior of their children, the women completed the Japanese Child Behavior Checklist for ages two to three years. The researchers compared the behaviors of the children of the women who took vitamin A supplementation to the children of the women who did not take the supplementation. The researchers found that there was an inverse association between the prenatal vitamin A supplementation and the behavior patterns of the young children. The mothers who took the supplementation had children with more negative behavior patterns at the age of three years. The researchers commented that excess vitamin A is stored in the body and may become toxic. Perhaps, they noted, it influenced the neural formation of the fetal brain during pregnancy. And, that, in turn, may result in "a deviation in child behavior at 3 years of age." They concluded that the intake of vitamin A before and/or during pregnancy "may worsen child behavior at 3 years of age."[7]

Vitamin A Supplementation May or May Not Be Useful for Very Low-Birth-Weight Infants

In an analysis published in 2016 in the *Cochrane Database of Systematic Reviews*, researchers examined the practice of giving low-birth-weight infants multiple doses of intramuscular vitamin A supplementation. They wanted to learn if it helped to prevent mortality and short- or long-term morbidity. Specifically, did vitamin A supplementation reduce the number problems associated with low birth weight, such as death, lung disease, abnormal development of the retina, bleeding in the brain, and neurodevelopmental disability? Eleven trials met the inclusion criteria. Ten of the trials, which had a total of 1,460 infants, compared vitamin A supplementation with a control. One trial, with 120 infants, compared different regimens of vitamin A supplementation. When compared to the controls, the researchers found that vitamin A supplementation slightly reduced the risk of death and the need for oxygen. It also lowered the risk of chronic lung disease. In one trial that examined neurodevelopmental status, the researchers found no evidence that vitamin A was either beneficial or harmful. While there were no reported adverse effects of the supplementation, it was noted that intramuscular injections of vitamin A were painful. The researchers concluded that the use of this vitamin A supplementation "may depend on the local incidence of this outcome and the value attached to achieving a modest reduction in the outcome balanced against the lack of other proven benefits and the acceptability of treatment."[8]

Types of Household Food Expenditures May Play a Key Role in Vitamin A Deficiency

In a cross-sectional study published in 2009 in the journal *Nutritional Research*, researchers from several locations throughout the world investigated the association between household food expenditures and night blindness among nonpregnant women of childbearing age in poor families in Jakarta, Indonesia. The researchers used data from the Indonesian Nutrition Surveillance System, which included 42,974 households. Food expenditures were divided into five major categories: plant-based foods, animal-based foods, eggs, other nongrain foods, and grain foods (primarily rice). The proportion of households with night blindness in nonpregnant women, which was used as a clinical indicator of vitamin A deficiency, was calculated to be 309 households or 0.72 percent. Plant-based foods, animal-based foods, and eggs were associated with a reduced risk of night blindness. Grain foods were related to an increased risk of night blindness. According to the researchers, their findings "suggest that nonpregnant women are at greater risk of clinical vitamin deficiency where families spend more on rice and less on animal and plant-based foods, a situation that is more typical when food prices are high."[9]

Vitamin A May Lower the Risk of Primary Liver Cancer

In a study published in 2016 in the journal *Nutrients*, researchers from China wanted to learn more about the consumption of vitamin A and the risk of developing primary liver cancer. The researchers noted that past studies of this topic have yielded inconsistent results. That is why they recruited 644 subjects with primary liver cancer and 644 age- and gender-matched controls in Guangzhou, China. The subjects with primary liver cancer ranged in age from 18 to 80 years; the median age of all the subjects was about 54 years. Dietary intake was assessed using a food frequency questionnaire. The study began in September 2013 and continued until January 2016. The researchers found that those with higher intakes of retinol, carotenes, and total vitamin A had a decreased risk of primary liver cancer. Thus, a "moderate" intake of vitamin A "could be beneficial for the prevention of PLC."[10]

Carotenoid Intake May Reduce Benign Breast Disease in Adolescents

In a case-controlled study published in 2014 in the journal *Pediatrics*, researchers from St. Louis, Missouri, and several locations in Boston wanted to learn more about the association between adolescent carotenoid intake and benign breast disease in adolescents. Benign breast disease is known to be an independent risk factor for breast cancer. Exposure to carotenoids during adolescence may be important, because that is when the tissue is still developing. The cohort consisted of 6,593 female adolescent teens, who were in the prospective Growing Up Today Study. The participants completed food frequency questionnaires, and they reported biopsy-confirmed benign breast disease. At baseline, the mean age of the cohort was 12.0 years. The researchers found that the teens who consumed more carotenoids had a lower incidence of benign breast disease. However, their findings were not statistically significant. Still, the researchers commented that their "data provide intriguing preliminary evidence that carrots and other carotenoid-rich vegetables may help to protect against BBD."[11]

There May Be an Association between Vitamin A and Type 2 Diabetes

In a study published in 2015 in the journal *Nutrition, Metabolism & Cardiovascular Diseases*, researchers from the Netherlands wanted to determine if there was any association between the intake of six different types of carotenoids and the risk of type 2 diabetes. The cohort consisted of data from the 37,846 participants in the European Prospective Investigation into Cancer and Nutrition—Netherlands. The study population had a mean age of 49.1 years, and 74 percent were female. A food frequency questionnaire was used to assess the intake of carotenoids; the incidence of type 2 diabetes was self-reported and verified against general practitioner information. During a mean follow-up of 10 years, there were 915 incident cases of type 2 diabetes. The researchers found an inverse association between two types of carotenoids—beta-carotene and alpha-carotene—and risk of type 2 diabetes; higher intake of these carotenoids lowered the risk of type 2 diabetes. "Dietary intakes of other individual carotenoids were not associated with diabetes risk." With the other carotenoids, the researchers found a tendency toward a reduced risk of diabetes, but it was not statistically significant.[12]

Low-Dose Vitamin A May Be Useful for Acne in Teens and Young Adults

In an open-label study published in the journal *Medical Archives*, a researcher from Kosovo examined the use of a low-dose vitamin A supplement for acne vulgaris, the common form of acne seen in teens and young adults. The researcher enrolled 50 patients and divided them into two groups—those between the ages of 12 and 20 years and those who were between 21 and 35 years. All of the subjects, who had moderate acne, were treated with low-dose vitamin A for three months. They were evaluated every two months. At the end of the treatment, 90.8 percent of the subjects in the younger group and 89.6 percent in the older group had "good results." During a two-year follow-up, researchers learned that relapses of acne occurred in 3.9 percent of the younger group and 5.9 percent of the older group.[13]

Serious Gastrointestinal Problems, Such As Crohn's Disease, May Increase the Risk of Vitamin A Deficiency and Night Blindness

In a report published in 2014 in the journal *International Ophthalmology*, researchers from the Cleveland Clinic Cole Eye Institute noted that profound gastrointestinal problems, such as Crohn's disease, requiring bowel resection, may result in vitamin deficiencies, including vitamin A deficiency. And the deficiency may well result in night blindness, a condition known as nyctalopia. In their report, the researchers described a 60-year-old man with a long history of Crohn's disease and multiple resections. During an eye examination, he complained that he was progressively losing his night vision. Laboratory studies determined that the man's vitamin A levels were "markedly depleted." Supplementation was initiated. In time, the "patient demonstrated both subjective and objective high vision improvement." However, the symptoms recurred, which was possibly a result of his numerous resections. And the researchers suggested that the patient might better benefit from parenteral rather than oral vitamin supplement.[14]

Bariatric Surgery May Trigger Vitamin A Deficiency

It is not uncommon for people who undergo weight loss surgery, also known as bariatric surgery, to experience nutrient deficiencies, such as vitamin A deficiency. In an article published in 2013 in the journal *Nutrición Hospitalaria*, researchers from Spain described a 48-year-old woman who had three bariatric surgeries over a multiyear period of time. After the third surgery, she began to lose serious amounts of weight, but she also had a number of health problems, including the loss of strength and energy (asthenia), generalized weakness, lower limb edema, skin dryness, loss of hearing, dry and itchy eyes, and visual problems, especially at night. The researchers determined that the woman had several vitamin deficiencies, but she was most seriously deficient in vitamin A. The woman was treated with multiple modalities, including high doses of vitamin A. By the end of six months, the "signs and symptoms of nutrient deficiencies disappeared completely." The researchers commented that "vitamin A plays an important role in several human functions, such as visual acuity, immunological activity, and cellular proliferation and differentiation."[15]

NOTES

1. The George Mateljan Foundation. "Vitamin A." December 29, 2017. http://whfoods.com/genpage.php?tname=nutrient&dbid=106.

2. Office of Dietary Supplements, National Institutes of Health. "Vitamin A." December 29, 2017. https://ods.od.nih.gov/factsheets/VitaminA-Consumer/.

3. The George Mateljan Foundation. "Vitamin A." December 29, 2017. http://whfoods.com/genpage.php?tname=nutrient&dbid=106.

4. Bitarafan, S., A. Saboor-Yaraghi, M. A. Sahraian, et al. "Effect of Vitamin A Supplementation on Fatigue and Depression in Multiple Sclerosis: A Double-Blind Placebo-Controlled Clinical Trial." *Iranian Journal of Allergy, Asthma and Immunology* 15, no. 1 (February 2016): 13–19.

5. Neves, Paulo Augusto Ribeiro, Cláudia Saunders, Denise Cavalcante de Barros, and Andréa Ramalho. "Vitamin A Supplementation in Brazilian Pregnant and Postpartum Women: A Systematic Review." *Revista Brasileira de Epidemiologia (Brazilian Journal of Epidemiology)* 18, no. 4 (October–December 2015): 824–836.

6. Oliveira, Julicristie M., Roman Allert, and Christine E. East. "Vitamin A Supplementation for Postpartum Women." *Cochrane Database of Systematic Reviews* 3 (2016): CD005944.

7. Ishikawa, Yohei, Haruka Tanaka, Taisuke Akutsu, et al. "Prenatal Vitamin A Supplementation Associated with Adverse Child Behavior at 3 Years in a Prospective Birth Cohort in Japan." *Pediatrics International* 58, no. 9 (September 2016): 855–861.

8. Darlow, B. A., P. J. Graham, and M. X. Rojas-Reyes. "Vitamin A Supplementation to Prevent Mortality and Short- and Long-Term Morbidity in Very Low Birth Weight Infants." *Cochrane Database of Systematic Reviews* 8 (August 22, 2016): CD000501.

9. Campbell, Ashley A., Andrew Thorne-Lyman, Kai Sun, et al. "Indonesian Women of Childbearing Age Are at Greater Risk of Clinical Vitamin A Deficiency in Families That Spend More on Rice and Less on Fruits/Vegetables and Animal-Based Foods." *Nutrition Research* 29 (2009): 75–81.

10. Lan, Qiu-Ye, Yao-Jun Zhang, Gong-Cheng Liao, et al. "The Association between Dietary Vitamin A and Carotenes and the Risk of Primary Live Cancer: A Case-Control Study." *Nutrients* 8 (2016): 624+.

11. Boeke, C. E., R. M. Tamimi, C. S. Berkey, et al. "Adolescent Carotenoid Intake and Benign Breast Disease." *Pediatrics* 133, no. 5 (May 2014): e1292–e1298.
12. Sluijs, I., E. Cadier, J. W. J. Beulens, et al. "Dietary Intake of Carotenoids and Risk of Type 2 Diabetes." *Nutrition, Metabolism & Cardiovascular Diseases* 25, no. 4 (April 2015): 376–381.
13. Kotori, M. G. "Low-Dose Vitamin 'A' Tablets—Treatment of Acne Vulgaris." *Medical Archives* 69, no. 1 (February 2015): 28–30.
14. da Rocha Lima, B., F. Pichi, and C. Y. Lowder. "Night Blindness and Crohn's Disease." *International Ophthalmology* 34, no. 5 (October 2014): 1141–1144.
15. Ramos-Levi, Ana M., Natalia Pérez-Ferre, Andrés Sánchez-Pernaute, et al. "Severe Vitamin A Deficiency after Malabsorptive Bariatric Surgery." *Nutrición Hospitalaria* 28, no. 4 (2013): 1337–1340.

REFERENCES AND FURTHER READINGS

Bitarafan, S., A. Saboor-Yaraghi, M. A. Sahraian, et al. "Effect of Vitamin A Supplementation on Fatigue and Depression in Multiple Sclerosis Patients: A Double-Blind Placebo-Controlled Clinical Trial." *Iranian Journal of Allergy, Asthma and Immunology* 15, no. 1 (February 2016): 13–19.

Boeke, C. E., R. M. Tamimi, C. S. Berkey, et al. "Adolescent Carotenoid Intake and Benign Breast Disease." *Pediatrics* 133, no. 5 (May 2014): e1292–e1298.

Campbell, Ashley A., Andrew Thorne-Lyman, Kai Sun, et al. "Indonesian Women of Childbearing Age Are at Greater Risk of Clinical Vitamin A Deficiency in Families That Spend More on Rice and Less on Fruits/Vegetables and Animal-Based Foods." *Nutrition Research* 29 (2009): 75–81.

da Rocha Lima, B., F. Pichi, and C. Y. Lowder. "Night Blindness and Crohn's Disease." *International Ophthalmology* 34, no. 5 (October 2014): 1141–1144.

Darlow, B. A., P. J. Graham, and M. X. Rojas-Reyes. "Vitamin A Supplementation to Prevent Mortality and Short- and Long-Term Morbidity in Very Low Birth Weight Infants." *Cochrane Database of Systematic Reviews* 8 (August 22, 2016): CD000501.

The George Mateljan Foundation. "Vitamin A." December 29, 2017. http://whfoods.com/genpage.php?tname=nutrient&dbid=106.

Ishikawa, Yohei, Haruka Tanaka, Taisuke Akutsu, et al. "Prenatal Vitamin A Supplementation Associated with Adverse Child Behavior at 3 Years in a Prospective Birth Cohort in Japan." *Pediatrics International* 58, no. 9 (September 2016): 855–861.

Kotori, M. G. "Low-Dose Vitamin 'A' Tablets—Treatment of Acne Vulgaris." *Medical Archives* 69, no. 1 (February 2015): 28–30.

Lan, Qiu-Ye, Yao-Jun Zhang, Gong-Cheng Liao, et al. "The Association between Dietary Vitamin A and Carotenes and the Risk of Primary Liver Cancer: A Case-Control Study." *Nutrients* 8 (2016): 624+.

Neves, Paulo Augusto Ribeiro, Cláudia Saunders, Denise Cavalcante de Barros, and Andréa Ramalho. "Vitamin A Supplementation in Brazilian Pregnant and Postpartum Women: A Systematic Review." *Revista Brasileira de Epidemiologia* (*Brazilian Journal of Epidemiology*) 18, no. 4 (October–December 2015): 824–836.

Office of Dietary Supplements, National Institutes of Health. "Vitamin A." December 29, 2017. https://ods.od.nih.gov/factsheets/VitaminA-Consumer/.

Oliveira, Julicristie M., Roman Allert, and Christine E. East. "Vitamin A Supplementation for Postpartum Women." *Cochrane Database of Systematic Reviews* 3 (2016): CD005944.
Ramos-Levi, Ana M., Natalia Pérez-Ferre, Andrés Sánchez-Pernaute, et al. "Severe Vitamin A Deficiency after Malabsorptive Bariatric Surgery." *Nutrición Hospitalaria* 28, no. 4 (2013): 1337–1340.
Sluijs, I., E. Cadier, J.W.J. Beulens, et al. "Dietary Intake of Carotenoids and Risk of Type 2 Diabetes." *Nutrition, Metabolism & Cardiovascular Diseases* 25, no. 4 (April 2015): 376–381.

Vitamin B1 (Thiamin)

Also known as thiamin or thiamine, vitamin B1, which plays an essential role in the production of energy from dietary fats and carbohydrates, is found in small amounts in almost all foods. Yet much of the vitamin B1 in foods is destroyed during storage, refining, and food processing. Vitamin B1, which is water soluble, is also easily damaged by heat from the stove or oven, as well as warming in a microwave. As a result, it is relatively easy, especially among those who eat a good deal of processed food, to become vitamin B1 deficient.

Vitamin B1 is a strong supporter of the nervous system, and it plays a key role in the structure and integrity of the cells in the brain. Because it strengthens the immune system and improves the body's ability to cope with stress, vitamin B1 is sometimes referred to as an anti-stress vitamin.[1] The body is unable to produce any vitamin B1; it must be obtained from food and/or supplementation.

FOOD SOURCES AND SUPPLEMENTS

Asparagus is an excellent source of vitamin B1. Very good sources of vitamin B1 include sunflower seeds, green peas, flaxseeds, Brussels sprouts, beet greens, spinach, cabbage, eggplant, romaine lettuce, and crimini mushrooms. There are countless good sources of vitamin B1. These include navy beans, black beans, barley, dried peas, lentils, oats, sesame seeds, peanuts, sweet potatoes, tofu, tuna, pineapple, oranges, broccoli, green beans, onions, summer squash, carrots, tomatoes, cantaloupe, kale, Swiss chard, bok choy, watermelon, bell peppers, cauliflower, grapefruit, garlic, cucumbers, and sea vegetables.[2] Vitamin B1 is generally included in multivitamins and B-complex vitamins, and it is sold as an individual supplement.

INTAKE RECOMMENDATIONS

The Office of Dietary Supplements of the National Institutes of Health cites the following recommendations for vitamin B1. Lactating women should take in

1.4 mg per day, while pregnant women should take in 1.1 mg per day. Males who are 19 years or older should take in 1.2 mg per day, while females who are 19 years or older should take in 1.1 mg per day. Males between the ages of 14 and 18 years should take in 1.2 mg per day, while females between the ages of 14 and 18 years should take in 1.0 mg per day. Children between the ages of 9 and 13 years should take in 0.9 mg per day, while children between the ages of 4 and 8 years should take in 0.6 mg per day. Children between the ages of 1 and 3 years should take in 0.5 mg per day, while infants between the ages of 6 and 12 months should take in 0.3 mg per day. From birth to six months, infants should take in 0.2 mg per day. There are no tolerable upper intake levels for vitamin B1.[3]

DEFICIENCY AND EXCESS

In the United States, almost 20 percent of the population over the age of two years is believed to be deficient in vitamin B1. In fact, if not for the enrichment of wheat flour, that figure would be much higher. People with certain medical problems, such as heart failure, gastrointestinal disease, diabetes, and/or a dependence on alcohol, have an increased risk for vitamin B1 deficiency. And because of a reduction in the ability to absorb vitamin B1, the elderly may be deficient. People who have had bariatric surgery to lose weight or are living with HIV/AIDS may easily be deficient. People who are deficient in other B vitamins, especially folic acid and vitamin B12, may have problems absorbing vitamin B1. People who eat a good deal of raw freshwater fish or shellfish may be at risk for deficiency. The raw fish contain chemicals the kill vitamin B1. (Cooking the fish destroys these chemicals.)

Medical concerns associated with vitamin B1 deficiency include loss of weight and appetite, headache, nausea, vomiting, fatigue, irritability, depression, abdominal discomfort, confusion, memory loss, muscle weakness, and heart problems. Severe vitamin B1 deficiency may result in diarrhea and the compromised absorption of other nutrients. Though rare in the United States, severe vitamin B1 deficiency may lead to an illness called beriberi, which causes tingling and numbness in the feet and hands, loss of muscle, and poor reflexes. A more common vitamin B1 deficiency illness in the United States is Wernicke-Korsakoff syndrome, which may affect people with alcoholism and other chronic health problems. It causes tingling and numbness in the hands and feet, severe memory loss, disorientation, and confusion.

There does not appear to be any toxicity associated with the excess consumption of vitamin B1; excess vitamin B1 is excreted in the urine.[4]

In a case report published in 2013 in the *American Journal of Emergency Medicine*, two physicians from Jerusalem commented that vitamin B1 deficiency is always considered when dealing with patients with chronic alcoholism. However, with other patients, "its recognition in developed countries is often poor and delayed." Medical providers may fail to connect the myriad of symptoms associated with vitamin B1 deficiency. "Timely treatment may be curative, whereas poor awareness of the multiple predisposing circumstances and the many guises of the syndrome . . . lead to the common delays in diagnosis."[5]

KEY RESEARCH FINDINGS

Vitamin B1 Supplementation May Be Useful for the Fatigue Associated with Inflammatory Bowel Diseases

In a pilot study published in 2013 in *The Journal of Alternative and Complementary Medicine*, researchers from Italy noted that people who live with inflammatory bowel diseases often experience fatigue. They wanted to learn if higher doses of vitamin B1 supplementation would be useful for this ongoing medical problem. The cohort consisted of 12 patients—8 with ulcerative colitis and 4 with Crohn's disease. Levels of fatigue were measured using a chronic fatigue syndrome scale, and blood tests measured levels of vitamin B1. Measurements were taken 20 days after the beginning of the therapy. Of the 12 subjects, 10 experienced "complete regression" of fatigue. The remaining two subjects "showed nearly complete regression of fatigue." The researchers commented that their findings "present a simple remedy for what is a significant, complex problem of fatigue in IBD patients."[6]

Vitamin B1 Deficiency May Play a Role in Heart Failure

In a meta-analysis published in 2015 in the *Journal of Cardiac Failure*, researchers from Florida noted that about 5.7 million Americans have been diagnosed with heart failure, a condition that may be associated with frequent hospitalization, poor quality of life, and a mortality of up to 50 percent. As a result, heart failure is a "major health care burden." Do inadequate amounts of vitamin B1 play a role in this serious health condition? The researchers conducted a review of nine relevant observational studies. They learned that vitamin B1 deficiency was more common in the subjects with heart failure than the controls. The researchers identified three potential explanations for this occurrence—diuretic use, changes in dietary habits, and altered vitamin B1 absorption and metabolism. While vitamin B1 supplementation did not improve mortality, most of the subjects with vitamin B1 deficiency treated with long-term supplementation had significant improvements in quality of life issues "as measured by appetite, energy, weight changes, and sleep pattern."[7]

Low Levels of Vitamin B1 May Be Associated with Cancer

In an exploratory study published in 2017 in the journal *Psycho-Oncology*, researchers from Canada and New York City wanted to learn more about the association between cancer and vitamin B1. Their cohort consisted of 217 patients with various types of cancer, who were admitted to the hospital between July 2013 and December 2014; a striking 55.3 percent were found to be deficient in vitamin B1. Of these, 49.8 percent did not receive treatment with vitamin B1; among those who did receive treatment, it was delayed in 59.6 percent of the cases. Generally, the oncologists did not initiate treatment with vitamin B1. "Given that patients were admitted to medical, surgical, intensive care, and neurology services," the researchers' findings "may have wide implications for many clinicians treating cancer patients." Vitamin B1 deficiency was seen even in subjects who had normal or greater than normal body weights, and in subjects who had adequate amounts of other vitamins in their blood. Vitamin B1 deficiency was "highly prevalent and clinically relevant among inpatients with a variety of cancer types and receiving a variety of cancer treatments."[8]

Vitamin B1 Supplementation May Be Useful for People Who Suffer from Migraine Headaches

In a brief report published in 2016 in the journal *Headache*, researchers from India described two female patients who suffered from chronic migraine headaches and a host of other symptoms, including nausea, vomiting, cognitive impairment, ocular abnormality, cerebellar dysfunction, weight loss, and anorexia. Their symptoms made it difficult for them to maintain proper nutrition; both women had a history of nutritional deficiencies and low levels of serum vitamin B1. For them, vitamin B1 supplementation appeared to be the solution. Vitamin B1 supplementation led to the improvement in severity and frequency of the headaches and the associated symptoms. "Breaking of this cycle by thiamine supplementation might be promising therapy in a subset of patients with chronic migraine."[9]

Older Adults Tend to Be Deficient in Vitamin B1

In a systematic review published in 2015 in the *British Journal of Nutrition*, researchers from the Netherlands noted that micronutrient deficiencies among community-dwelling elders may be associated with "functional decline, frailty, and difficulties with independent living." That is why it is important to know which micronutrients are more likely to be deficient in the elderly. The analysis consisted of 37 published studies that included more than 28,000 subjects. Fifty-seven percent of the subjects were female, and they lived in 20 different Western countries. In total, 20 nutrients were examined. The researchers determined that six of the nutrients were considered "possible public health concern." Vitamin B1 was among the six. In fact, more than 30 percent of the populations studied were at risk for inadequate intake of vitamin B1 from food alone. While a notable half of the males studied were at risk for inadequate intake of vitamin B1, women also had inadequate amounts. Low levels of vitamin B1 "were of concern for both men and women."[10]

In a study published a few years earlier, in 2011, in *The Journal of Nutrition, Health & Aging*, researchers from Italy examined the vitamin intakes of "successfully aging" elders over a period of 10 years. The cohort consisted of 78 "free-living and still well-functioning" subjects (34 males and 44 females) from the city of Padua, Italy. At baseline, they were all between the ages of 70 and 75 years. Data were collected at baseline and after 10 years by means of a modified validated dietary history. The researchers learned that 44 percent of the men and 60 percent of the women were vitamin B1 deficient when the study began. It soon became evident that people who appear to be healthy may still be seriously deficient in vitamin B1. According to the researchers, many elderly may require supplementation, "even in healthy individuals, to ensure an adequate micronutrient intake."[11]

Many Obese People Are Deficient in Vitamin B1

In an article published in 2015 in the journal *Advances in Nutrition*, researchers from Washington, DC, and Bethesda, Maryland, wanted to learn more about the relationship between vitamin B1 and obesity. According to these researchers, vitamin B1 deficiency has been found in 15.5 to 29 percent of obese people seeking bariatric surgery. Was obesity less a function of the consumption of excess amounts of nutrition and more a result of malnutrition? The researchers noted that people who are obese often consume a diet that is high in simple sugars and low in whole grains, legumes, and other whole foods that naturally contain vitamin B1. Meanwhile, the metabolism of food with larger amounts of sugar requires high amounts of vitamin B1. That may further deplete levels of vitamin B1. People who are obese may need far more than the recommended levels of vitamin B1. "Current RDAs for micronutrients apply to normal, healthy adults but may not meet the metabolic needs of overweight or obese adults. . . . Understanding the impact of obesity on micronutrient status is an important public health issue."[12]

Males Addicted to Alcohol May Benefit from Vitamin B1 Supplementation

In a pilot study published in 2015 in the journal *Drug and Alcohol Dependence*, researchers from Kansas City, Kansas, wanted to learn if men addicted to alcohol would benefit from high-dose vitamin B1 supplementation. Vitamin B1 deficiency is a common condition among people addicted to alcohol. In fact, 30 to 80 percent of inpatients admitted for alcohol treatment are deficient in vitamin B1. The cohort consisted of 85 adult men, with a mean age of 48.5 years. (They ranged in age from 21 to 59 years.) Seventy-one percent were African American, and 82 percent reported a family history of alcoholism among first-degree relatives and/or grandparents. They all met the criteria for current alcohol use disorder—they were actively abusing alcohol over the 30 days prior to entering the study. The men were randomly assigned to take a high-dose vitamin B1 supplement or a placebo for six months. The researchers measured mood, anxiety, and impulsive tendencies, as well as the men's drinking patterns at baseline and after six months. Based on the severity of their alcoholism, the 50 men who completed the study were divided into two groups. When compared to the controls, the men in the high-alcoholism severity group who took the supplementation experienced significant reductions in anxiety and phobia symptoms. In addition, after six months, above-normal levels of vitamin B1 in the blood were associated with reductions in depression among a subset of the treated men. "The results suggest that thiamine deficiency contributes significantly to psychiatric distress in severe alcoholism and supports a possible benefit of thiamine supplementation for the alleviation of acute and chronic thiamine deficiency and psychiatric symptomatology in alcoholism."[13]

Gastrointestinal Surgery for Cancer Increases the Risk of Severe Vitamin B1 Deficiency

In a study published in 2016 in the journal *Support Care Cancer*, researchers from Italy investigated the association between gastrointestinal surgery for cancer and the risk of severe vitamin B1 deficiency, such as a diagnosis of Wernicke's encephalopathy. (Wernicke's encephalopathy is a debilitating neuropsychiatric syndrome caused by profound vitamin B1 deficiency. Some common symptoms include mental status changes, ocular abnormalities, and ataxia.) The initial cohort consisted of 45 patients, who had a median hospital stay of 20 days. At discharge from the hospital, 4.4 percent of the patients had signs of Wernicke's encephalopathy. After six months, 21 patients were interviewed. Of these, 90.4 percent had signs of Wernicke's encephalopathy. None of the patients received vitamin B1 supplementation during hospitalization, and only five received this treatment after discharge, but in suboptimal doses. The researchers concluded that the majority of patients with Wernicke's encephalopathy do not receive adequate vitamin B1 treatment. That is why all people who have gastrointestinal surgery for cancer should be considered at risk for vitamin B1 deficiency and should take vitamin B1 supplementation. People who demonstrate symptoms of Wernicke's encephalopathy should be treated with high doses of vitamin B1. "Overtreatment is preferable in these patients, as side effects are rare and [the] consequences of misdiagnosis can be severe."[14]

Insufficient Vitamin B1 May Be Associated with Adiposity in Mexican American Children

In a study published in 2014 in *The Journal of Nutrition*, researchers from Australia and Switzerland examined the relationship between four vitamins, including vitamin B1, and obesity in Mexican American children. Obesity among Mexican American children has become a major public health concern. The cohort consisted of 1,131 Mexican American children between the ages of 8 and 15 years. Obtained from the National Health and Nutrition Examination Survey (2001–2004), the data were collected on the children's body mass index, trunk fat mass, and total body fat mass. Intake of vitamin B1 was measured via a 24-hour dietary recall. The researchers found an inverse association between levels of vitamin B1 and body mass index and trunk fat mass. Children with higher intakes of vitamin B1 were more likely to have a healthy body mass index and lower body trunk fat mass. Vitamin B1 status "may play a role in reducing adiposity and fat mass among children."[15]

NOTES

1. University of Maryland Medical Center. "Vitamin B1 (Thiamin)." December 30, 2017. http://www.umm.edu/health/medical/altmed/supplement/vitamin-b1-thiamine.

2. The George Mateljan Foundation. "Vitamin B1-Thiamin." December 30, 2017. http://whfoods.com/genpage.php?tname=nutrient&dbid=100.

3. Office of Dietary Supplements, National Institutes of Health. "Thiamin." December 30, 2017. https://ods.od.nih.gov/factsheets/Thiamin-Consumer/.

4. Ibid.

5. Schattner, Ami and Asaf Kedar. "An Unlikely Culprit—The Many Guises of Thiamine Deficiency." *American Journal of Emergency Medicine* 31 (2013): 635.e5–635.e6.

6. Costantini, Antonio, and Maria Immacolata Pala. "Thiamine and Fatigue in Inflammatory Bowel Diseases: An Open-Label Pilot Study." *The Journal of Alternative and Complementary Medicine* 19, no. 8 (2013): 704–708.

7. Jain, A., R. Mehta, M. Al-Ani, et al. "Determining the Role of Thiamine Deficiency in Systolic Heart Failure: A Meta-Analysis and Systematic Review." *Journal of Cardiac Failure* 21, no. 12 (December 2015): 1000–1007.

8. Isenberg-Grzeda, E., M. J. Shen, Y. Alici, et al. "High Rate of Thiamine Deficiency among Inpatients with Cancer Referred for Psychiatric Consultation: Results of a Single Site Prevalence Study." *Psycho-Oncology* 26, no. 9 (September 2017): 1384–1389.

9. Prakash, Sanjay, Ajai Kumar Singh, and Chaturbhuj Rathore. "Chronic Migraine Responding to Intravenous Thiamine: A Report of Two Cases." *Headache* 56, no. 7 (July 2016): 1204–1209.

10. ter Borg, Sovianne, Sjors Verlaan, Jaimie Hemsworth, et al. "Micronutrient Intakes and Potential Inadequacies of Community-Dwelling Older Adults: A Systematic Review." *British Journal of Nutrition* 113 (2015): 1195–1206.

11. Toffanello, E. D., E. M. Inelmen, N. Minicuci, et al. "Ten-Year Trends in Vitamin Intake in Free-Living Healthy Elderly People: The Risk of Subclinical Malnutrition." *The Journal of Nutrition, Health & Aging* 15, no. 2 (2011): 99–103.

12. Kerns, Jennifer C., Cherinne Arundel, and Lakhmir S. Chawla. "Thiamin Deficiency in People with Obesity." *Advances in Nutrition* 6 (March 2015): 147–153.

13. Manzardo, Ann M., Tiffany Pendleton, Albert Poje, et al. "Change in Psychiatric Symptomatology after Benfotiamine Treatment in Males Is Related to Lifetime Alcoholism Severity." *Drug and Alcohol Dependence* 152 (July 1, 2015): 257–263.

14. Restivo, Angelo, Mauro Giovanni Carta, Anna Maria Giulia Farci, et al. "Risk of Thiamine Deficiency and Wernicke's Encephalopathy after Gastrointestinal Surgery for Cancer." *Support Care Cancer* 24, no. 1 (January 2016): 77–82.

15. Gunanti, Inong R., Geoffrey C. Marks, Abdullah Al-Mamun, and Kurt Z. Long. "Low Serum Vitamin B-12 and Folate Concentrations and Low Thiamin and Riboflavin Intakes Are Inversely Associated with Greater Adiposity in Mexican American Children." *The Journal of Nutrition* 144, no. 12 (December 2014): 2027–2033.

REFERENCES AND FURTHER READINGS

Costantini, Antonio and Maria Immacolata Pala. "Thiamine and Fatigue in Inflammatory Bowel Diseases: An Open-Panel Pilot Study." *The Journal of Alternative and Complementary Medicine* 19, no. 8 (2013): 704–708.

The George Mateljan Foundation. "Vitamin B1-Thiamin." December 30, 2017. http://whfoods.com/genpage.php?tname=nutrient&dbid=100.

Gunanti, Inong R., Geoffrey C. Marks, Abdullah Al-Mamun, and Kurt Z. Long. "Low Serum Vitamin B-12 and Folate Concentrations and Low Thiamin and Riboflavin Intakes Are Inversely Associated with Greater Adiposity in Mexican American Children." *The Journal of Nutrition* 144, no. 12 (December 2014): 2027–2033.

Isenberg-Grzeda, E., M. J. Shen, Y. Alici, et al. "High Rate of Thiamine Deficiency among Inpatients with Cancer Referred for Psychiatric Consultation: Results of a Single Site Prevalence Study." *Psycho-Oncology* 26, no. 9 (September 2017): 1384–1389.

Jain, A., R. Mehta, M. Al-Ani, et al. "Determining the Role of Thiamine Deficiency in Systolic Heart Failure: A Meta-Analysis and Systematic Review." *Journal of Cardiac Failure* 21, no. 12 (December 2015): 1000–1007.

Kerns, Jennifer C., Cherinne Arundel, and Lakhmir S. Chawla. "Thiamin Deficiency in People with Obesity." *Advances in Nutrition* 6 (March 2015): 147–153.

Manzardo, Ann M., Tiffany Pendleton, Albert Poje, et al. "Change in Psychiatric Symptomatology after Benfotiamine Treatment in Males Is Related to Lifetime Alcoholism Severity." *Drug and Alcohol Dependence* 152 (July 1, 2015): 257–263.

Office of Dietary Supplements, National Institutes of Health. "Thiamin." December 30, 2017. https://ods.od.nih.gov/factsheets/Thiamin-Consumer/.

Prakash, Sanjay, Ajai Kumar Singh, and Chaturbhuj Rathore. "Chronic Migraine Responding to Intravenous Thiamine: A Report of Two Cases." *Headache* 56, no. 7 (July 2016): 1204–1209.

Restivo, Angelo, Mauro Giovanni Carta, Anna Maria Giulia Farci, et al. "Risk of Thiamine Deficiency and Wernicke's Encephalopathy after Gastrointestinal Surgery for Cancer." *Support Care Cancer* 24, no. 1 (January 2016): 77–82.

Schattner, Ami and Asaf Kedar. "An Unlikely Culprit—The Many Guises of Thiamine Deficiency." *American Journal of Emergency Medicine* 31 (2013): 635.e5–635.e6.

ter Borg, Sovianne, Sjors Verlaan, Jaimie Hemsworth, et al. "Micronutrient Intakes and Potential Inadequacies of Community-Dwelling Older Adults: A Systematic Review." *British Journal of Nutrition* 113 (2015): 1195–1206.

Toffanello, E. D., E. M. Inelmen, N. Minicuci, et al. "Ten-Year Trends in Vitamin Intake in Free-Living Healthy Elderly People: The Risk of Subclinical Malnutrition." *The Journal of Nutrition, Health & Aging* 15, no. 2 (2011): 99–103.

University of Maryland Medical Center. "Vitamin B1 (Thiamin)." December 30, 2017. http://www.umm.edu/health/medical/altmed/supplement/vitamin-b1-thiamine.

Vitamin B2 (Riboflavin)

Also known as riboflavin, vitamin B2 is water soluble, which means that it is not stored in the body. It is important to consume vitamin B2 every day. Like the other B vitamins, vitamin B2 helps the body convert carbohydrates into glucose, which the body uses to produce energy. It is an integral component of energy metabolism.

Vitamin B2 also functions as an antioxidant, fighting free radicals, which damage cells and DNA. Why is this important? Free radicals support the aging process and contribute to the development of health conditions such as heart disease and cancer. Vitamin B2 is important for growth and the production of red blood cells.

Vitamin B2 is the only vitamin that people can actually see passing through their bodies. People who consume lots of vitamin B2 or take vitamin B2 supplements tend to have bright yellow urine. The *flavin* in riboflavin comes from the Latin word *flavus*, which means yellow.

The potency of vitamin B2 is diminished by exposure to light. Thus, when vitamin B2 in milk, cheese, yogurt, and other dairy products is placed in lighted areas, the strength of the vitamin may be compromised. When possible, it is best to purchase these dairy products in opaque containers.[1]

FOOD SOURCES AND SUPPLEMENTS

Excellent sources of vitamin B2 include spinach, beet greens, crimini mushrooms, asparagus, and sea vegetables. Very good sources of vitamin B2 include eggs, cow's milk, collard greens, broccoli, Swiss chard, green beans, shiitake mushrooms, bok choy, turnip greens, kale, mustard greens, and bell peppers. Many foods are good sources of vitamin B2. These include soybeans, tempeh, yogurt, almonds, turkey, green peas, sweet potatoes, sardines, tuna, summer and winter squash, Brussels sprouts, grapes, cabbage, carrots, romaine lettuce, celery, chili peppers, and miso.[2]

Vitamin B2 is found in multivitamins, B-complex dietary supplements, and supplements with only vitamin B2. Some vitamin B2 supplements contain very high doses, but the body is unable to absorb more than about 27 mg at any one time.

INTAKE RECOMMENDATIONS

The Office of Dietary Supplements of the National Institutes of Health cites the following recommendations for vitamin B2. Breastfeeding teens and women should take in 1.6 mg per day, while pregnant teens and women should take in 1.4 mg per day. Adult women should take in 1.1 mg per day, while adult men should take in 1.3 mg per day. Teen females between the ages of 14 and 18 years should take in 1 mg per day, while teen males between the ages of 14 and 18 should take in 1.3 mg per day. Children between the ages of 9 and 13 years should take in

0.9 mg per day, while children between the ages of 4 and 8 years should take in 0.6 mg per day. Children between the ages of one and three years should take in 0.5 mg per day. Infants between the ages of 7 and 12 months should take in 0.4 mg per day, while infants from birth to six months should take in 0.3 mg per day.[3] There are no tolerable upper intake levels for vitamin B2.

DEFICIENCY AND EXCESS

Most healthy people who eat a well-balanced diet obtain sufficient amounts of vitamin B2. However, older people and those who consume large amounts of alcohol may need to take supplementation. Also at increased risk are people who are vegan, pregnant and breastfeeding women, people who do not eat dairy foods, and people with a genetic disorder that causes vitamin B2 deficiency, such as Infantile Brown-Vialetto-Van Laere syndrome. Symptoms of vitamin B2 deficiency include fatigue; slowed growth; digestive problems; cracks and sores around the corners of the mouth (angular cheilitis); cracked lips; dry skin; mouth ulcers; red lips; eye fatigue; hair loss; liver disorders; reproductive problems; nervous system problems; scrotal dermatitis; fluid in mucous membranes; iron-deficiency anemia; swelling and soreness in the throat; sensitivity to light; itchy, watery, and/or bloodshot eyes; and swollen magenta-colored tongue. Severe long-term vitamin B2 deficiency causes a shortage of red blood cells and the clouding of the lens in the eyes (cataracts).

There is no evidence that the intake of excess amounts of vitamin B2 is harmful. Extremely high doses have been associated with itching, numbness, and sensitivity to light.

KEY RESEARCH FINDINGS

Vitamin B2 May Be Useful for Some People Who Suffer from Migraines

In a randomized, double-blind, multicenter study published in 2015 in *The Journal of Headache and Pain*, researchers from Germany wanted to determine if a supplement containing vitamin B2, magnesium, and coenzyme Q10 would be useful for the symptoms associated with migraines, such as throbbing headaches, nausea, and a hypersensitivity to sounds and light. While acute attacks are usually treated with analgesics or triptans, only a minority of migraine sufferers take medication or supplements to attempt to prevent attacks. Would the supplement, known as Migravent® in Germany or Dolovent® in the United States, be useful for this painful, debilitating disorder? The researchers recruited 130 adults between the ages of 18 and 65 years who had three or more migraines per month. They were divided into two groups—one group took the supplement for three months and the other group took a placebo for the same period of time. The subjects in both groups experienced reductions in migraine days per month.

The subjects in the treatment group, who previously averaged 6.2 days of migraines per month, dropped to 4.4 days per month. Though not statistically significant, the reduction was considered "clinically relevant." The subjects in the placebo group went from 6.2 days to 5.2 days per month. The subjects in the treatment group also had significant reductions in migraine pain. Moreover, "patients rated the efficacy of the treatment significantly superior to placebo."[4]

In a study published a few years earlier, in 2009, in *The Journal of Headache and Pain*, researchers from Bologna, Italy, reported on their experiences using vitamin B2 supplementation for migraine prevention in 41 pediatric and adolescent patients (16 males and 25 females). Their mean age was 13 years, 7 months. All the patients kept journals to record the number and intensity of the migraine attacks, type of symptoms, and the degree of efficacy of the symptomatic medication. The patients took 200 or 400 mg per day of oral vitamin B2 for three, four, or six months. During follow-up, the researchers learned that 68.4 percent of the patients had a 50 percent or greater reduction in the frequency of attacks and 21 percent reduction in intensity. The researchers determined that vitamin B2 supplementation significantly reduced the frequency and intensity of migraines. The vitamin B2 supplementation was well-tolerated, and the compliance rate was "excellent." In addition, vitamin B2 "is devoid of adverse effects, so it is easy to recommend its use as a therapeutic option to parents of younger patients, who often had reservations about pharmacological therapy."[5]

Another study on the topic was published in 2010 in the journal *Cephalalgia*. The researchers from the Netherlands assembled a cohort that included 42 children between the ages of 6 and 13 years who suffered from migraines. Of these, 14 children also suffered from tension-type headaches. Following a 4-week baseline period, all the children received a placebo for 16 weeks and then vitamin B2 for 16 weeks or vice versa, with a 4-week washout period in-between. Parents kept a detailed headache diary during all stages of the study, which documented the date and severity of every headache. Though the researchers did not observe any significant differences between the frequency of migraine attacks during the last month of treatment, there was a significant difference in the reduction of frequency of tension-type headaches during the same time period. According to the researchers, there is some evidence that vitamin B2 "may have a prophylactic effect on interval headaches that may correspond to mild migraine or tension-type headaches attacks in children with migraine."[6]

Vitamin B2 Deficiency May Be More Common Than Many People Realize

In a study published in 2015 in the journal *Nutrients*, researchers from Korea wanted to learn more about the prevalence of vitamin B2 deficiency among adults in the Seoul metropolitan area. The researchers collected three consecutive 24-hour food recalls from 412 healthy adults (145 men and 267 women) between the ages of 20 and 64 years, with a mean age of 38.8 years. Urine samples were obtained from 149 subjects, and the researchers calculated the dietary and total vitamin B2 intakes. The 10 top major dietary sources of vitamin B2 consumed by the subjects were whole eggs, citrus fruit, whole milk, Korean instant noodles, Kimchi, pork loin, mackerel, spinach, chicken, and pork belly. Cereal was the only vitamin B2–fortified food that the subjects consumed. The researchers found that 28 percent of the subjects consumed less than the recommended amounts of vitamin B2. And one-third of the subjects had "inadequate riboflavin status." As a result, the consumption of foods high in vitamin B2 among this population "should be encouraged."[7]

Vitamin B2 May or May Not Play a Role in the Prevention of Colorectal Cancer

In a study published in 2013 in the *American Journal of Clinical Nutrition*, researchers from Germany and multiple locations in the United States examined the association between four different B vitamins, including vitamin B2, and the incidence of colorectal cancer. The cohort consisted of 88,045 postmenopausal women who were part of the Women's Health Initiative Observational Study. More than 1,000 cases of colorectal cancer were diagnosed. The researchers learned that the total intake of vitamin B2, from diet and supplements, was associated with a significant reduction in the risk of colorectal cancer. The researchers commented that suboptimal vitamin B2 status leads to the accumulation of homocysteine, a metabolite that has been strongly linked to colorectal cancer. The researchers emphasized that a major strength of their study was the large sample size "that allowed subgroup analysis."[8]

On the other hand, in a study published in 2016 in the *International Journal of Cancer*, researchers from several locations in the United States found a different association between vitamin B2 and colorectal cancer. They used data obtained from the Nurses' Health Study and the Health Professionals Follow-Up Study. Among the 100,033 in the Nurses' Health Study and the 44,007 men in the Health Professionals Follow-Up Study, there were a total of 3,037 incident cases of colorectal cancer during 24 to 26 years of follow-up. Dietary intakes were assessed using a food frequency questionnaire. The researchers were unable to find a significant association between intake of vitamin B2 and risk of colorectal cancer. The researchers commented that the cohort studies had relatively high intakes of vitamin B2. It is possible that the high intakes "masked the effect of dietary vitamin B2 intake on CRC [colorectal cancer] risk." Obviously, there is the need for additional studies on this topic.[9]

Young Adults with Attention Deficit Hyperactivity Disorder (ADHD) May Well Have Low Levels of Vitamin B2

In a study published in 2016 in the psychiatry journal *BJPsych Open*, researchers from Norway noted that people who have attention-deficit attention disorder, a neurodevelopmental disorder characterized by hyperactivity, impulsivity and inattention, sometimes experience improvements when they consume micronutrient vitamins. However, data on vitamin levels in people with ADHD tend to be "sparse." The researchers analyzed the serum levels of eight vitamins, including vitamin B2, in 133 people with ADHD and 131 controls. All of the participants were between the ages of 18 and 40 years; males represented 46.6 percent of the people with ADHD and 42.7 percent of the control group. The researchers determined that the concentrations of vitamin B2 were significantly lower in the ADHD subjects, and lower levels of vitamin B2 were significantly associated with high ADHD symptom scores. And the researchers suggested that "it may be hypothesized that vitamin deficiency could contribute to ADHD symptoms." Likewise, the "identification and correction of low vitamin levels could be beneficial in treatment of ADHD."[10]

Inadequate Vitamin B2 Intake Is Associated with Anemia

In a prospective study published in 2014 in the online journal *PLoS ONE*, researchers from China and Australia wanted to learn more about the association between vitamin B2 and anemia. The researchers used data from 1,253 men and women who participated in two waves of the Jiangsu Nutrition Study, five years apart, in 2002 and 2007. The data contained information on vitamin B2 intake, hemoglobin, dietary patterns, lifestyle factors, and sociodemographic and health-related factors. At baseline, a striking 97.2 percent of the participants had inadequate intake of vitamin B2, which, in turn, was positively associated with an increased risk for persistent anemia. Among those subjects who were anemic at baseline, low vitamin B2 intake was associated with increased risk of anemia at follow-up. According to the researchers, animal studies have found that vitamin B2 increases the absorption of iron. The researchers commented that "correcting riboflavin deficiency may therefore be one of the components in the prevention of anemia."[11]

There May or May Not Be an Association between Vitamin B2 and Risk of Breast Cancer

In a systematic review and meta-analysis published in 2017 in the journal *Archives of Gynecology and Obstetrics*, researchers from China noted that studies on the relationship between dietary vitamin B2 and risk of breast cancer have produced inconsistent results. Why is that important? The researchers noted that the cause of many cases of breast cancer "is still obscure," and many people believe that dietary factors may play a role. If dietary factors are found to cause breast cancer, then the diet may be modified. That is why the researchers conducted a review of 10 studies that included a total of 12,268 breast cancer patients who ranged in age from 20 to 80 years. The five case-control studies and five cohort studies were published between 1996 and 2015. Overall, the researchers learned that dietary vitamin B2 intake "could weakly reduce the risk of breast cancer." Before firm conclusions may be made, more studies need to be completed and published. Still, the researchers commented that their findings "indicated that dietary vitamin B2 intake could slightly decrease breast cancer risk."[12]

In a study published in 2013 in the journal *Cancer Causes & Control*, researchers from Australia examined the association between several B vitamins, including vitamin B2, an amino acid (methionine), and the risk of breast cancer. The cohort consisted of 20,756 women from the Melbourne Collaborative Cohort Study, who were followed for an average of 16 years. During that time, 936 incident cases of breast cancer were identified. The mean age at diagnosis was 64 years. Dietary intakes were estimated with a 121-item food frequency questionnaire. The researchers found only "weak" evidence for an inverse association between intake of vitamin B2 and breast cancer. There was "suggestive evidence of a weak inverse association between riboflavin intake and breast cancer risk."[13]

Children and Teens with Type 1 Diabetes May Benefit from More Nutritious Foods, Including Foods with Vitamin B2

In a study published in 2015 in the *Asian Pacific Journal of Clinical Nutrition*, researchers from India underscored the importance of proper nutrition in children and teens with type 1 diabetes. Because of the limitations placed on their diets, these children and teens are "likely to become deficient in certain nutrients." As a result, the researchers decided to investigate the possible dietary nutritional deficiencies of Indian children and teens with type 1 diabetes. The cohort consisted of 24 males and 46 females, who had a mean age of 10.6 years. Dietary food intakes were assessed by 24-hour recalls on three random and nonconsecutive days of a week. The researchers even recorded the recipes of food items. As expected, the children and teens were deficient in a number of nutrients. In fact, the mean intake of vitamin B2 was less than 50 percent of the recommended amount. The researchers recommended the inclusion of foods with enhanced micronutrients, and they provided a number of newly developed recipes.[14]

Low Intake of B Vitamins, Including Vitamin B2, May Be Associated with Adolescent Psychiatric and Behavior Problems

In a study published in 2012 in the journal *Preventive Medicine*, researchers from Australia noted that about 20 percent of Western populations have mental health problems, and about half of these originate during the adolescent years. Diet plays a key role in "modulating psychological wellbeing," and the B vitamins, including vitamin B2, are essential "for the synthesis of neurotransmitters such as serotonin." Data were obtained from the West Australian Pregnancy Cohort Study, which compiled statistics on food frequency consumption and intake of the various B vitamins for 17 years. Mental health issues were assessed using the Youth Self Report, which measures withdrawn/depressed and aggressive/

delinquent behaviors. There were more than 700 participants in the analysis. The researchers found an association between a lower intake of several B vitamins, including vitamin B2, and aggressive and delinquent behaviors. "The rapidly developing young brain may be more susceptible to nutrient insufficiency." Moreover, people who develop these problems during adolescence have higher rates of offending and substance abuse later in life. "Diet is modifiable and it is plausible that certain foods or vitamin supplements may ensure optimal biochemical performance and improve mood and mental functioning, particularly where biochemical deficiencies exist."[15]

Like Other B Vitamins, Vitamin B2 Appears to Reduce Incident Premenstrual Syndrome

In a study published in 2011 in the *American Journal of Clinical Nutrition*, researchers from Massachusetts and Iowa wanted to learn more about the association between intake of B vitamins, including vitamin B2, from food and supplements and the initial development of premenstrual syndrome. The researchers used data from the Nurses' Health Study II cohort. In 1991, all of the participants did not have premenstrual syndrome. After 10 years of follow-up, 1,057 women were confirmed as cases and 1,968 were confirmed as controls. Using food frequency questionnaires, dietary information was collected in 1991, 1995, and 1999; the researchers determined that intake of dietary vitamin B2 was inversely associated with incident premenstrual syndrome. When compared to the women with the lowest intake of vitamin B2, women who had the highest dietary intake of vitamin B2 during the two to four years before they developed symptoms of premenstrual syndrome had a 35 percent lower risk of having the medical problem. And it does not require huge amounts of food to have a high intake of vitamin B2. "This level of intake can be achieved with 1–2 servings of fortified cereal per day or 6–7 servings of riboflavin-rich foods such as cow milk or soy milk, spinach, and red meats." Foods that many people eat everyday contain effective amounts of vitamin B2.[16]

NOTES

1. The George Mateljan Foundation. "Vitamin B2-Riboflavin." December 30, 2017. http://whfoods.com/genpage.php?tname=nutrient&dbid=93.

2. Ibid.

3. Office of Dietary Supplements, National Institutes of Health. "Riboflavin." December 30, 2017. https://ods.od.nih.gov/factsheets/Riboflavin-Consumer/.

4. Gaul, Charly, Hans-Christoph Diener, Ulrich Danesch, and On Behalf of the Migravent® Study Group. "Improvement of Migraine Symptoms with a Proprietary Supplement Containing Riboflavin, Magnesium and Q10: A Randomized, Placebo-Controlled, Double-Blind, Multicenter Trial." *The Journal of Headache and Pain* 16 (2015): 32+.

5. Condò, Maria, Annio Posar, Annalisa Arbizzani, and Antonia Parmeggiani. "Riboflavin Prophylaxis in Pediatric and Adolescent Migraine." *The Journal of Headache and Pain* 10 (2009): 361–365.

6. Bruijn, Jacques, Hugo Duivenvoorden, Jan Passchier, et al. "Medium-Dose Riboflavin as a Prophylactic agent in Children with Migraine: A Preliminary Placebo-Controlled, Randomised, Double-Blind, Cross-Over Trial." *Cephalalgia* 30, no. 12 (2010): 1426–1434.

7. Choi, Ji Young, Young-Nam Kim, and Young-OK Cho. "Evaluation of Riboflavin Intakes and Status of 20–64-Year-Old Adults in South Korea." *Nutrients* 7, no. 1 (2015): 253–264.

8. Zschäbitz, S., T.Y. Cheng, M.L. Neuhouser, et al. "B Vitamin Intakes and Incidence of Colorectal Cancer: Results from the Women's Health Initiative Observational Study Cohort." *American Journal of Clinical Nutrition* 97, no. 2 (February 2013): 332–343.

9. Yoon, Yeong Sook, Seungyoun Jung, Xuehong Zhang, et al. "Vitamin B2 Intake and Colorectal Cancer Risk: Results from the Nurses' Health Study and the Health Professionals Follow-Up Study Cohort." *International Journal of Cancer* 139, no. 5 (September 1, 2016): 996–1008.

10. Landaas, E.T., T.I. Aarsland, A. Ulvik, et al. "Vitamin Levels in Adults with ADHD." *BJPsych Open* 2, no. 6 (November 2016): 377–384.

11. Shi, Zumin, Shiqi Zhen, Gary A. Wittert, et al. "Inadequate Riboflavin Intake and Anemia Risk in a Chinese Population: Five-Year Follow Up of the Jiangsu Nutrition Study." *PLoS ONE* 9, no. 2 (February 2014): e88862.

12. Yu, Lanting, Yuyan Tan, and Lin Zhu. "Dietary Vitamin B2 Intake and Breast Cancer Risk: A Systematic Review and Meta-Analysis." *Archives of Gynecology and Obstetrics* 295, no. 3 (2017): 721–729.

13. Bassett, J.K., L. Baglietto, A.M. Hodge, et al. "Dietary Intake of B Vitamins and Methionine and Breast Cancer Risk." *Cancer Causes & Control* 24, no. 8 (August 2013): 1555–1563.

14. Parthasarathy, Lavanya S., Shashi A. Chiplonkar, Anuradha V. Khadilkar, and Vaman V. Khadilkar. "Dietary Modifications to Improve Micronutrient Status of Indian Children and Adolescents with Type 1 Diabetes." *Asian Pacific Journal of Clinical Nutrition* 24, no. 1 (2015): 73–82.

15. Herbison, Carly E., Siobhan Hickling, Karina L. Allen, et al. "Low Intake of B-Vitamins Is Associated with Poor Adolescent Mental Health and Behaviour." *Preventive Medicine* 55 (2012): 634–638.

16. Chocano-Bedoya, P.O., J.E. Manson, S.E. Hankinson, et al. "Dietary B Vitamin Intake and Incident Premenstrual Syndrome." *American Journal of Clinical Nutrition* 93, no. 5 (May 2011): 1080–1086.

REFERENCES AND FURTHER READINGS

Bassett, J.K., L. Baglietto, A.M. Hodge, et al. "Dietary Intake of B Vitamins and Methionine and Breast Cancer Risk." *Cancer Causes & Control* 24, no. 8 (August 2013): 1555–1563.

Bruijn, Jacques, Hugo Duivenvoorden, Jan Passchier, et al. "Medium-Dose Riboflavin as a Prophylactic Agent in Children with Migraine: A Preliminary Placebo-Controlled, Randomised, Double-Blind, Cross-Over Trial." *Cephalalgia* 30, no. 12 (2010): 1426–1434.

Chocano-Bedoya, P.O., J.E. Manson, S.E. Hankinson, et al. "Dietary B Vitamin Intake and Incident Premenstrual Syndrome." *American Journal of Clinical Nutrition* 93, no. 5 (May 2011): 1080–1086.

Choi, Ji Young, Young-Nam Kim, and Young-OK Cho. "Evaluation of Riboflavin Intakes and Status of 20–64-Year-Old Adults in South Korea." *Nutrients* 7, no. 1 (2015): 253–264.

Condò, Maria, Annio Posar, Annalisa Arbizzani, and Antonia Parmeggiani. "Riboflavin Prophylaxis in Pediatric and Adolescent Medicine." *The Journal of Headache and Pain* 10 (2009): 361–365.

Gaul, Charly, Hans-Christoph Diener, Ulrich Danesch, and on Behalf of the Migravent® Study Group. "Improvement of Migraine Symptoms with a Proprietary Supplement Containing Riboflavin, Magnesium and Q10: A Randomized, Placebo-Controlled, Double-Blind, Multicenter Trial." *The Journal of Headache and Pain* 16 (2015): 32+.

The George Mateljan Foundation. "Vitamin B2-Riboflavin." December 30, 2017. http://whfoods.com/genpage.php?tname=nutrient&dbid=93.

Herbison, Carly E., Siobhan Hickling, Karina L. Allen, et al. "Low Intake of B-Vitamins Is Associated with Poor Adolescent Mental Health and Behaviour." *Preventive Medicine* 55 (2012): 634–638.

Landaas, E. T., T. I. Aarsland, A. Ulvik, et al. "Vitamin Levels in Adults with ADHD." *BJPsych Open* 2, no. 6 (November 2016): 377–384.

Office of Dietary Supplements, National Institutes of Health. "Riboflavin." December 30, 2017. https://ods.od.nih.gov/factsheets/Riboflavin-Consumer/.

Parthasarathy, Lavanya S., Shashi A. Chiplonkar, Anuradha V. Khadilkar, and Vaman V. Khadilkar. "Dietary Modifications to Improve Micronutrient Status of Indian Children and Adolescents with Type 1 Diabetes." *Asian Pacific Journal of Clinical Nutrition* 24, no. 1 (2015): 73–82.

Shi, Zumin, Shiqi Zhen, Gary A. Wittert, et al. "Inadequate Riboflavin Intake and Anemia Risk in a Chinese Population: Five-Year Follow Up of the Jiangsu Nutrition Study." *PLoS ONE* 9, no. 2 (February 2014): e88862.

Yoon, Yeong Sook, Seungyoun Jung, Xuehong Zhang, et al. "Vitamin B2 Intake and Colorectal Cancer Risk: Results from the Nurses' Health Study and the Health Professionals Follow-Up Study Cohort." *International Journal of Cancer* 139, no. 5 (September 1, 2016): 996–1008.

Yu, Lanting, Yuyan Tan, and Lin Zhu. "Dietary Vitamin B2 Intake and Breast Cancer Risk: A Systematic Review and Meta-Analysis." *Archives of Gynecology and Obstetrics* 295, no. 3 (2017): 721–729.

Zschäbitz, S., T. Y. Cheng, M. L. Neuhouser, et al. "B Vitamin Intakes and Incidence of Colorectal Cancer: Results from the Women's Health Initiative Observational Study Cohort." *American Journal of Clinical Nutrition* 97, no. 2 (February 2013): 332–343.

Vitamin B3 (Niacin)

There are two main forms of vitamin B3—niacin (nicotinic acid) and niacinamide (nicotinamide). For most everyday purposes, these water-soluble vitamins are very similar and tend to be used interchangeably, as they will be in this entry. The human body is able to convert niacin into niacinamide, and it is able to make niacinamide from tryptophan, an amino acid found in animal foods. Medical professionals sometimes note that there are a few differences between niacin and niacinamide. Higher doses of niacin widen blood vessels, resulting in skin flushing; this does not occur with niacinamide. On the other hand, niacin is considered useful for elevated levels of cholesterol; niacinamide is not believed to be effective for this medical problem. Both niacin and niacinamide are thought to help psychiatric disorders such as depression and anxiety as well as cognitive problems, memory loss, motion sickness, edema, acne, attention deficit hyperactivity disorder, premenstrual headache, digestive problems, toxins and pollutants, elevated blood pressure, niacin deficiency and related conditions, and cataracts.

Niacin plays an important role in the production of energy. Two types of niacin, nicotinamide adenine dinucleotide (NAD) and nicotinamide adenine dinucleotide phosphate (NADP), are essential components in the conversion of dietary proteins, fats, and carbohydrates to usable energy. NAD and NADP also stop free radicals and protect the body against tissue damage. Niacin is required to synthesize starch that is stored in muscles and the liver, enabling the starch to become an energy source.

FOOD SOURCES AND SUPPLEMENTS

Tuna, chicken, turkey, and crimini mushrooms are excellent sources of niacin. Very good sources of niacin include salmon, lamb, beef, asparagus, tomatoes, and bell peppers. Many foods are considered a good source of niacin. Among these are shrimp, cod, brown rice, barley, green peas, potatoes, corn, carrots, cantaloupe, summer and winter squash, spinach, broccoli, bok choy, eggplant, cabbage, and shiitake mushrooms. Niacin and niacinamide are both sold as tablets and capsules. To reduce the risk of flushing, niacin is also sold in a slow release form. Many multivitamins contain niacin.

INTAKE RECOMMENDATIONS

The Food and Nutrition Board at the Institute of Medicine has developed dietary reference intakes for vitamin B3 for adults and children and adequate intake levels for infants. Females 14 years and older should take in 14 mg per day. But females 14 years and older should take in 18 mg per day during pregnancy and 17 mg per day during lactation. Males 14 years and older should take in 16 mg per day. Children between the ages of 9 and 13 years should take in 12 mg per day, while children between the ages of 4 and 8 years should take in 8 mg per day. Children between the ages of one and three years should take in 6 mg per day. The adequate intake for infants between the ages of 7 and 12 months is 4 mg per day, while the adequate intake for infants from birth to 6 months is 2 mg per day.[1]

DEFICIENCY AND EXCESS

Since vitamin B3 is found in so many common foods, the body's needs may be easily met through diet. Today, true vitamin B3 deficiency is rare in the developed world. In the United States, the primary cause of vitamin B3 deficiency is alcoholism. The symptoms of vitamin B3 deficiency include indigestion, fatigue, canker sores, vomiting, poor circulation, depression, burning in the mouth, and a bright red tongue. Severe vitamin B3 deficiency is the cause of a condition known as pellagra. Symptoms of pellagra include cracked, scaly skin, diarrhea, and dementia. It is treated with a nutritionally balanced diet and niacin supplementation.

While it is thought to be almost impossible to obtain too much vitamin B3 from food, excessive amounts of the vitamin may be obtained from supplementation, especially with the very high doses available by prescription. Side effects associated with very high doses include nausea, jaundice, and elevated liver enzymes. In addition, very high-dose vitamin B3 may cause liver damage and stomach ulcers.

KEY RESEARCH FINDINGS

Niacinamide Appears to Be Useful for the Prevention of Nonmelanoma Skin Cancers

In a phase 3, double-blind, randomized, controlled trial published in 2015 in the *New England Journal of Medicine*, researchers from several locations in Sydney, Australia, noted that nonmelanoma skin cancers, such as basal-cell carcinoma and squamous-cell carcinoma, are common types of cancer that are primarily caused by ultraviolet radiation. They wondered if vitamin B3 supplementation would offer a degree of protection against these cancers. The cohort consisted of 386 participants, 18 years or older, who had at least two histologically confirmed nonmelanoma skin cancers during the previous five years. For 12 months, the subjects took either 500 mg of niacinamide twice each day or a placebo. During an 18-month period, every 3 months, the subjects were evaluated by dermatologists. The researchers found that after 12 months, the rate of new nonmelanoma skins cancers was 23 percent lower in the subjects taking supplementation. This finding was statistically significant. The supplementation appeared to be most useful for the subjects who had the highest number of skin cancers. Moreover, people taking the supplementation had 11 percent fewer actinic keratoses or rough, scaly patches of skin that have the potential to develop into skin cancer. But after the supplement was discontinued, the effect was not maintained. The researchers concluded that niacinamide "is widely accessible as an inexpensive over-the-counter vitamin supplement and presents a new opportunity for the chemoprevention of nonmelanoma skin cancers that is readily translatable into clinical practice."[2]

Niacin May Help Prevent Vascular Disease in People with Metabolic Syndrome

In a study published in 2016 in the journal *Pharmacology Research & Perspectives*, researchers from various locations in Ontario, Canada, tested the ability of niacin supplementation to improve vascular functioning in mice bred to have metabolic syndrome. The researchers divided five-week-old mice into two main groups. One group of mice was fed a Western diet containing 42 percent of calories from animal fat; the goal was to have these mice experience the symptoms of metabolic syndrome. The second group of mice, the control group, was maintained on a chow diet with 14 percent of calories from fat. After 15 weeks on these diets, the mice were anesthetized, and the researchers made incisions in their femoral arteries. For the next 14 days, the mice in the treatment group received daily injections of low-dose niacin. The treatment mice experienced improvements in the use of their hind limbs, enhanced revascularization, and decreases in inflammation. The researchers commented that their findings "may have implications for the use of low dose niacin in the treatment of peripheral ischemic vascular disease in the setting of obesity and metabolic syndrome."[3]

Dietary Niacin Appears to Improve Vascular Health

In a study published in 2014 in the *Journal of Applied Physiology*, researchers from Boulder, Colorado, wanted to learn more about the association between the intake of dietary niacin and vascular health. The cohort consisted of 127 healthy subjects between the ages of 48 and 77 years. The subjects participated in a variety of clinical tests; dietary niacin intake was estimated from food frequency questionnaires. Among the evaluations completed were tests for vascular endothelial functioning and oxidative stress. The researchers determined that the subjects with above-average intakes of dietary niacin had better results on several different vascular tests than those with below-average intakes of dietary niacin. And they commented that their findings "support the hypothesis that higher dietary niacin intake is associated with greater vascular endothelial function related to lower systemic and vascular oxidative stress among healthy middle-aged and older adults."[4]

Niacin Seems to Be Useful for the Prevention of Cardiovascular Disease

In a meta-analysis published in 2013 in the *Journal of the American College of Cardiology*, researchers from Boston, Massachusetts, wanted to assess the ability of niacin to reduce cardiovascular disease. The researchers identified 11 relevant niacin trials, published in English-language literature between January 1966 and December 2011, that included a total of 9,959 subjects. The eligible studies were randomized and controlled, reporting clinical cardiovascular disease data with a minimum of six months follow-up. The researchers found strong evidence in the efficacy of niacin as an agent to reduce the risk of cardiovascular disease. And they concluded that "taking in aggregate the cumulative body of relevant empirical clinical data . . . continues to support that niacin is an effective agent to reduce CVD [cardiovascular disease] risk."[5]

Slow-Release Niacin Effectively Lowers Levels of Cholesterol

In a study published in 2013 in the *Journal of Clinical Lipidology*, a researcher from the University of Minnesota compared the use of three different products—extended-release niacin, inositol hexanicotinate (a compound that contains niacin and inositol), and a placebo—on people with mild to moderate levels of elevated cholesterol. The cohort consisted of 120 subjects between the ages of 18 and 75 years; each of the three test groups had 40 randomly placed subjects. No subject was on any medication or supplement that altered cholesterol levels. After an initial four-week diet lean-in period, the subjects took one of the supplements for six weeks. The subjects in all three groups had good medication compliance. At the end of the trial, the subjects taking the extended-release niacin had significant improvements in total cholesterol, low-density lipoprotein, and high-density lipoprotein. Even the six subjects who took reduced doses saw improvements and "good lipid results." There were no significant improvements in the subjects taking inositol hexanicotinate or the placebo. The researchers noted that their findings should enable clinicians to make more informed recommendations to their patients. Only the extended-release niacin was "an effective niacin delivery agent."[6]

Low Levels of Niacin May Play a Role in Depression

In a study published in 2016 in the journal *Clinical Nutrition Research*, researchers from Korea compared the nutritional status of adult Korean women who were not depressed to adult Korean women who were depressed. Among the nutrients examined was niacin. The cohort consisted of 2,236 women between the ages of 19 and 64 years, who participated in the 2013 Korea National Health and Nutrition Examination Survey. There were 315 women in the depressed group and 1,921 in the not-depressed group. The women in the depressed group, who were between the ages of 19 and 29 years, had a lower intake of certain nutrients, including niacin. In addition, the women in the depressed group, who were between the ages of 50 and 64 years, had a lower niacin "nutritional quality." It was very evident to the researchers that depressed women had poorer nutritional health, and that included a less-than-desirable intake of niacin.[7]

In Some Patients, Niacin Supplementation May Improve the Symptoms of Schizophrenia

In an article published in 2015 in the *European Review for Medical and Pharmacological Sciences*, researchers from China noted that it is well known that niacin deficiencies may have "psychiatric manifestations." And it is also known that niacin has been used successfully to treat schizophrenia. The researchers wanted to further examine the topic and uncover more information. They presented studies showing dramatic improvements following niacin supplementation. For example, in one study, 75 percent of the treatment group achieved a 10-year cure rate compared to 37 percent of a control group. In another study, 31 people with acute schizophrenia were randomized to receive niacin, niacinamide, or a placebo for 30 days. After one year, the treated subjects had an 80 percent recovery rate versus 33 percent for the placebo group. In still another study, there were 39 subjects in the treatment group and 43 in the placebo group. After 33 days, 79.5 percent of the niacin subjects improved compared to 41.9 percent in the placebo group. The researchers concluded that niacin deficiency appears to be an important contributor to the development of at least some cases of schizophrenia. "Studies and sparse case reports indicate that niacin augmentation could help a subset of patients suffering from schizophrenia."[8]

Still, Some People Should Probably Avoid Niacin

In a study published in 2014 in the *New England Journal of Medicine*, researchers based in the United Kingdom examined the use of niacin with laropiprant, another cholesterol-reducing medication, in people with vascular disease. The initial cohort consisted of 25,673 adults, with a mean age of 64.9 years, who had been diagnosed with atherosclerotic vascular disease—cerebrovascular disease, peripheral artery disease, myocardial infarction, or diabetes mellitus with evidence of symptomatic coronary disease. The subjects, who were 82.7 percent men, were randomly assigned to take 2 g of extended-release niacin and 40 mg of laropiprant or a matching placebo once each day. During a median follow-up of 3.9 years, the researchers learned that the treatment did not reduce the risk of heart attack or stroke in people with vascular disease. Of even more concern was the fact that the treatment appeared to have some dangerous side effects, including a potential increased risk of death. Other side effects included a 55 percent increase in the loss of blood sugar control among people with diabetes and a 32 percent increase in new diabetes diagnoses. People also experienced excess bleeding and infections, diarrhea, gout, and skin and liver problems. And though the treatment seemed to trigger modest improvements in the levels of "good" HDL cholesterol, it did not appear to benefit cardiovascular health. According to the researchers, "Although niacin might still be relevant for particular patient groups (e.g., patients at high risk for vascular events who have high levels of LDL cholesterol), any potential benefits should be considered in the context of the observed hazards."[9]

Two years later, in 2016, the journal *Circulation: Cardiovascular Quality and Outcomes* published another study of this same cohort. This time, a few of the UK researchers on the previous study wanted to learn more about the effect the extended-release niacin and laropiprant had on quality-of-life issues and healthcare costs. No one should be surprised that the researchers determined that the incidences of strokes, heart failure, musculoskeletal events, gastrointestinal problems, and infections associated with taking the niacin and laropiprant supplement significantly decreased the quality of life during the effective time period and subsequent years. Moreover, all of the serious medical events were associated with high hospital costs. The subjects on the treatment had worse health and higher health-care costs than those on the placebo.[10] It is evident that people who are already dealing with a cardiovascular problem should use niacin with extreme care and caution.

NOTES

1. Medlineplus. "Niacin." December 30, 2017. https://medlineplus.gov/druginfo/natural/924.html.

2. Chen, Andrew C., Andrew J. Martin, Bonita Choy, et al. "A Phase 3 Randomized Trial of Nicotinamide for Skin-Cancer Chemoprevention." *New England Journal of Medicine* 373, no. 17 (October 22, 2015): 1618–1626.

3. Pang, Dominic K. T., Zengxuan Nong, Brian G. Sutherland, et al. "Niacin Promotes Revascularization and Recovery of Limb Function in Diet-Induced Obese Mice with Peripheral Ischemia." *Pharmacology Research & Perspectives* 4, no. 3 (2016): e00233.

4. Kaplon, Rachelle E., Lindsey B. Gano, and Douglas R. Seals. "Vascular Endothelial Function and Oxidative Stress Are Related to Dietary Niacin Intake among Healthy Middle-Aged and Older Adults." *Journal of Applied Physiology* 116, no. 2 (January 15, 2014): 156–163.

5. Lavigne, Paul M. and Richard H. Karas. "The Current State of Niacin in Cardiovascular Disease Prevention: A Systematic Review and Meta-Regression." *Journal of the American College of Cardiology* 61, no. 4 (2013): 440–446.

6. Keenan, Joseph M. "Wax-Matrix Extended-Release Niacin vs Inositol Hexanicotinate: A Comparison of Wax-Matrix, Extended-Release Niacin to Inositol Hexanicotinate 'No-Flush' Niacin in Persons with Mild to Moderate Dyslipidemia." *Journal of Clinical Lipidology* 7, no. 1 (January–February 2013): 14–23.

7. Won, Myeong Suk, Sunghee Kim, and Yoon Jung Yang. "Comparison of Health Status and Nutrient Intake between Depressed Women and Non-Depressed Women: Based on the 2013 Korea National Health and Nutrition Examination Survey." *Clinical Nutrition Research* 5, no. 2 (April 2016): 112–125.

8. Xu, X. J. and G. S. Jiang. "Niacin-Respondent Subset of Schizophrenia—A Therapeutic Review." *European Review for Medical and Pharmacological Sciences* 19, no. 6 (2015): 988–997.

9. HPS2-THRIVE Collaborative Group, Landray, M. J., R. Haynes, J. C. Hopewell, et al. "Effects of Extended-Release Niacin with Laropiprant in High-Risk Patients." *New England Journal of Medicine* 371, no. 3 (July 17, 2014): 203–212.

10. Kent, Seamus, Richard Haynes, Jemma C. Hopewell, et al. "Effects of Vascular and Nonvascular Adverse Events and of Extended-Release Niacin with Laropiprant on Health and Healthcare Costs." *Circulation: Cardiovascular Quality and Outcomes* 9, no. 4 (July 2016): 348–354.

REFERENCES AND FURTHER READINGS

Chen, Andrew C., Andrew J. Martin, Bonita Choy, et al. "A Phase 3 Randomized Trial of Nicotinamide for Skin-Cancer Chemoprevention." *New England Journal of Medicine* 373, no. 17 (October 22, 2015): 1618–1626.

HPS2-THRIVE Collaborative Group, Landray, M.J., R. Haynes, J.C. Hopewell, et al. "Effects of Extended-Release Niacin with Laropiprant in High-Risk Patients." *New England Journal of Medicine* 371, no. 3 (July 17, 2014): 203–212.

Kaplon, Rachelle E., Lindsey B. Gano, and Douglas R. Seals. "Vascular Endothelial Function and Oxidative Stress Are Related to Dietary Niacin Intake among Healthy Middle-Aged and Older Adults." *Journal of Applied Physiology* 116, no. 2 (January 15, 2014): 156–163.

Keenan, Joseph M. "Wax-Matrix Extended-Release Niacin vs Inositol Hexanicotinate: A Comparison of Wax-Matrix, Extended-Release Niacin to Inositol Hexanicotinate 'No-Flush' Niacin in Persons with Mild to Moderate Dyslipidemia." *Journal of Clinical Lipidology* 7, no. 1 (January–February 2013): 14–23.

Kent, Seamus, Richard Haynes, Jemma C. Hopewell, et al. "Effects of Vascular and Nonvascular Adverse Events and of Extended-Release Niacin with Laropiprant on Health and Healthcare Costs." *Circulation: Cardiovascular Quality and Outcomes* 9, no. 4 (July 2016): 348–354.

Lavigne, Paul M. and Richard H. Karas. "The Current State of Niacin in Cardiovascular Disease Prevention: A Systematic Review and Meta-Regression." *Journal of the American College of Cardiology* 61, no. 4 (2013): 440–446.

Medlineplus. "Niacin." December 30, 2017. https://medlineplus.gov/druginfo/natural/924.html.

Pang, Dominic K.T., Zengxuan Nong, Brian G. Sutherland, et al. "Niacin Promotes Revascularization and Recovery of Limb Function in Diet-Induced Obese Mice with Peripheral Ischemia." *Pharmacology Research & Perspectives* 4, no. 3 (2016): e00233.

Won, Myeong Suk, Sunghee Kim, and Yoon Jung Yang. "Comparison of Health Status and Nutrient Intake between Depressed Women and Non-Depressed Women: Based on the 2013 Korea National Health and Nutrition Examination Survey." *Clinical Nutrition Research* 5, no. 2 (April 2016): 112–125.

Xu, X.J. and G.S. Jiang. "Niacin-Respondent Subset of Schizophrenia—A Therapeutic Review." *European Review for Medical and Pharmacological Sciences* 19, no. 6 (2015): 988–997.

Vitamin B5 (Pantothenic Acid)

Also known as pantothenic acid, vitamin B5 enables people to transfer fats, carbohydrates, and proteins into sources of energy. The body needs vitamin B5 to make hormones and red blood cells, and vitamin B5 supports the body's immune system and helps the nervous system function properly. The digestive tract requires vitamin B5 to function, and vitamin B5 strengthens other vitamins, especially vitamin B2. Like the other B vitamins, vitamin B5 is water soluble; it is not stored in the body.

While the actual amount of vitamin B5 varies from food to food, vitamin B5 is found in almost all foods. The name pantothenic references that fact. The Greek word *pantothen* means "on all sides" or "from all quarters," and the Greek work *pantos* means "everywhere."[1]

Vitamin B5 is more stable than some of the other B vitamins, even during the cooking process. Still, over time, it does degrade.

FOOD SOURCES AND SUPPLEMENTS

Excellent sources of vitamin B5 include shiitake and crimini mushrooms and cauliflower. Very good sources of vitamin B5 include sweet potatoes, broccoli, beet greens, asparagus, turnip greens, bell peppers, cucumbers, and celery. Good sources of vitamin B5 include avocado, lentils, dried peas, chicken, turkey, yogurt, salmon, rye, beef, eggs, potatoes, wheat, corn, shrimp, papaya, winter and summer squash, cow's milk, cod, collard greens, raspberries, Brussels sprouts, grapefruit, pineapple, watermelon, carrots, oranges, cranberries, Swiss chard, spinach, cabbage, mustard greens, tomatoes, sea vegetables, figs, romaine lettuce, and bok choy.[2] Vitamin B5 is found in multivitamins, B-complex dietary supplements, and supplements with only vitamin B5.

INTAKE RECOMMENDATIONS

The National Academy of Sciences has established adequate intake amounts for vitamin B5. Lactating women should take in 7 mg per day, while pregnant women should take in 6 mg per day. Males and females 14 years and older should take in 5 mg per day, while children between the ages of 9 and 13 years should take in 4 mg per day. Children between the ages of four and eight years should take in 3 mg per day, while children between the ages of one and three years should take in 2 mg per day. Infants between the ages of six months and one year should take in 1.8 mg per day, while newborns until six months should take in 1.7 mg per day. The National Academy of Sciences did not establish a tolerable upper intake level for the vitamin.[3]

DEFICIENCY AND EXCESS

Because vitamin B5 is found in so many foods, true deficiency is thought to be rare. But slight deficiencies do occur, especially among children, teens, women who are pregnant, and the elderly.[4] Symptoms of vitamin B5 deficiency include fatigue, insomnia, depression, irritability, vomiting, stomach pains, burning feet, and upper respiratory infections. In all probability, true vitamin B5 toxicity may be created only in a laboratory setting. "In research settings, use of supplemental pantothenic acid at daily doses more than 1000 times the Adequate Intake (AI) of 5 mg did not lead to any discernible side effects."[5]

KEY RESEARCH FINDING

Pantethine, a Derivative of Vitamin B5, Appears to Support Cardiovascular Health

In a study published in 2014 in the journal *Vascular Health and Risk Management*, researchers from Canada, Japan, New York City, and Allentown, Pennsylvania, noted that high serum concentrations of low-density lipoprotein (LDL) is a major risk factor for coronary heart disease. While there are a number of prescription medications that are useful in lowering LDL levels, they tend to have side effects. That is why the researchers wanted to determine if pantethine, a derivative of vitamin B5, would be useful in lowering LDL levels in people at low to moderate risk of cardiovascular disease. The researchers recruited 32 people to participate in a triple-blinded, placebo-controlled trial. The participants were instructed how to follow a Therapeutic Lifestyle Change diet, or a diet that would help lower levels of cholesterol, which they began four weeks before the trial started. Then, the participants were randomly assigned to take pantethine 600 mg per day from weeks 1 to 8 and 900 mg per day from weeks 9 to 16 or a placebo. Twenty-four participants completed the entire trial. The researchers determined that pantethine significantly lowered levels of LDL at 8 and 16 weeks. In fact, LDL levels were lowered by 11 percent. This was in contrast to the participants on the placebo, who had 3 percent increases in their LDL levels. The researchers also found that pantethine significantly lowered total cholesterol levels at 16 weeks. "Supplementation with pantethine may therefore be considered as an optional adjunctive therapy for patients with low to moderate CVD [cardiovascular disease] risk."[6]

Vitamin B5 May Be Useful for Mild to Moderate Facial Acne

In a randomized, double-blind, placebo-controlled study published in 2014 in the journal *Dermatology and Therapy*, researchers from New York City wanted to learn if the daily oral intake of vitamin B5 would be useful for men and women with facial acne lesions. The study was conducted from August 2012 to November 2013, and the initial cohort consisted of 51 adults who had facial acne. For 12 weeks, the participants took a daily pantothenic acid–based dietary supplement or a placebo, which did not contain any active ingredients. The researchers evaluated the study based on findings from 41 participants. They found that the participants taking the supplement had a statistically significant decrease in the number of total facial lesions. After 12 weeks, the subjects taking the supplement experienced a more than 67 percent reduction in the number of total facial lesions. The researchers concluded that "the administration of a pantothenic-based dietary supplement in healthy human adults with facial lesions is safe, well-tolerated and reduces total facial lesion count."[7]

Another study examined the use of a topical cream that contains 4 percent D-panthenol (an alcohol analogue of vitamin B5), hydrogen peroxide, and salicylic acid. In this study, which was published in 2016 in the *European Review for Medical and Pharmacological Sciences*, researchers from Rome, Italy, treated 30 patients with mild to moderate acne from April to November 2012 with this cream. Evaluations of the 15 males and 15 females were made after 30 and 60 days of treatment. The researchers found that the cream resulted in statistically significant reductions in acne. There were only infrequent side effects, such as dryness and abnormal redness. The cream with vitamin B5 had "a good skin tolerability and efficacy in reducing acne lesions."[8]

Postmenopausal Women May Be Taking in Too Little Vitamin B5

In a study published in 2014 in the *Journal of Diabetes & Metabolic Disorders*, researchers from Iran wanted to learn more about the energy and nutrient intake of postmenopausal women. A cohort of 30 postmenopausal women, with a mean age of 55 years, were followed for one year. Dietary assessments were made by three-day food records that were collected during each season. Among the assessments were intakes of vitamins, including vitamin B5. The researchers determined that the mean daily intake of vitamin B5 was significantly lower than the Recommended Dietary Allowance. And it remained low in all the seasons. However, the researchers commented that the study was limited by the "small sample size."[9]

Teens with Eating Disorders Have a High Risk of Nutritional Deficiencies, Including Vitamin B5 Deficiency

In a study published in 2014 in the journal *Public Health Nutrition*, researchers from Spain wanted to learn more about the nutritional status of adolescents who have eating disorders. In addition, they hoped to determine what happened to the nutritional status if the illness worsened. Vitamin B5 was among the nutritional components they examined. The cohort consisted of 495 teens with a mean age of 14.2 years; there were 120 males and 375 females. The researchers used the Eating Attitudes Test and structured interviews to identify the teens at risk for eating disorders. Dietary intake was quantified using 24-hour recalls over a three-day period of time. The researchers learned that the female teens had more severe levels of illness, and they had lower intakes of nutrients, including vitamin B5. According to the researchers, the "risk of micronutrient deficiency becomes evident as soon as the first symptoms [of the eating disorder] appear and may be sufficiently severe to interfere in the optimum development of the adolescent."[10]

There Appears to Be an Association between Vitamin B5 and Depressive Symptoms

In a study published in 2016 in the *International Journal of Environmental Research and Public Health*, researchers from Spain investigated the association between several nutrients, including vitamin B5, and depressive symptoms in children. During the 2013–2014 academic year, 710 children (372 girls and 338 boys) between the ages of six and nine years were randomly selected from 11 primary schools in Valencia, Spain. Three-day food records detailed the children's dietary intake, and depressive symptoms were detected using the 20-item Center for Epidemiologic Studies Depression Scale for Children. Almost 21 percent of the children were found to have depressive symptoms. Children with more depressive symptoms had lower levels of several nutrients, including vitamin B5, and this association was statistically significant. The researchers commented that "nutrition possibly plays a decisive role in the onset of depression, and in its severity and duration." And they concluded that "nutritional inadequacy plays an important role in mental health and poor nutrition, and may contribute to the pathogenesis of depression."[11]

Puerto Rican Children Appear to Take in Too Little Vitamin B5

In a study published online in 2016 in the *International Journal for Vitamin and Nutrition Research*, researchers from Puerto Rico and Worcester, Massachusetts, wanted to learn more about the micronutrient intake of children in Puerto Rico. Their cohort consisted of 732 children, who were all 12 years old. The subjects were enrolled in an oral health study in which they completed 24-hour dietary recalls and multivitamin and multi-mineral assessments. The mean intake of several vitamins, including vitamin B5, was below the recommended Daily Reference Intakes. When compared to the girls, the boys had a significantly higher level of vitamin B5 intake. This is probably "related to the overall higher dietary intake among boys in this age range." As might be expected, the children who took multivitamin and multi-mineral supplements had significantly higher intakes of vitamin B5. Still, only "a very small proportion" of the children in this cohort actually took these supplements. The researchers concluded that "public health measures to improve micronutrient intake among children in Puerto Rico are needed."[12]

Topical Vitamin B5 Has Wound-Healing Properties

In a study published in 2016 in the *International Wound Journal*, researchers from Turkey wanted to learn more about the wound-healing properties of dexpanthenol, the stable alcohol analogue of vitamin B5. The researchers divided 30 albino rats into three groups of 10 and made linear incisions on the backs of all of the rats. The first group of 10 rats received no treatment; they served as controls. The second group of rats was treated with 5 percent dexpanthenol cream. And the third group of rats was treated with 5 percent nebivolol cream, a wound-healing product. The creams were applied so that they covered the entire wound area. The researchers measured how all of the wounds healed. After 21 days, the wounds were excised and histologically evaluated. The researchers determined that the wounds treated with both products healed at essentially the same rate; there was no statistical difference in their healing rates. Both creams healed the wounds faster than the control group. The researchers concluded that "dexpanthenol has been shown to improve wound healing and is widely used for various types of wounds."[13]

Vitamin B5 Appears to Help Moisturize the Skin

In a study published in 2011 in the *Journal of Cosmetic Science*, researchers from Brazil evaluated the skin moisturizing properties of formulations containing varying amounts of vitamin B5 (panthenol) or no vitamin B5. The cohort consisted of 40 healthy females between the ages of 20 and 35 years. They were told not to apply any topical products on the test sites—their arms—for two weeks before and during the study. The researchers tested formulations containing 0.5, 1.0, and 5.0 percent panthenol as well as no panthenol. Another group of 20 volunteers did not receive any formulation; they served as controls. All of the subjects were exposed to the same conditions and methods of evaluating water loss and skin moisture. The researchers found that the 1.0 and 5.0 percent formulations produced significant decreases in water loss. "This study emphasized the importance of adequate panthenol concentrations required in effective formulations for skin protection."[14]

The Topical Application of Vitamin B5 May Cause Dermatitis or Skin Inflammation

In a case report published in 2013 in the journal *Contact Dermatitis*, researchers from the United Kingdom described an 11-year-old girl who had a history of two episodes of facial eczema, which developed one day after the application of makeup that was removed with "hypoallergenic" facial wipes. The researchers were able to determine that the panthenol in the wipes triggered the reaction. They explained that panthenol is commonly used in hair preparations, wipes, cosmetic makeup, cleansers, and nail polish. They cautioned people to realize that "what has been used to remove make-up can be as important as what may have been originally applied."[15]

In another case report published in 2016 in *Contact Dermatitis*, researchers from Denmark described a reaction to the use of panthenol for aftercare treatment of a new tattoo. The researchers explained that tattooing "involves overcoming the skin barrier in order to deposit pigment intradermally, thus mechanically damaging the skin." Since it is believed that tattoo aftercare may reduce the incidence of complications, such treatment may be recommended. The researchers noted that the 40-year-old woman used a panthenol cream on the tattoo on her lower right arm. There was an intense reddening in the area around the tattoo, and the researchers concluded that the woman's skin reacted to the cream. The cream was discontinued, and the area was treated with topical corticosteroids. "The patient was advised to avoid panthenol in the future."[16]

Rats That Exercise and Eat a Higher-Fat Diet Need More Vitamin B5. This May Also Be True for Humans

In a study published in 2015 in the *Journal of Nutritional Science and Vitaminology*, researchers from Japan wanted to learn more about the association between vitamin B5, exercise, and regular and high-fat diets. The researchers fed rats a vitamin B5–sufficient diet or a vitamin B5–restricted diet that contained a regular amount of fat (5%) or an excessive amount of fat (20%). In addition, for 22 days, the rats were forced to swim until exhaustion every other day in a running water pool. The amount of vitamin B5 in the rats was determined by evaluated urinary excretions. While the excretion of vitamin B5 was not altered in the rats on a normal diet, the excretion of vitamin B5 in the rats on the high-fat diet was decreased. The researchers concluded that rats on a high-fat diet that exercised may require more vitamin B5. The findings suggested that the intake of vitamin B5 "should be increased in the presence of exercise or a high-fat diet, and especially when these conditions are combined."[17]

NOTES

1. The George Mateljan Foundation. "Pantothenic Acid." December 30, 2017. http://whfoods.com/genpage.php?tname=nutrient&dbid=87.

2. Ibid.

3. Ibid.

4. Kelly, Gregory S. "Pantothenic Acid." *Alternative Medicine Review* 16, no. 3 (2011): 263–274.

5. The George Mateljan Foundation. "Pantothenic Acid." December 30, 2017. http://whfoods.com/genpage.php?tname=nutrient&dbid=87.

6. Evans, Malkanthi, John A. Rumberger, Isao Azumano, et al. "Pantethine, a Derivative of Vitamin B5, Favorably Alters Total, LDL, and Non-HDL Cholesterol in Low to Moderate Cardiovascular Risk Subjects Eligible for Statin Therapy: A Triple-Blinded Placebo and Diet-Controlled Investigation." *Vascular Health and Risk Management* 10 (2014): 89–100.

7. Yang, Michael, Betsy Moclair, Virgil Hatcher, et al. "A Randomized, Double-Blind, Placebo-Controlled Study of a Novel Pantothenic Acid-Based Dietary Supplement in Subjects with Mild to Moderate Facial Acne." *Dermatology and Therapy* 4, no. 1 (June 2014): 93–101.

8. Ricci, F., F. Masini, B. Fossati, et al. "Combination Therapy with Hydrogen Peroxide (4%), Salicylic Acid (0.5%) and D-Panthenol (4%): Efficacy and Skin Tolerability

in Common *Acne Vulgaris* during Sun Exposure Period." *European Review for Medical and Pharmacological Sciences* 20, no. 2 (2016): 232–236.

9. Mansour, Asieh, Zeinab Ahadi, Mostafa Qorbani, and Saeed Hosseini. "Association between Dietary Intake and Seasonal Variations in Postmenopausal Women." *Journal of Diabetes & Metabolic Disorders* 13 (2014): 52+.

10. Aparicio, Estefania, Josefa Canals, Susana Pérez, and Victoria Arija. "Dietary Intake and Nutritional Risk in Mediterranean Adolescents in Relation to the Severity of the Eating Disorder." *Public Health Nutrition* 18, no. 8 (2014): 1461–1473.

11. Rubio-López, Nuria, María Morales-Suárez-Varela, Yolanda Pico, et al. "Nutrient Intake and Depressive Symptoms in Spanish Children: The ANIVA Study." *International Journal of Environmental Research and Public Health* 13, no. 3 (2016): 352+.

12. Lopez-Cepero, A., R. Torres, A. Elias, et al. "Micronutrient Intake among Children in Puerto Rico: Dietary and Multivitamin-Multimineral Supplement Sources." *International Journal for Vitamin and Nutrition Research*. Online, July 20, 2016.

13. Ulger, Burak V., Murat Kapan, Omer Uslukaya, et al. "Comparing the Effects of Nebivolol and Dexpanthenol on Wound Healing: An Experimental Study." *International Wound Journal* 13, no. 3 (June 2016): 367–371.

14. Camargo, F.B., Jr., L.R. Gaspar, and P.M.B.G. Maia Campos. "Skin Moisturizing Effects of Panthenol-Based Formulations." *Journal of Cosmetic Science* 62, no. 4 (July–August 2011): 361–369.

15. Chin, Mei Fong, Thomas M. Hughes, and Natalie M. Stone. "Allergic Contact Dermatitis Caused by Panthenol in a Child." *Contact Dermatitis* 69, no. 5 (November 2013): 321–322.

16. Bregnbak, David, Jeanne D. Johansen, and Claus Zachariae. "Contact Dermatitis Caused by Panthenol Used for Aftercare Treatment of a New Tattoo." *Contact Dermatitis* 75, no. 1 (July 2016): 50–52.

17. Takahashi, K., T. Fukuwatari, and K. Shibata. "Exercise and a High Fat Diet Synergistically Increase the Pantothenic Acid Requirement in Rats." *Journal of Nutritional Science and Vitaminology* 61, no. 3 (2015): 215–221.

REFERENCES AND FURTHER READINGS

Aparicio, Estefania, Josefa Canals, Susana Pérez, and Victoria Arija. "Dietary Intake and Nutritional Risk in Mediterranean Adolescents in Relation to the Severity of the Eating Disorder." *Public Health Nutrition* 18, no. 8 (2014): 1461–1473.

Bregnbak, David, Jeanne D. Johansen, and Claus Zachariae. "Contact Dermatitis Caused by Panthenol Used for Aftercare Treatment of a New Tattoo." *Contact Dermatitis* 75, no. 1 (July 2016): 50–52.

Camargo, F.B., Jr., L.R. Gaspar, and P.M.B.G. Maia Campos. "Skin Moisturizing Effects of Panthenol-Based Formulations." *Journal of Cosmetic Science* 62, no. 4 (July–August 2011): 361–369.

Chin, Mei Fong, Thomas M. Hughes, and Natalie M. Stone. "Allergic Contact Dermatitis Caused by Panthenol in a Child." *Contact Dermatitis* 69, no. 5 (November 2013): 321–322.

Evans, Malkanthi, John A. Rumberger, Isao Azumano, et al. "Pantethine, a Derivative of Vitamin B5, Favorably Alters Total, LDL, and Non-HDL Cholesterol in Low to Moderate Cardiovascular Risk Subjects Eligible for Statin Therapy: A Triple-Blinded Placebo and Diet-Controlled Investigation." *Vascular Health and Risk Management* 10 (2014): 89–100.

The George Mateljan Foundation. "Pantothenic Acid." December 30, 2017. http://whfoods.com/genpage.php?tname=nutrient&dbid=87.

Kelly, Gregory S. "Pantothenic Acid." *Alternative Medicine Review* 16, no. 3 (2011): 263–274.

Lopez-Cepero, A., R. Torres, A. Elias, et al. "Micronutrient Intake among Children in Puerto Rico: Dietary and Multivitamin-Multimineral Supplement Sources." *International Journal for Vitamin and Nutrition Research.* Online, July 20, 2016.

Mansour, Asieh, Zeinab Ahadi, Mostafa Qorbani, and Saeed Hosseini. "Association between Dietary Intake and Seasonal Variations in Postmenopausal Women." *Journal of Diabetes & Metabolic Disorders* 13 (2014): 52+.

Ricci, F., F. Masini, B. Fossati, et al. "Combination Therapy with Hydrogen Peroxide (4%), Salicylic Acid (0.5%), and D-Panthenol (4%): Efficacy and Skin Tolerability in Common *Acne Vulgaris* during Sun Exposure Period." *European Review for Medical and Pharmacological Sciences* 20, no. 2 (2016): 232–236.

Rubio-López, Nuria, María Morales-Suárez-Varela, Yolanda Pico, et al. "Nutrient Intake and Depressive Symptoms in Spanish Children: The ANIVA Study." *International Journal of Environmental Research and Public Health* 13, no. 3 (2016): 352+.

Takahashi, K., T. Fukuwatari, and K. Shibata. "Exercise and a High Fat Diet Synergistically Increase the Pantothenic Acid Requirement in Rats." *Journal of Nutritional Science and Vitaminology* 61, no. 3 (2015): 215–221.

Ulger, Burak V., Murat Kapan, Omer Uslukaya, et al. "Comparing the Effects of Nebivolol and Dexpanthenol on Wound Healing: An Experimental Study." *International Wound Journal* 13, no. 3 (June 2016): 367–371.

University of Maryland Medical Center. "Vitamin B5 (Pantothenic Acid)." December 30, 2017. http://www.umm.edu/health/medical/altmed/supplement/vitamin-b5-pantothenic-acid.

Yang, Michael, Betsy Moclair, Virgil Hatcher, et al. "A Randomized, Double-Blind, Placebo-Controlled Study of a Novel Pantothenic Acid-Based Dietary Supplement in Subjects with Mild to Moderate Facial Acne." *Dermatology and Therapy* 4, no. 1 (June 2014): 93–101.

Vitamin B6 (Pyridoxine)

Also known as pyridoxine, vitamin B6 helps the body convert food into fuel, which is needed to produce energy. Like other B vitamins, vitamin B6 is needed to metabolize fats and proteins and to have healthy skin, hair, eyes, and liver.

Vitamin B6 is integral to the proper functioning of the nervous system. The body requires vitamin B6 to carry signals from nerve cell to nerve cell, and it needs the vitamin for normal brain development and functioning. The body uses vitamin B6 to make certain hormones, such as serotonin and norepinephrine, which influence mood.

Working with vitamins B12 and B9 (folate), vitamin B6 controls levels of homocysteine in the blood. Homocysteine is an amino acid that has been associated with heart disease. In addition, the body uses vitamin B6 to absorb vitamin B12 and to make red blood cells and support the immune system.[1]

FOOD SOURCES AND SUPPLEMENTS

Excellent sources of vitamin B6 include tuna, spinach, cabbage, bok choy, bell peppers, turnip greens, garlic, and cauliflower. Very good sources of vitamin B6 include turkey, beef, chicken, salmon, sweet potatoes, potatoes, banana, winter and summer squash, broccoli, Brussels sprouts, collard greens, beet greens, kale, carrots, Swiss chard, asparagus, mustard greens, tomatoes, leeks, and chili peppers. Good sources of vitamin B6 include sunflower seeds, pinto beans, avocados, lentils, green peas, lima beans, onions, shrimp, pineapple, cod, shiitake and crimini mushrooms, cantaloupe, corn, beets, eggplant, green beans, celery, strawberries, watermelon, romaine lettuce, figs, and sea vegetables.[2] Vitamin B6 is usually contained in a multivitamin, and it may also be purchased in a B-complex vitamin or as a single supplement. It may be sold under several names, including pyridoxal, pyridoxamine, pyridoxine hydrochloride, and pyridoxal-5-phosphate.

INTAKE RECOMMENDATIONS

The National Academy of Sciences has established Recommended Dietary Allowances for vitamin B6 by age and gender. The recommendations for infants under one year are adequate intake standards. Lactating women should take in 2 mg per day, while pregnant women should take in 1.9 mg per day. Males 50 years and older should take in 1.7 mg per day, while females 50 years and older should take in 1.5 mg per day. Males and females between the ages of 19 and 50 years and males between the ages of 14 and 18 years should take in 1.3 mg per day, while females between the ages of 14 and 18 years should take in 1.2 mg per day. Children between the ages of 9 and 13 years should take in 1 mg per day, while children between the ages of 4 and 8 years should take in 0.6 mg per day. Children between the ages of one and three years should take in 0.5 mg per day. Infants between the ages of 6 and 12 months should take in 0.3 mg per day, while infants between birth and 6 months should take in 0.1 mg per day. The tolerable upper limit for vitamin B6 is set at 100 mg per day. Very high intake levels may be achieved only with supplementation.[3]

DEFICIENCY AND EXCESS

True serious vitamin B6 deficiency is believed to be rare. But mild vitamin B6 deficiency is thought to be more common, especially in children and the elderly. There are certain people who are at increased risk for vitamin B6 deficiency. People with autoimmune diseases, people with kidney problems, and people with alcohol dependence are all at increased risk, as are women on oral contraceptive pills. Some medications, such as steroids, antibiotics, and drugs for Parkinson's disease, may lower levels of vitamin B6. Diets very high in protein, which are sometimes used to lose weight, deplete levels of vitamin B6. Symptoms of serious deficiency include muscle weakness, nervousness, irritability, anemia, itchy rashes, scaly skin on the lips, cracks in the corners of the mouth, depression, difficulty concentrating, and short-term memory loss.

Taking very high doses of vitamin B6, such as more than 200 mg per day, may result in neurological problems, such as the loss of feeling in the legs and imbalance. There are rare reports of allergic reactions to high doses. Other side effects of excessive intake of vitamin B6 include sunlight sensitivity, headache, nausea, abdominal pain, and loss of appetite.

KEY RESEARCH FINDINGS

Higher Intake of Vitamin B6 Appears to Be Associated with a Lower Risk for Depression

In a study published in 2016 in the *European Journal of Clinical Nutrition*, researchers from Québec, Canada, examined the association between intake of vitamin B6, folate, and vitamin B12 and depression among generally healthy, community-dwelling older men and women. The cohort consisted of 1,368 men and women who participated in the Québec Longitudinal Study on Nutrition and Aging (NuAge). Slightly more than half of the participants were women, and they ranged in age from 67 to 84 years, with an average age of 74 years. At baseline, everyone was free of depression. Scores were obtained using a 30-item Geriatric Depression Scale. During a three-year follow-up, the researchers identified 170 participants (12.5%) who were depressed. Nutrient intake was obtained using multiple, nonconsecutive, 24-hour dietary recalls. Though it tended to be low, supplement use was also recorded. The researchers learned that the women with the highest intake of vitamin B6 from food were 43 percent less likely to become depressed. The researchers concluded that their findings "provided some evidence of decreased depression risk among women with higher intakes of vitamin B6 from food."[4]

In an earlier study published in 2013 in the same journal, researchers from Japan investigated the cross-sectional and prospective associations between serum vitamin B6 and depressive symptoms among Japanese workers. The cohort consisted of 422 municipal employees between the ages of 21 and 67 years. Of these, 159 employees (37.7%) were found to have depressive symptoms. The researchers determined that higher serum levels of vitamin B6 were associated with lower levels of depressive symptoms. Likewise, "depressive symptoms after three years tended to decrease with increasing levels of serum pyridoxal [vitamin B6]." The researchers concluded that "higher vitamin B6 status may prevent the development of depressive symptoms."[5]

Sufficient Levels of Serum Vitamin B6 May Reduce the Risk of Coronary Artery Disease

In a case-control study published in 2012 in the journal *Nutrition Research*, researchers from Taiwan noted that coronary artery disease is a leading cause of death throughout the world. That is why the researchers wanted to determine if serum levels of vitamin B6 and coenzyme Q10 were associated with the risk of coronary artery disease. The researchers recruited 45 patients from a hospital's cardiology clinic; all of the patients had at least 50 percent stenosis or blockage of one major coronary artery. The control group consisted of 89 healthy people with normal blood biochemistry test result. Blood samples of all of the participants were evaluated. The day before these samples were collected, the subjects completed a 24-hour dietary recall questionnaire. The researchers learned that compared to the control group, the blood samples of the subjects with coronary artery disease had significantly lower levels of vitamin B6, "but the relationship lost its statistical significance after adjusting for the risk factors for CAD [coronary artery disease]." The researchers concluded that future research should determine if people with CAD should take supplemental vitamin B6.[6]

There May Be an Association between Low Levels of Vitamin B6 and Parkinson's Disease

In a multihospital-based case-controlled study published in 2010 in the *British Journal of Nutrition*, researchers from Japan wanted to learn more about the association between B vitamins, including vitamin B6, and the risk of Parkinson's disease. (Parkinson's disease is an illness of the nervous system characterized by tremors, muscular rigidity, and slow imprecise movements.) The researchers recruited 249 patients with Parkinson's disease and 368 controls who did not have any neurodegenerative diseases. Dietary intake during the preceding month was assessed using a validated, self-administered, semiquantitative, comprehensive diet history questionnaire. The researchers found that a low intake of vitamin B6 was associated with an increased risk of Parkinson's disease. And they commented that "the importance of research on the possible role of dietary factors in PD [Parkinson's disease] is emphasized by the fact that diet is modifiable."[7]

Higher Vitamin B6 Intake May Slow Cognitive Decline in Older People

In a longitudinal study published in 2017 in the journal *Nutrients*, researchers from Northern Ireland noted that aging comes with an increased risk for cognitive dysfunction ranging from mild cognitive impairment to dementia. Would higher intake of the B vitamins, including vitamin B6, help slow cognitive decline? The baseline cohort consisted of 155 older adults between the ages of 60 and 88 years. They were screened for cognitive functioning and screened again at a three-and-a-half- to four-year follow-up. Blood tests were performed. Dietary intakes were assessed using a four-day food diary and a food frequency questionnaire. After the second screening, the researchers found that 27 percent of the participants demonstrated a greater-than-expected rate of cognitive decline. Moreover, a lower intake of vitamin B6 was associated with a 3.5 times higher risk of accelerated cognitive decline. The researchers concluded that vitamin B6 "may be an important (often overlooked) protective factor in helping maintain cognitive health in aging." Why is this finding so important? "Optimizing vitamin B6 status in older people, through the use of fortified foods or supplements, may have a positive impact on cognition."[8]

Higher Intake of Vitamin B6 May Reduce Levels of Oxidative DNA Damage

In a study published in 2013 in the journal *Nutrition*, researchers from Japan wanted to learn more about the association between vitamin B6, folate, homocysteine, and oxidative DNA damage. (Oxidative DNA damage may contribute to the development of cancer and other medical problems.) The cohort consisted of 500 men and women between the ages of 21 and 66 years who were employed at two municipal offices in Japan. Blood samples provided information on levels of vitamin B6, folate, and homocysteine, and a urinary test detected levels of a marker for DNA damage. The researchers determined that in nonsmoking men who consumed less than 20 g per day of alcohol, higher levels of vitamin B6 were associated with significantly lower levels of DNA damage. This association was not seen in women. The researchers concluded that vitamin B6 "plays a role against oxidative damage in Japanese men." Still, "intervention studies are required to confirm whether increase of vitamin B6 can decrease oxidative DNA damage."[9]

Vitamin B6 May or May Not Reduce the Risk of Cancer

In an article published in 2017 in the *Journal of the National Cancer Institute*, researchers from Italy described their systematic review of both observational and intervention studies on the association between vitamin B6 and the risk of any type of cancer. The researchers identified 121 observational studies, with close to 2 million participants, and 9 randomized, controlled trials, with almost 35,000 participants. The researchers found that a higher dietary intake of vitamin B6 was associated with a lower risk of all cancers. However, when total intake of vitamin B6 was considered—through food and supplements—the associations were weaker or null. According to the researchers, their findings "raise the question of whether vitamin B6 can exert a direct preventive effect against cancer development or if it rather represents an indicator of the presence of other protective micronutrients in a healthy diet."[10]

But Vitamin B6 May Be Useful in the Prevention of Breast Cancer

In a case-controlled study published in 2011 in the *Journal of Epidemiology*, researchers from Taiwan wanted to learn more about the association between dietary intake of vitamin B6 and breast cancer. The cohort consisted of 391 women, between the ages of 24 and 72 years, who were treated for breast cancer and 782 control subjects enrolled at the Tri-Service General Hospital in Taipei, Taiwan. The control subjects had no history of cancer. Of the women treated for breast cancer, 227 were premenopausal and 164 were postmenopausal. Information on the intake of vitamin B6 was derived from a food frequency questionnaire. The researchers found that for all women a higher dietary intake of vitamin B6 was associated with a significantly lower risk of breast cancer. This association was most evident among premenopausal women. The researchers commented that "there is a substantial body of data supporting the biological plausibility of a protective effect of vitamin B6 on breast cancer risk."[11]

Vitamin B6 Helps Control Symptoms of Premenstrual Syndrome

In a double-blind, randomized, and controlled study published in 2016 in the *Journal of Caring Sciences*, researchers from Iran explained that premenstrual syndrome is one of the most common disorders in women, and it includes a variety of physical and psychological symptoms such as breast tenderness, abdominal cramps, bloating, crying, mood swings, and irritability. It has been estimated that as many as 85 percent of women experience at least one symptom of premenstrual syndrome. That is why the researchers wanted to learn if vitamin B6 and calcium would have any impact on these symptoms. The cohort consisted of 76 students who attended the Hamadan University of Medical Sciences and had symptoms of premenstrual syndrome. For two consecutive months, 38 students took calcium and vitamin B6 supplementation and 38 students in a second group took only vitamin B6 supplementation during specific times of the month. Different methods were used to assess symptoms. While the researchers found that the severity of the symptoms was reduced in both groups, the reduction was significantly greater in the women taking both vitamin B6 and calcium. "It seems that the combination of calcium and vitamin B6 can be used for better controlling of the premenstrual syndrome symptoms."[12]

Vitamin B6 May Be Useful for the Nausea and Vomiting Associated with Pregnancy

In a study published in 2015 in the journal *BMC Pregnancy & Childbirth*, researchers from Toronto, Canada, Jerusalem, Israel, and multiple locations in the United States commented that nausea and vomiting are very common during pregnancy. It has been estimated that up to 80 percent of expectant women suffer from these problems. In April 2013, the U.S. Food and Drug Administration approved Diclegis, which contains vitamin B6 and a delayed released antihistamine known as doxylamine, for pregnant women with nausea and vomiting. The researchers wanted to learn more about its safety. Previous studies have proven the treatment to be efficacious. The cohort consisted of 256 women, in the gestational age range of 7 to 14 weeks, who suffered from nausea and vomiting. None of the women responded to the more traditional treatments such as dietary and lifestyle changes. For 14 days, 131 women took different doses of Diclegis; 125 women took a placebo. When the researchers compared the women taking Diclegis to the control women, they learned that Diclegis was not associated with any adverse effects. When taken at the recommended dose of up to four tablets per day, Diclegis "is safe and well tolerated by pregnant women."[13]

Vitamin B6 May Be Useful for the Side Effects of Oral Contraception

In a longitudinal study published in 2014 in the journal *Nutrients*, researchers from Cambodia and New Orleans, Louisiana, noted that some women experience negative side effects from oral contraceptives, including nausea/no appetite, dizziness, headache, hot flashes, depression, and menstrual changes. As a result, in some instances, women avoid using them as a method of family planning. Would vitamin B6 supplementation help these women remain on oral contraception? The cohort consisted of 1,011 women with a mean age of 29 years. The women obtained oral contraception through the public health system in rural Cambodia. They were placed in a vitamin B6 supplementation group (577 women) or a control group (434 women) in which the participants did not take vitamin B6 supplementation. All of the women were enrolled in the study for at least six months. Demographic data were obtained using a standardized questionnaire during in-person interviews. The researchers learned that the most commonly reported side effects were nausea/no appetite, headache, and depression. When compared to the women in the control group, the women taking the supplementation had statistically lower rates of nausea/no appetite, headache, and depression. The researchers concluded that some of the side effects of oral contraception "may be ameliorated through the administration of vitamin B6."[14]

NOTES

1. The George Mateljan Foundation. "Vitamin B6-Pyridoxine." December 30, 2017. http://whfoods.com/genpage.php?tname=nutrient&dbid=108.
2. Ibid.
3. Ibid.
4. Gougeon, L., H. Payette, J. A. Morais, et al. "Intakes of Folate, Vitamin B6 and B12 and Risk of Depression in Community-Dwelling Older Adults: The Quebec

Longitudinal Study on Nutrition and Aging." *European Journal of Clinical Nutrition* 70, no. 3 (March 2016): 380–385.

5. Nanri, A., N.M. Pham, K. Kurotani, et al. "Serum Pyridoxal Concentrations and Depressive Symptoms among Japanese Adults: Results from a Prospective Study." *European Journal of Clinical Nutrition* 67 (2013): 1060–1065.

6. Lee, Bor-Jen, Chi-Hua Yen, Hui-Chen Hsu, et al. "A Significant Correlation between Plasma Levels of Coenzyme Q10 and Vitamin B-6 and a Reduced Risk of Coronary Artery Disease." *Nutrition Research* 32 (2012): 751–756.

7. Murakami, Kentaro, Yoshihiro Miyake, Satoshi Sasaki, et al. "Dietary Intake of Folate, Vitamin B6, Vitamin B12 and Riboflavin and Risk of Parkinson's Disease: A Case-Control Study in Japan." *British Journal of Nutrition* 104 (2010): 757–764.

8. Hughes, Catherine F., Mary Ward, Fergal Tracey, et al. "B-Vitamin Intake and Biomarker Status in Relation to Cognitive Decline in Healthy Older Adults in a 4-Year Follow-Up Study." *Nutrients* 9, no. 1 (2017): 53+.

9. Kuwahara, K., A. Nanri, N.M. Pham, et al. "Serum Vitamin B6, Folate, and Homocysteine Concentrations and Oxidative DNA Damage in Japanese Men and Women." *Nutrition* 29, no. 10 (October 2013): 1219–1223.

10. Mocellin, Simone, Marta Briarava, and Pierluigi Pilati. "Vitamin B6 and Cancer Risk: A Field Synopsis and Meta-Analysis." *Journal of the National Cancer Institute* 109, no. 3 (March 2017): djw230.

11. Chou, Yu-Ching, Chi-Hong Chu, Mei-Hsuan Wu, et al. "Dietary Intake of Vitamin B6 and Risk of Breast Cancer in Taiwanese Women." *Journal of Epidemiology* 21, no. 5 (2011): 329–336.

12. Masoumi, S.Z., M. Ataollahi, and K. Oshvandi. "Effect of Combined Use of Calcium and Vitamin B6 on Premenstrual Syndrome Symptoms: A Randomized Clinical Trial." *Journal of Caring Sciences* 5, no. 1 (March 1, 2016): 67–73.

13. Koren, G., S. Clark, G.D. Hankins, et al. "Maternal Safety of the Delayed-Release Doxylamine and Pyridoxine Combination for Nausea and Vomiting of Pregnancy: A Randomized Placebo Controlled Trial." *BMC Pregnancy & Childbirth* 15 (2015): 59+.

14. Var, Chivorn, Sheryl Keller, Rathavy Tung, et al. "Supplementation with Vitamin B6 Reduces Side Effects in Cambodian Women Using Oral Contraceptives." *Nutrients* 6 (2014): 3353–3362.

REFERENCES AND FURTHER READINGS

Chou, Yu-Ching, Chi-Hong Chu, Mei-Hsuan Wu, et al. "Dietary Intake of Vitamin B6 and Risk of Breast Cancer in Taiwanese Women." *Journal of Epidemiology* 21, no. 5 (2011): 329–336.

The George Mateljan Foundation. "Vitamin B6-Pyridoxine." December 30, 2017. http://whfoods.com/genpage.php?tname=nutrient&dbid=108.

Gougeon, L., H. Payette, J.A. Morais, et al. "Intakes of Folate, Vitamin B6 and B12 and Risk of Depression in Community-Dwelling Older Adults: The Quebec Longitudinal Study on Nutrition and Aging." *European Journal of Clinical Nutrition* 70, no. 3 (March 2016): 380–385.

Hughes, Catherine F., Mary Ward, Fergal Tracey, et al. "B-Vitamin Intake and Biomarker Status in Relation to Cognitive Decline in Healthy Older Adults in a 4-Year Follow-Up Study." *Nutrients* 9, no. 1 (2017): 53+.

Koren, G., S. Clark, G.D. Hankins, et al. "Maternal Safety of the Delayed-Release Doxylamine and Pyridoxine Combination for Nausea and Vomiting of Pregnancy: A Randomized Placebo Controlled Trial." *BMC Pregnancy & Childbirth* 15 (2015): 59+.

Kuwahara, K., A. Nanri, N.M. Pham, et al. "Serum Vitamin B6, Folate, and Homocysteine Concentrations and Oxidative DNA Damage in Japanese Men and Women." *Nutrition* 29, no. 10 (October 2013): 1219–1223.

Lee, Bor-Jen, Chi-Hua Yen, Hui-Chen Hsu, et al. "A Significant Correlation between Plasma Levels of Coenzyme Q10 and Vitamin B-6 and a Reduced Risk of Coronary Artery Disease." *Nutrition Research* 32 (2012): 751–756.

Masoumi, S.Z., M. Ataollahi, and K. Oshvandi. "Effect of Combined Use of Calcium and Vitamin B6 on Premenstrual Syndrome Symptoms: A Randomized Clinical Trial." *Journal of Caring Sciences* 5, no. 1 (March 1, 2016): 67–73.

Mocellin, Simone, Marta Briarava, and Pierluigi Pilati. "Vitamin B6 and Cancer Risk: A Field Synopsis and Meta-Analysis." *Journal of the National Cancer Institute* 109, no. 3 (March 2017): djw230.

Murakami, Kentaro, Yoshihiro Miyake, Satoshi Sasaki, et al. "Dietary Intake of Folate, Vitamin B6, Vitamin B12 and Riboflavin and Risk of Parkinson's Disease: A Case-Control Study in Japan." *British Journal of Nutrition* 104 (2010): 757–764.

Nanri, A., N. M. Pham, K. Kurotani, et al. "Serum Pyridoxal Concentrations and Depressive Symptoms among Japanese Adults: Results from a Prospective Study." *European Journal of Clinical Nutrition* 67 (2013): 1060–1065.

Var, Chivorn, Sheryl Keller, Rathavy Tung, et al. "Supplementation with Vitamin B6 Reduces Side Effects in Cambodian Women Using Oral Contraceptives." *Nutrients* 6 (2014): 3353–3362.

Vitamin B7 (Biotin)

Biotin (also known as vitamin B7 or vitamin H) is a vitamin that is part of the B-complex group of vitamins. All the B vitamins help the body convert carbohydrates into glucose—or food into fuel—which the body requires to function. The B vitamins also metabolize fats and proteins. The B vitamins are useful for healthy skin, hair, eyes, and liver, and they play a role in the proper functioning of the nervous system. In the body, biotin functions as a coenzyme. That means that certain enzymes in the body need biotin in order to function properly. These enzymes are primarily involved in the functioning of the skin, intestinal tract, and the nervous system. Biotin is especially important during pregnancy; it supports normal fetal development.

Like all the B vitamins, biotin is water soluble, which means that it is not stored in the body. But bacteria in the intestine have the potential to make biotin. Still, one needs to consume biotin, which is found in small amounts in a large number of foods, fairly often. And because biotin supports hair and nails, biotin is found in a number of cosmetic products.

FOOD SOURCES AND SUPPLEMENTS

There are numerous food sources of biotin. These include brewer's yeast, cooked eggs, especially egg yolks, sardines, salmon, carrots, almonds, peanuts, pecans, walnuts, nut butters, soybeans, beans, blackeye peas, whole grains, cauliflower, bananas, and mushrooms. On the other hand, raw egg whites contain a protein called avidin that interferes with the body's absorption of biotin. Less-processed foods contain more biotin than highly processed foods. Biotin is sold in vitamin B complex supplements, in multivitamins, and as individual supplements, mostly in tablets, capsules, and lozenges.

INTAKE RECOMMENDATIONS

There are no Recommended Dietary Allowance levels established for biotin. The following are the adequate intake levels for biotin: Breastfeeding women should take in 35 mcg per day, while adults over 18 years and pregnant women should take in 30 mcg per day. Teens between 14 and 18 years should take in 25 mcg per day, while children between 9 and 13 years should take in 20 mcg per day. Children between four and eight years should take in 12 mcg per day, and children between one and three years should take in 8 mcg per day. Infants under 12 months should take in 7 mcg per day.[1]

DEFICIENCY AND EXCESS

A severe biotin deficiency is believed to be exceedingly rare. Symptoms of biotin deficiency include hair loss, dry scaly skin, cracking in the corners of the mouth (cheilitis), a tongue that is swollen, painful, and magenta in color (glossitis), dry eyes, loss of appetite, fatigue, insomnia, and depression. Certain people are at increased risk for biotin deficiency. These include women who are pregnant, people with poor nutrition, and those who have experienced rapid weight loss. Others at increased risk for biotin deficiency include people who have been on intravenous nutrition (parenteral nutrition) for a long period of time, people taking long-term anti-seizure medications or antibiotics, and people with gastrointestinal conditions, such as Crohn's disease, who have a problem absorbing nutrients. People on dialysis and who smoke cigarettes also have an increased risk for biotin deficiency. Infants with deficient levels of biotin are at risk for cradle cap, a scaly scalp condition. Yet there are no studies showing that biotin supplementation effectively treats cradle cap.

Biotin is generally safe, even in larger-than-recommended doses. There are no reported cases of adverse effects from taking high doses of biotin. Still, higher doses may lead to the slower release of insulin, a skin rash, lower levels of vitamin C and B6, and higher blood sugar levels.

KEY RESEARCH FINDINGS

Some Infant Formulas May Not Contain Sufficient Amounts of Biotin

In a study published in 2016 in the journal *Pediatrics International,* researchers from Japan observed that some infant formulas were not providing adequate amounts of biotin, thus placing infants at risk for biotin deficiency. The researchers measured the biotin levels in 54 types of formulas, including hydrolysate formula for milk allergy, and they also tested the serum levels of 27 infants fed with these formulas. The researchers determined that the biotin content reached the recommended value in only five formulas. All of the hydrolysate formulas and more than half of the other formulas had insufficient amounts of biotin. The researchers found that the serum biotin levels were low in the infants who were fed only the hydrolysate formula, and one of the infants had alopecia or hair loss related to the biotin deficiency. The infants fed the formulas with higher levels of biotin or treated with biotin supplement had higher amounts of biotin in their blood. The researchers commented that "the infants fed with formulas devoid of biotin are subject to the risk of developing symptomatic disease."[2]

Biotin Appears to Have Antidiabetic Properties

In a study published in 2013 in the *British Journal of Nutrition,* researchers from Turkey and Purchase, New York, investigated the antidiabetic properties of biotin alone and in combination with chromium picolinate. The researchers began by dividing rats into five groups. One group of rats was fed a regular diet; this group served as the control. The other rats were fed various combinations of food and biotin and chromium picolinate. To induce type 2 diabetes, some rats were fed a high-fat diet and low doses of a chemical (streptozotocin). The researchers learned that both biotin alone and in combination with chromium picolinate had antidiabetic properties such as reducing insulin resistance and lowering the pathological changes in the liver, kidneys, and pancreas. The researchers commented that their findings "clearly showed that supplementing CrPi [chromium picolinate] or biotin alone or in a combination exerts antioxidant, anti-hyperlipidaemic, anti-inflammatory and anti-hyperglycaemic effects, and increases the level of insulin in diabetic rats."[3]

Marginal Biotin Deficiency May Be Induced in Humans

In a study published in 2012 in *The Journal of Nutrition,* researchers from Arkansas wanted to determine if they could use a simplified outpatient design to induce marginal biotin deficiency in humans. They decided to test three different models. Two of the designs were based on the addition of different doses of oral avidin to the diet. The first design had four participants and the second had two. In the third design, the five participants consumed egg white beverages that contained avidin. While the first two designs did not effectively induce marginal biotin deficiency, the third was as effective as previously completed during inpatient protocols. The researchers commented that their egg white beverage method "should be useful to the broader nutritional research community."[4]

Biotin May Be Useful for Chronic Progressive Multiple Sclerosis

In an open-label pilot study published in 2015 in the journal *Multiple Sclerosis and Related Disorders*, researchers from France noted that no medication has been found to be effective for progressive multiple sclerosis. As a result, they wanted to determine if high doses of biotin would be useful for people with this serious neurological problem. The cohort consisted of 23 patients, between the ages of 26 and 75 years, who have been dealing with primary or secondary progressive multiple sclerosis for at least 12 months. All of participants were treated with high doses (100 to 600 mg per day) of biotin for 2 to 36 months, with a mean of 9.2 months. The patients experienced a number of improvements. For example, four of the patients who had prominent visual impairment from optic nerve injury had significant improvements in visual acuity. Of the 18 patients with spinal cord problems, 16 improved. Improvements were also experienced in fatigue, swallowing difficulty, speech, sensory signs, gait, and urinary dysfunction. Of the 23 participants, 21 (91.3%) exhibited some degree of qualitative or quantitative clinical improvement. The dose of 300 mg per day was believed to be associated with the best clinical responses. According to the researchers, "High doses of biotin have never been hypothesized as a potential treatment for MS." Yet "these preliminary data suggest that high doses of biotin might have an impact on disability and progression in progressive MS."[5]

High Doses of Biotin May Be Useful for the Loss of Taste Sensation

In a study published in 2011 in the *Journal of the American College of Nutrition*, researchers from Louisiana and Florida described two patients who lost their sense of taste. In both instance, taste was returned by the intake of high doses of biotin. The first person was a 67-year-old Caucasian woman, who lost her sense of taste after taking an herbal supplement. The second person was a 60-year-old Caucasian male, who lost his sense of taste after a gastrectomy, a surgery for obesity. Both patients did not respond to the initial 5 mg per day doses of biotin. Once the woman was placed on a dose of 10 mg per day and the man was placed on a dose of 20 mg per day, they experienced a restoration of taste. Additional testing showed that neither of these patients exhibited any typical form of biotin deficiency. The researchers commented that more research is needed to understand how these high doses of biotin were able to restore the taste sensation and to determine if other people dealing with a loss of taste might benefit from this treatment.

The researchers encouraged other medical providers treating patients with a loss of taste "that defies an obvious explanation" to attempt a trial of high doses of biotin.[6]

NOTES

1. U.S. National Library of Medicine. "Biotin." December 30, 2017. https://medlineplus.gov/druginfo/natural/313.html.
2. Sato, Y., K. Wakabayashi, E. Ogawa, et al. "Low Serum Biotin Levels in Japanese Children Fed with Hydrolysate Formula." *Pediatrics International* 58 (2016): 867–871.
3. Sahin, Kazim, Mehmet Tuzcu, Cemal Orhan, et al. "Anti-Diabetic Activity of Chromium Picolinate and Biotin in Rats with Type 2 Diabetes Induced by High-Fat Diet and Streptozotocin." *British Journal of Nutrition* 110, no. 2 (2013): 197–205.
4. Stratton, Shawna L., Cindy L. Henrich, Nell I. Matthews, et al. "Marginal Biotin Deficiency Can Be Induced Experimentally in Humans Using a Cost-Effective Outpatient Design." *The Journal of Nutrition* 142, no. 1 (January 1, 2012): 22–26.
5. Sedel, F., C. Papeix, A. Bellanger, et al. "High Doses of Biotin in Chronic Progressive Multiple Sclerosis: A Pilot Study." *Multiple Sclerosis and Related Disorders* 4, no. 2 (March 2015): 159–169.
6. Greenway, Frank L., Donald K. Ingram, Eric Ravussin, et al. "Loss of Taste Responds to High-Dose Biotin Treatment." *Journal of the American College of Nutrition* 30, no. 3 (2011): 178–181.

REFERENCES AND FURTHER READINGS

Greenway, Frank L., Donald K. Ingram, Eric Ravussin, et al. "Loss of Taste Responds to High-Dose Biotin Treatment." *Journal of the American College of Nutrition* 30, no. 3 (2011): 178–181.
Sahin, Kazim, Mehmet Tuzcu, Cemal Orhan, et al. "Anti-Diabetic Activity of Chromium Picolinate and Biotin in Rats with Type 2 Diabetes Induced by High-Fat Diet and Streptozotocin." *British Journal of Nutrition* 110, no. 2 (2013): 197–205.
Sato, Y., K. Wakabayashi, E. Ogawa, et al. "Low Serum Biotin Levels in Japanese Children Fed with Hydrolysate Formula." *Pediatrics International* 58 (2016): 867–871.
Sedel, F., C. Papeix, A. Bellanger, et al. "High Doses of Biotin in Chronic Progressive Multiple Sclerosis: A Pilot Study." *Multiple Sclerosis and Related Disorders* 4, no. 2 (March 2015): 159–169.
Stratton, Shawna L., Cindy L. Henrich, Nell I. Matthews, et al. "Marginal Biotin Deficiency Can Be Induced Experimentally in Humans Using a Cost-Effective Outpatient Design." *The Journal of Nutrition* 142, no. 1 (January 1, 2012): 22–26.
U.S. National Library of Medicine. "Biotin." December 30, 2017. https://medlineplus.gov/druginfo/natural/313.html.

Vitamin B9 (Folate)

Also known as folic acid, folacin, vitamin B9, and pteroylglutamic acid, folate is a water-soluble B vitamin that occurs naturally in food. Helping the body make healthy new cells, folate plays an essential role in the creation of DNA and RNA.

Folate is necessary for the production of normal red blood cells, the metabolism of homocysteine, the maintenance of amino acid levels, and the preventions of changes to DNA that could trigger the development of cancerous cells.

While everyone needs folate, it is especially important for women who may become pregnant. Adequate amounts of folate are required to prevent major birth defects in a baby's brain and spinal cord. Since 1998, the U.S. Food and Drug Administration has mandated that food companies add folate to enriched breads, cereals, flour, cornmeal, rice, and other grain products. This has resulted in a reduction in the number of babies born with neural tube defects.

FOOD SOURCES AND SUPPLEMENTS

There are a number of sources of folate, including lentils, pinto beans, garbanzo beans, asparagus, leafy green vegetables, avocados, bananas, melons, lemons, peas, mushrooms, organ meats, orange juice, tomato juice, and enriched bread, pasta, cereals, and other grain-based foods. Folate supplements, which are generally referred to as folic acid, are available as a single-ingredient supplement, but folate is often combined with other B vitamins. In order to prevent birth defects, women who are pregnant or may become pregnant are often advised take folate supplementation. Folate is commonly added to multivitamins for adults and children.

INTAKE RECOMMENDATIONS

The Food and Nutrition Board has issued the following Recommended Dietary Allowances for folate. Males and females 14 years and older should take in 400 mcg per day, while children between the ages of 9 and 13 years should take in 300 mcg per day. Children between the ages of four and eight years should take in 200 mcg per day, while children between the ages of one and three years should take in 150 mcg per day. The adequate intake level for children seven months to one year is 80 mcg, and the adequate intake level for infants up to six months is 65 mcg. There are also tolerable upper intake levels for folate. Males and females 19 years and older should not take in more than 1,000 mcg per day, while teens between the ages of 14 and 18 years should take in no more than 800 mcg per day. Children between the ages of 9 and 13 years should take in no more than 600 mcg per day, while children between the ages of 4 and 8 should take in no more than 400 mcg per day. Children between the ages of one and three years should take in no more than 300 mcg per day. No upper limits have been established for infants.[1]

DEFICIENCY AND EXCESS

It is generally believed that most adults and children in the United States take in adequate amounts of folate. However, there are some groups that are at increased risk for deficiency, including women of childbearing age and non-Hispanic black women. One of the medical problems associated with folate deficiency is a condition known as megaloblastic anemia, which is characterized by weakness, fatigue, difficulty concentrating, irritability, headache, heart palpitations, and shortness of breath. Other symptoms associated with folate deficiency include soreness and shallow ulcerations on the tongue and in the mouth, changes in skin, hair, and fingernail pigmentation, and elevated levels of homocysteine in the blood. In addition to increasing the risk of neural tube defects, women of childbearing age who have insufficient levels of folate have a higher rate of babies born with lower birth weights, preterm deliveries, and fetal growth retardation.

It is considered impossible to consume excess amounts of folate from food. Still, in the United States, people over the age of 50 who consume lots of folate-fortified foods and folate supplements may take in too much folate. Signs and symptoms of excessive folate intake include digestive problems, nausea, loss of appetite, bloating, gas, a bitter taste in the mouth, depression, sleep problems, excessive excitability, irritability, and zinc deficiency. More serious signs of excessive levels of folate include psychotic behavior, numbness, tingling, mouth pain, weakness, problems with concentration, confusion, fatigue, and seizures.

KEY RESEARCH FINDINGS

When Used at Specific Times, Folic Acid Supplements Appear to Have Prenatal Benefits

In a study published in 2016 in the *British Journal of Nutrition*, researchers from China wanted to learn about the relationship between folic acid supplementation and infants who are born preterm and small for their gestational age. The trial included 231,179 pregnant women from the Jiaxing Birth Cohort. Information on these women was collected during in-person interviews. The researchers learned that one-fourth of the women took folic acid supplementation. The prevalence of preterm birth and small-for-gestational-age birth was, respectively, 3.48 and 9.2 percent. Preconception folic acid supplementation was associated with an 8 percent lower risk of preterm birth and a 19 percent lower risk of small-for-gestational-age birth. No significant association between postconception initiation of folic acid supplementation with either outcome was observed. The researchers commented that their trial provided "important and valuable information for the prevention of PTB [preterm birth] and SGA [small-for-gestational-age] in the Chinese populations."[2]

In a study published in 2014 in the *International Journal of Epidemiology*, researchers from China examined the association between the intake of folic acid around the time of conception and the incidence of preterm birth. The data were derived from a large population-based cohort conducted in China to evaluate the prevention of neural tube defects with folic acid supplementation. The cohort consisted of 207,936 singleton live births delivered at gestational ages of 20 to 42 weeks to women from two provinces in southern China. Of the total number of women, slightly more than half took folic acid around the time their babies were conceived. The total incidence of preterm birth, or birth before 37 weeks, was 5.67 percent. The researchers determined that the incidence of preterm birth was significantly lower among folic acid users (5.28%) than among nonusers (6.10%). Overall, folic acid use reduced the rate of preterm delivery by 14 percent. The researchers concluded that they found "strong clinical support for folic acid usage in the prevention of preterm birth."[3]

Folic Acid Supplementation in Early Pregnancy May Increase the Risk of Gestational Diabetes

In an article published in 2016 in the journal *Diabetes Care*, researchers from China and Australia described the China-Anhui Birth Cohort study, a population-based study that recruited 3,474 pregnant women from the Anhui Province of China from May 2013 to September 2014. At approximately 28 weeks of gestation, the women had glucose tolerance tests. An analysis was conducted of the 1,938 women who had either used folic acid supplement or never used any vitamin supplements. Diabetes was diagnosed in 249 or 12.8 percent of these women. The researchers learned that daily folic acid supplementation during the first trimester was associated with an increased risk of gestational diabetes. Heavier women who took the folic acid supplementation had a much higher risk than normal-sized women who were not taking the supplement. This increased risk was not observed in women who used folic acid before pregnancy or who used folic acid only in the second trimester. The researchers noted that there is a need for further studies with larger cohorts.[4]

Folate May Provide a Degree of Protection from Cancer

In a study published in 2016 in the online journal *PLoS ONE*, researchers from College Park, Maryland, noted that since the addition of folate to cereal-grain products began some have raised concern that such fortification would increase the risk of certain types of cancer. The researchers reviewed data from about 1,400 participants in the National Health and Nutrition Examination Survey (NHANES) 1999–2002, which included people 57 years and older. The participants answered questions about health and nutrition. Non-Hispanic white men with higher levels of education and more physical activity had higher intakes of folate. During the 8,114 person-years of follow-up, at least 125 cases of cancer were identified. No significant associations were found between the presence of unmetabolized folic acid, intake of naturally occurring food folate or folic acid, and the incidence of cancer. In fact, "high total folate intake and biomarkers in older adults appeared to be protective against cancer in post-folic acid fortification years."[5]

In a prospective study published in 2011 in the *American Journal of Clinical Nutrition*, researchers from New Haven, Connecticut, Rockville, Maryland, and

Washington, DC, wanted to determine if the consumption of folate offered a degree of protection from colorectal cancer. The researchers obtained their data from the NIH-AARP Diet and Health Study, a U.S. cohort study of 525,488 individuals between the ages of 50 and 71 years. Data were collected before and after the folate fortification was implemented in 1998. More than half of the subjects reported an intake of supplemental folate through the use of multivitamins. During a mean follow-up period of more than nine years, 7,212 incident colorectal cases were identified. Higher intake of folate was associated with a decreased risk of colorectal cancer. Nevertheless, since it is known that colorectal cancer may take 10 or more years to develop, the researchers cautioned that "additional follow-up time is needed to fully examine the effect of folic acid fortification."[6]

High Levels of Folate May Promote the Growth of Prostate Cancer Cells

In a study published in 2011 in the journal *The Prostate*, researchers from Pittsburgh and Boston reported that a previous laboratory study had found that folate supported the growth of prostate cancer cells. They wanted to determine if that also occurred in humans. The cohort consisted of 87 randomly selected men who were undergoing surgery for prostate cancer and 25 cancer-free controls. Tests were completed to determine levels of serum folate and/or prostate tissue folate. The researchers found a positive correlation between serum folate levels and prostate tumor tissue folate content. Men with prostate cancer had significantly higher serum folate levels than men who were cancer free. The top quartile of patients had serum folate levels six times the level considered adequate. Yet nearly half of these men reported no use of folate-containing supplements. The researchers wondered if the body stores excess amounts of folate. "Although folate is considered a water-soluble vitamin and therefore expected to be excreted when in excess, this may not be true in practice." The researchers underscored the need for more research on folate. "Given widespread dietary folate supplementation the relationship between folate intake and prostate cancer should be better defined."[7]

Then Again, Folic Acid May Not Increase or Decrease the Incidence of Site-Specific Cancer

In a meta-analysis published in 2013 in the journal *Lancet*, researchers from many locations throughout the world but based in Norway explained that some countries do not fortify foods with folate because they fear that such supplementation increases the risk of cancer. To test that theory, the researchers conducted a meta-analysis of the site-specific cancer rates in the randomized trials of folic acid supplementation, at doses higher than those used in fortification. Their cohort consisted of 13 trials that included almost 50,000 subjects. The researchers compared the cancer rates among the subjects allocated folic acid to the cancer rates among the subjects who received placebos. The average treatment period was more than five years. The researchers determined that folic acid supplementation appeared to have no significant effect on overall cancer incidence, even by those who took folic acid for longer periods of time. The researchers concluded that during the first five years of supplementation, folic acid "does not substantially increase or decrease incidence of site-specific cancer." Likewise, "both hopes for rapid cancer prevention and the fears about rapidly increased cancer risk from folic acid supplementation were not confirmed by this meta-analysis."[8]

Folic Acid Supplementation May Improve Cognitive Functioning in the Elderly with Depressive Symptoms

In a random, placebo-controlled trial published in 2012 in the *American Journal of Clinical Nutrition*, researchers based in Australia wanted to learn if supplementation with folic acid and vitamin B12 would help prevent cognitive decline in a cohort of community-dwelling older adults with depressive symptoms. The cohort consisted of 900 adults between the ages of 60 and 74 years. Cognitive function was assessed during telephone interviews. After two years, the researchers found that the supplementation improved some aspects of cognition, but the overall results were modest. The researchers commented that their findings "suggest that there may be a role for combined FA [folic acid] and vitamin B-12 in lowering the risk of cognitive decline."[9]

Certain People Who Take Folic Acid Supplementation Are More Likely to Exceed the Tolerable Upper Intake Level of Folate

In a study published in 2016 in the journal *Nutrients*, researchers from Georgia, California, and Iowa wanted to learn more about the people who routinely exceeded recommended upper limit for the intake of folate. The cohort consisted of data from NHANES, 2003–2010, with 18,321 nonpregnant adults, 19 years and older. NHANES is a stratified multistage probability survey designed to represent the civilian, noninstitutionalized U.S. population. The researchers learned that 2.7 percent of the cohort consumed more than the upper limit of folate. Of these, 62.2 percent were women, 86.3 percent were non-Hispanic whites, and 98.5 percent took supplements that contained folic acid. They are likely to have at least one chronic medical condition and to be between the ages of 19 and 39 years or 60 years or older. The researchers concluded that "voluntary consumption of supplements containing folic acid is the main factor associated with usual daily intake exceeding the folic acid UL [upper level]."[10]

NOTES

1. Office of Dietary Supplements, National Institutes of Health. "Folate." December 30, 2017. https://ods.od.nih.gov/factsheets/Folate-Consumer/.

2. Zheng, Ju-Sheng, Yuhong Guan, Yimin Zhao, et al. "Pre-Conceptional Intake of Folic Acid Supplements Is Inversely Associated with Risk of Preterm Birth and

Small-for-Gestational-Age Birth: A Prospective Cohort Study." *British Journal of Nutrition* 115, no. 3 (February 2016): 509–516.

3. Li, Zhiwen, Rongwei Ye, Le Zhang, et al. "Periconceptional Folic Acid Supplementation and the Risk of Preterm Births in China: A Large Prospective Cohort Study." *International Journal of Epidemiology* 43, no. 4 (2014): 1132–1139.

4. Zhu, Beibei, Xing Ge, Kun Huang, et al. "Folic Acid Supplement Intake in Early Pregnancy Increases Risk of Gestational Diabetes Mellitus: Evidence from a Prospective Cohort Study." *Diabetes Care* 39 (March 2016): e36–e37.

5. Hu, Jing, WenYen Juan, and Nadine R. Sahyoun. "Intake and Biomarkers of Folate and Risk of Cancer Morbidity in Older Adults, NHANES 1999–2002 with Medicare Linkage." *PLoS ONE* 11, no. 2 (February 10, 2016): e0148697.

6. Gibson, Todd M., Stephanie J. Weinstein, Ruth M. Pfeiffer, et al. "Pre- and Postfortification Intake of Folate and Risk of Colorectal Cancer in a Large Prospective Cohort Study in the United States." *American Journal of Clinical Nutrition* 94 (2011): 1053–1062.

7. Tomaszewski, Jeffrey J., Jessica L. Cummings, Anil V. Parwani, et al. "Increased Cancer Cell Proliferation in Prostate Cancer Patients with High Levels of Serum Folate." *The Prostate* 71 (2011): 1287–1293.

8. Vollset, Stein Emil, Robert Clarke, Sarah Lewington, et al. "Effects of Folic Acid Supplementation on Overall and Site-Specific Cancer Incidence during the Randomised Trials: Meta-Analysis of Data on 50,000 Individuals." *Lancet* 381 (March 23, 2013): 1029–1036.

9. Walker, Janine G., Philip J. Batterham, Andrew J. Mackinnon, et al. "Oral Folic Acid and Vitamin B-12 Supplementation to Prevent Cognitive Decline in Community-Dwelling Older Adults with Depressive Symptoms—The Beyond Ageing Project: A Randomized Controlled Trial." *American Journal of Clinical Nutrition* 95 (2012): 194–203.

10. Orozco, Angela M., Lorraine F. Yeung, Jing Guo, et al. "Characteristics of U.S. Adults with Usual Daily Folic Acid Intake Above the Tolerable Upper Intake Levels: National Health and Nutrition Examination Survey, 2003–2010." *Nutrients* 8 (April 1, 2016): 195+.

REFERENCES AND FURTHER READINGS

Gibson, Todd M., Stephanie J. Weinstein, Ruth M. Pfeiffer, et al. "Pre- and Postfortification Intake of Folate and Risk of Colorectal Cancer in a Large Prospective Cohort Study in the United States." *American Journal of Clinical Nutrition* 94 (2011): 1053–1062.

Hu, Jing, WenYen Juan, and Nadine R. Sahyoun. "Intake and Biomarkers of Folate and Risk of Cancer Morbidity in Older Adults, NHANES 1999–2002 with Medicare Linkage." *PLoS ONE* 11, no. 2 (February 10, 2016): e0148697.

Li, Zhiwen, Rongwei Ye, Le Zhang, et al. "Periconceptional Folic Acid Supplementation and the Risk of Preterm Births in China: A Large Prospective Cohort Study." *International Journal of Epidemiology* 43, no. 4 (2014): 1132–1139.

Office of Dietary Supplements, National Institutes of Health. "Folate." December 30, 2017. https://ods.od.nih.gov/factsheets/Folate-Consumer/.

Orozco, Angela M., Lorraine F. Yeung, Jing Guo, et al. "Characteristics of U.S. Adults with Usual Daily Folic Acid Intake above the Tolerable Upper Intake Level: National Health and Nutrition Examination Survey, 2003–2010." *Nutrients* 8 (April 1, 2016): 195+.

Tomaszewski, Jeffrey J., Jessica L. Cummings, Anil V. Parwani, et al. "Increased Cancer Cell Proliferation in Prostate Cancer Patients with High Levels of Serum Folate." *The Prostate* 71 (2011): 1287–1293.

Vollset, Stein Emil, Robert Clarke, Sarah Lewington, et al. "Effects of Folic Acid Supplementation on Overall and Site-Specific Cancer Incidence during the Randomised Trials: Meta-Analysis of Data on 50,000 Individuals." *Lancet* 381 (March 23, 2013): 1029–1036.

Walker, Janine G., Philip J. Batterham, Andrew J. Mackinnon, et al. "Oral Folic Acid and Vitamin B-12 Supplementation to Prevent Cognitive Decline in Community-Dwelling Older Adults with Depressive Symptoms—The Beyond Ageing Project: A Randomized Controlled Trial." *American Journal of Clinical Nutrition* 95 (2012): 194–203.

Zheng, Ju-Sheng, Yuhong Guan, Yimin Zhao, et al. "Pre-Conceptional Intake of Folic Acid Supplements Is Inversely Associated with Risk of Preterm Birth and Small-for-Gestational-Age Birth: A Prospective Cohort Study." *British Journal of Nutrition* 115, no. 3 (February 2016): 509–516.

Zhu, Beibei, Xing Ge, Kun Huang, et al. "Folic Acid Supplement Intake in Early Pregnancy Increases Risk of Gestational Diabetes Mellitus: Evidence from a Prospective Cohort Study." *Diabetes Care* 39 (March 2016): e36–e37.

Vitamin B12 (Cobalamin)

Also known as cobalamin, vitamin B12 is one of the B-complex vitamins. Like the other B vitamins, vitamin B12 is water soluble and helps the body convert carbohydrates into glucose, which gives the body energy. In addition, the body needs vitamin B12 to use fats and proteins and to have healthy skin, hair, eyes, and liver. Without the B vitamins, especially vitamin B12, the nervous system is unable to function properly. Vitamin B12 is not stored by the body.

Vitamin B12 is required to produce DNA and RNA, the body's genetic material, and it works together with folate to make red blood cells, improve the body's iron, and produce S-adenosylmethionine, a compound involved in immune function and mood.

Moreover, vitamin B12 works with folate and vitamin B6 to control levels of the amino acid homocysteine. High levels of homocysteine are associated with heart disease and other related medical problems.[1]

FOOD SOURCES AND SUPPLEMENTS

Excellent sources of vitamin B12 include sardines, salmon, tuna, cod, lamb, scallops, and shrimp. Very good sources of vitamin B12 include beef, yogurt, cow's milk, and eggs. Good sources of vitamin B12 include turkey, chicken, cheese, and crimini mushrooms.[2] Some cereals are fortified with vitamin B12. Vitamin B12 is generally included in multivitamins as well as in B-complex vitamins. It may also be purchased as a single-ingredient supplement. Some types of vitamin B12 are sold in sublingual forms; these should be dissolved under the tongue. A prescription form of vitamin B12 may be administered as a shot; another prescription form is sold as a nasal gel. Medical providers recommend the prescription forms when higher doses are required.

INTAKE RECOMMENDATIONS

The National Academy of Sciences has the following Recommended Dietary Allowances for vitamin B12. Values for infants under the age of one year are adequate intake levels. Lactating women should take in 2.8 mcg per day, while pregnant women should take in 2.6 mcg per day. Men and women over the age of 14 years should take in 2.4 mcg per day, while children between the ages of 9 and 13 years should take in 1.8 mcg per day. Children between the ages of four and eight years should take in 1.2 mcg per day, while children between the ages of one and three years should take in 0.9 mcg per day. Infants from six months to one year should take in 0.5 mcg per day, while infants from birth to six months should take in 0.4 mcg per day.[3]

DEFICIENCY AND EXCESS

Severe vitamin B12 deficiency is thought to be rare. However, it is not uncommon for older people to be mildly deficient. As people age, they have reduced levels of stomach acid, which is needed to absorb vitamin B12. Since they do not consume any animal products, vegans are at increased risk. Other conditions that place people at increased risk include gastrointestinal malabsorption problems, such as Crohn's disease, pancreatic disease, weight loss surgery, *Helicobacter pylori* infection, eating disorders, HIV, and diabetes. Since vitamin B12 plays a key role in red cell production, low levels of vitamin B12 may cause a type of anemia known as B12 deficiency anemia. But this condition is thought to be rare.

Another type of anemia, pernicious anemia, is more common. People who have this condition are unable to make intrinsic factor, a protein made by the stomach. Without this protein, they have trouble absorbing vitamin B12. Symptoms of pernicious anemia include weakness, pale skin, diarrhea, weight loss, fever, numbness or tingling in the hands and feet, loss of balance, confusion, memory loss, and moodiness.[4]

Low levels of vitamin B12 have been associated with fatigue, shortness of breath, diarrhea, nervousness, numbness, weakness, constipation, loss of appetite, weight loss, balance problems, depression, confusion, dementia, poor memory, soreness of the mouth and tongue, and tingling sensation in the fingers and toes. Severe vitamin B12 deficiency may cause nerve damage. In infants, signs of vitamin B12 deficiency include the failure to thrive, problems with movement, anemia, and delays in reaching developmental goals.

There is no known risk of toxicity from the dietary intake of vitamin B12. Even people on higher doses of supplemental vitamin B12 do not experience any known negative side effects.

KEY RESEARCH FINDINGS

Vegetarians Have an Increased Risk for Vitamin B12 Deficiency

In a systematic literature search published in 2014 in the *European Journal of Clinical Nutrition*, researchers from North Carolina (Unites States) wanted to learn more about the association between vegetarian diets and vitamin B12. Were vegetarians at increased risk for vitamin B12 deficiency? The researchers included 40 studies in their review. Subjects came from many different countries and varying ethnic and cultural backgrounds. Almost all of the studies found serious vitamin B12 deficiencies among vegetarians, especially vegans, who consume no animal products. In infants, the deficiency prevalence was 45 percent; among children and teens it ranged from 0 to 33.3 percent. Deficiency among pregnant women ranged from 17 to 39 percent, depending on the trimester. Adults and the elderly had deficiencies ranging from 0 to 86.5 percent. Vegans who were not deficient ate foods that were fortified with vitamin B12. The researchers commented that "including vitamin B12 supplements even when food fortified with vitamin B12 are ingested is the most reliable way of preventing vitamin B12 deficiency among vegetarians, especially vegans."[5]

Use of Oral Contraceptives May Impact Levels of Vitamin B12 in the Body

In a study published in 2013 in the journal *Nutrients*, researchers from Australia wanted to learn more about the effect oral contraceptives have on serum levels of several B vitamins, including vitamin B12. The cohort consisted of 22 healthy women between the ages of 18 and 35 years who took no medication other than oral contraceptives. Blood samples were collected at baseline and then every four weeks until week 12. On two occasions, food frequency questionnaires were completed. When compared to the 13 women who did not take oral contraceptives, the researchers found that the 9 women taking oral contraceptives consistently had low levels of vitamin B12. While the findings in this study are certainly interesting, the sample size is small. There is clearly a need for further investigation of this potential association.[6]

The Elderly Are at Risk for Vitamin B12 Deficiency

In a retrospective study published in 2016 in the journal *Applied Physiology, Nutrition & Metabolism*, researchers from Ontario, Canada, evaluated the prevalence of vitamin B12 deficiency among the elderly, who were recently admitted to long-term care residences. The cohort consisted of 412 elders over the age of 65 years. The mean age at admission was 83 years. Sixty-nine percent were female. Admission to the residences required a vitamin B12 screening. Once admitted, the residents were screened every year. At admission, 13.8 percent had vitamin B12 deficiency. Subclinical deficiency was much higher—38.3 percent. Meanwhile, 47.6 percent had normal B12 status. Better levels of vitamin B12 were significantly associated with the use of B12 supplementation. One year after admission, the deficiency rate dropped to 4 percent. The researchers concluded that their findings "provide evidence that B12 status is amenable to treatment."[7]

Long-Term Use of Acid-Lowering Agents May Reduce Serum Levels of Vitamin B12

In a systematic search and meta-analysis published in 2015 in *Internal Medicine Journal*, researchers from Australia examined the association between the long-term use of acid-lowering agents and levels of serum vitamin B12. The researchers reviewed four case-controlled studies with 4,254 cases and 19,228 controls and one observational study that were published between 2001 and 2013. They learned that the long-term use of acid-lowering agents was significantly and positively associated with the development of a vitamin B12 deficiency. People who take acid-lowering agents for 10 or more months are at increased risk for a deficiency. In addition, higher doses of these agents are more likely than lower doses to trigger deficiencies. Once a vitamin B12 deficiency is diagnosed, it may be "easily treated with supplements, preventing dire consequences, such as irreversible neurological pathology."[8]

People with Depression May Have Low Levels of Vitamin B12

In a study published in 2015 in the journal *BioMed Research International*, researchers from Turkey wanted to learn more about the nutritional status of people with depression. The study included 59 people, between the ages of 18 and 60 years. Twenty-nine people, with a mean age of 37 years, were diagnosed with depression; 30 healthy volunteers, with a mean age of 33 years, were in a control group. There were more females than males in both groups. A 24-hour dietary recall enabled the researchers to learn more about their nutrient intake, and blood tests were performed. The researchers found that the intake of vitamin B12 was significantly lower in the depression group than the control group. The researchers commented that larger-scale studies are needed to confirm their findings.[9]

Older Adults Who Appear to Have a Normal Nutritional Status May Be Deficient in Vitamin B12

In a study published in 2016 in the *European Journal of Clinical Nutrition*, researchers from Portugal evaluated the vitamin B12 serum levels of elders who appeared, according to the Mini Nutritional Assessment (MNA), to take in adequate amounts of the nutrient. The cohort consisted of 97 elders between the ages of 65 and 101 years; there were 65 women and 32 men. Following an overnight fast, blood samples were collected. Surprisingly, 11.8 percent of the participants had vitamin B12 deficiency and 32.4 percent had low serum levels. There were no statistical differences between the sexes. "Study results showed that low serum levels of vitamin B12 are highly prevalent in subjects who have a nutritional status categorized as normal by MNA." That is why there is a "need to diagnose vitamin B12 deficiencies independent of the MNA result."[10]

Low Levels of Vitamin B12 May Increase the Risk of Fractures

In a population-based study published in 2014 in the journal *Osteoporosis International*, researchers from Sweden and San Francisco examined the association between vitamin B12 and the incidence of fractures in elderly community-dwelling men. At baseline, the cohort consisted of 790 men, between the ages of 70 and 81 years. All the subjects were interviewed by questionnaire. During a mean follow-up of 5.9 years, 110 men sustained at least one X-ray-verified fracture, including 45 men with clinical vertebral fractures. The researchers found that the men with the lowest intake of vitamin B12 had a much higher risk for all fractures. The researchers underscored the need for more research on the interaction between vitamin B12 and bone tissue. In addition, researchers should address whether low levels of serum vitamin B12 should be considered a risk factor for fractures in the elderly.[11]

Vitamin B12 Supplementation May Be Useful for the Cardiovascular Health of Vegetarians and Vegans

In a study published in 2012 in *The Journal of Nutrition, Health & Aging*, researchers based in Hong Kong noted that vegetarians take in lower levels of vitamin B12, which is primarily found in animal products. According to some data, that places vegetarians at increased risk for atherosclerosis or the hardening and narrowing of the arteries. The cohort consisted of 43 healthy vegetarians with an average age of 45 years. The participants completed food frequency questionnaires. Then, for 12 weeks, the participants took a vitamin B12 supplement or a placebo. After a 10-week wash-out period, the participants who took the supplement were placed on a placebo, and the placebo-taking participants were placed on the supplement. The researchers determined that the people taking the supplementation experienced significant increases in vitamin B12 serum levels. They also had improvements in their blood vessels, such as better arterial endothelial function and reduction in the thickness of their carotid artery walls. The researchers concluded that "vitamin B12 supplementation improved arterial function in vegetarians with subnormal vitamin B12 levels, proposing a novel strategy for atherosclerosis prevention."[12]

Healthy Obese Women May Have Low Levels of Serum Vitamin B12

In a cross-sectional study published in 2017 in the *Nigerian Journal of Clinical Practice*, researchers from Turkey and Macedonia investigated the association between serum vitamin B12, body mass index (BMI), and the nutritional status of obese women. Data were collected between January 2014 and June 2014; the cohort included females between the ages of 18 and 65 years. Based on their BMI values, the women were assigned to nonobese or obese groups. Blood samples were obtained for every subject, and nutritional information was gathered during face-to-face interviews. The researchers learned that the nonobese women had significantly higher levels of serum vitamin B12 than the obese women, and the levels of vitamin B12 "negatively correlated with BMI." In addition, levels of serum vitamin B12 were "closely associated with amount of nutrition containing animal protein except fish."[13]

Vitamin B12 Deficiency Is More Common in Morbidly Obese Men and Women

In a retrospective, randomized study published in 2013 in the *International Journal of Food and Nutritional Sciences*, researchers from India wanted to learn more about the association between morbid obesity and vitamin B12. The cohort consisted of 65 randomly selected morbidly obese men and women who were treated at a tertiary care hospital; all of the participants had BMI values over 35. (BMI is a measure of body fat based on height and weight.) The average age of the subjects was 38 years. There were almost equal numbers of vegetarian and nonvegetarian subjects. Forty-two of the subjects (65%) were vitamin B12 deficient; of these, 14 were male and 28 were female. The researchers commented that the "prevalence observed in the present study was found to be highly significant and consistent with several other studies addressing the problem with vitamin B12 deficiency."[14]

Pernicious Anemia May Be Treated with Oral Vitamin B12 Instead of Intramuscular Vitamin B12

In a research review published in 2016 in *Frontiers in Medicine*, researchers from Singapore wanted to learn if people with pernicious anemia could be treated with oral vitamin B12 instead of intramuscular vitamin B12. Would people respond as well to oral supplementation as they do to shots? (Once diagnosed, people with pernicious anemia require vitamin B12 for the remainder of their lives.) The researchers identified several relevant articles published from January 1, 1980, to March 31, 2016. Included in the review were two randomized, controlled trials, three prospective papers, one systematic review, and six clinical reviews. The participants in these studies ranged in age from 23 to 92 years. The researchers determined that oral vitamin B12, at a daily dose of 1,000 mcg, was an effective replacement treatment for pernicious anemia. Still, the researchers advised people with symptoms from severe vitamin B12 deficiency to begin with intramuscular treatments. "Subsequently, patients may be able to convert to oral replacement with close monitoring."[15]

Low Levels of Vitamin B12 during Pregnancy Appear to Increase the Risk of Preterm Birth and Low Birth Weight

In a systematic review and meta-analysis published in 2017 in the *American Journal of Epidemiology*, researchers from a number of different countries, but based in Norway, examined the association between low levels of vitamin B12 during pregnancy and risk of preterm birth and low birth weight. The analysis included 18 studies from 11 countries with 11,216 pregnancies. The researchers found evidence that lower maternal B12 levels were associated with a higher risk of preterm birth, especially in the cases of B12 deficiency. In fact, women who had B12 deficiency were 21 percent more likely to have a preterm birth. Why is this important? Preterm birth is the leading cause of neonatal death. Levels of vitamin B12 did not appear to affect birth weight. The researchers concluded that there is a "need to conduct randomized controlled trials to evaluate whether maternal B12 supplementation in pregnancy reduces the risk of preterm birth."[16]

Vitamin B12 Supplementation May Not Provide Significant Neurological or Cognitive Benefits to the Elderly

In a double-blind, randomized, placebo-controlled study published in 2016 in the *American Journal of Clinical Nutrition*, researchers from the United Kingdom wanted to determine if vitamin B12 supplementation would be useful for the elderly with moderate—not severe—vitamin B12 deficiency. The researchers used data from the Older People and Enhanced Neurological Function study conducted in Southeast England. The cohort consisted of 201 participants who were 75 years old or older; they had a mean age of 80 years. Forty-seven percent of the participants were men. For one year, the elders took either a vitamin B12 supplement or a placebo. When compared to those on the placebo, the people taking the supplement demonstrated no evidence of improved neurological or cognitive function. While research has proven that elders with severe deficiency benefit from supplementation, in this study, people with moderate deficiency did not experience the same improvements. The researchers commented that their findings "are unlikely to be generalizable to a less healthy older population with more severe vitamin B12 deficiency."[17]

In a multicenter, double-blind, randomized, placebo-controlled trial, published in 2014 in the journal *Neurology*, researchers based in the Netherlands examined the ability of vitamin B12 and folic acid to benefit thinking and memory in elders. The cohort consisted of 2,919 men and women with a mean age of 74.1 years, who participated in the B-Vitamins for the Prevention of Osteoporotic Fractures study. All of the subjects had elevated homocysteine levels, which placed them at increased risk for cognitive decline and dementia. For two years, the participants took daily vitamin B12 and folate supplementation or a placebo. Cognitive functioning was determined by using the Mini-Mental State Examination; the test evaluated episodic memory, attention and working memory, information processing speed, and executive function. The researchers had initially theorized that the elders on supplementation would experience less cognitive decline than those on the placebo. However, the researchers found that the cognitive domain scores of the two groups had only the negligible differences. The researchers concluded that vitamin B12 "may slightly slow the rate of decline of global cognition, but the reported small difference may be attributable to chance."[18]

NOTES

1. University of Maryland Medical Center. "Vitamin B12 (Cobalamin)." December 30, 2017. http://www.umm.edu/health/medical/altmed/supplement/vitamin-b12-cobalamin.

2. The George Mateljan Foundation. "Vitamin B12-Cobalamin." December 30, 2017. http://whfoods.com/genpage.php?tname=nutrient&dbid=107.

3. Ibid.

4. University of Maryland Medical Center. "Vitamin B12 (Cobalamin)." December 30, 2017. http://www.umm.edu/health/medical/altmed/supplement/vitamin-b12-cobalamin.

5. Pawlak, R., S. E. Lester, and T. Babatunde. "The Prevalence of Cobalamin Deficiency among Vegetarians Assessed by Serum Vitamin B12: A Review of Literature." *European Journal of Clinical Nutrition* 68 (2014): 541–548.

6. McArthur, Jennifer O., HoMan Tang, Peter Petocz, and Samir Samman. "Biological Variability and Impact of Oral Contraceptives on Vitamins B6, B12 and Folate Status in Women of Reproductive Age." *Nutrients* 5 (2013): 3634–3645.

7. Pfisterer, Kaylen J., Mike T. Sharratt, George G. Heckman, and Heather H. Keller. "Vitamin B12 Status in Older Adults Living in Ontario Long-Term Care Homes: Prevalence and Incidence of Deficiency with Supplementation as a Protective Factor." *Applied Physiology, Nutrition & Metabolism* 41, no. 2 (February 2016): 219–222.

8. Jung, S. B., V. Nagaraja, A. Kapur, and G. D. Eslick. "Association between Vitamin B12 Deficiency and Long-Term Use of Acid-Lowering Agents: A Systematic Review and Meta-Analysis." *Internal Medicine Journal* 45, no. 4 (2015): 409–416.

9. Kaner, G., M. Soylu, N. Yüksel, et al. "Evaluation of Nutritional Status of Patients with Depression." *BioMed Research International.* Article ID 521481 (2015): nine pages.

10. Araújo, D. A., M. B. Noronha, N. A. Cunha, et al. "Low Serum Levels of Vitamin B12 in Older Adults with Normal Nutritional Status by Mini Nutritional Assessment." *European Journal of Clinical Nutrition* 70, no. 7 (July 2016): 859–862.

11. Lewerin, C., H. Nilsson-Ehle, S. Jacobsson, et al. "Low Holotranscobalamin and Cobalamins Predict Incident Fractures in Elderly Men: The MrOS Sweden." *Osteoporosis International* 25 (2014): 131–140.

12. Kwok, T., P. Chook, M. Qiao, et al. "Vitamin B-12 Supplementation Improves Arterial Function in Vegetarians with Subnormal Vitamin B-12 Status." *The Journal of Nutrition, Health & Aging* 16, no. 6 (2012): 569–573.

13. Baltaci, D., M. H. Deler, Y. Turker, et al. "Evaluation of Serum Vitamin B12 Level and Related Nutritional Status among Apparently Healthy Obese Female Individuals." *Nigerian Journal of Clinical Practice* 20, no. 1 (January 2017): 99–105.

14. Goyal, Raksha, Sanjay Dhanuka, Vishwesh Mehta, et al. "To Study the Vitamin B12 Status in Morbidly Obese Patients." *International Journal of Food and Nutritional Sciences* 2, no. 2 (April–June 2013): 73–76.

15. Chan, C.Q., L.L. Low, and K.H. Lee. "Oral Vitamin B12 Replacement for the Treatment of Pernicious Anemia." *Frontiers in Medicine* 3 (August 2016): Article 38.

16. Rogne, Tormod, Myrte J. Tielemans, Mary Foong-Fong Chong, et al. "Associations of Maternal Vitamin B12 Concentration in Pregnancy with the Risks of Preterm Birth and Low Birth Weight: A Systematic Review and Meta-Analysis of Individual Participant Data." *American Journal of Epidemiology* 185, no. 3 (January 20, 2017): 212–223.

17. Miles, Lisa M., Elizabeth Allen, Kerry Mills, et al. "Vitamin B-12 Status and Neurologic Function in Older People: A Cross-Sectional Analysis of Baseline Trial Data from the Older People and Enhanced Neurological Function (OPEN) Study." *American Journal of Clinical Nutrition* 104 (2016): 790–796.

18. van der Zwaluw, Nikita L., Rosalie A. M. Dhonukshe-Rutten, Janneke P. van Wijngaarden, et al. "Results of Two-Year Vitamin B Treatment on Cognitive Performance." *Neurology* 83 (2014): 2158–2166.

REFERENCES AND FURTHER READINGS

Araújo, D. A., M. B. Noronha, N. A. Cunha, et al. "Low Serum Levels of Vitamin B12 in Older Adults with Normal Nutritional Status by Mini Nutritional Assessment." *European Journal of Clinical Nutrition* 70, no. 7 (July 2016): 859–862.

Baltaci, D., M.H. Deler, Y. Turker, et al. "Evaluation of Serum Vitamin B12 Level and Related Nutritional Status among Apparently Healthy Obese Female Individuals." *Nigerian Journal of Clinical Practice* 20, no. 1 (January 2017): 99–105.

Chan, C.Q., L.L. Low, and K.H. Lee. "Oral Vitamin B12 Replacement for the Treatment of Pernicious Anemia." *Frontiers in Medicine* 3 (August 2016): Article 38.

The George Mateljan Foundation. "Vitamin B12-Cobalamin." December 30, 2017. http://whfoods.com/genpage.php?tname=nutrient&dbid=107.

Goyal, Raksha, Sanjay Dhanuka, Vishwesh Mehta, et al. "To Study the Vitamin B12 Status in Morbidly Obese Patients." *International Journal of Food and Nutritional Sciences* 2, no. 2 (April–June 2013): 73–76.

Jung, S.B., V. Nagaraja, A. Kapur, and G.D. Eslick. "Association between Vitamin B12 Deficiency and Long-Term Use of Acid-Lowering Agents: A Systematic Review and Meta-Analysis." *Internal Medicine Journal* 45, no. 4 (2015): 409–416.

Kaner, G., M. Soylu, N. Yüksel, et al. "Evaluation of Nutritional Status of Patients with Depression." *BioMed Research International*. Article ID 521481 (2015): nine pages.

Kwok, T., P. Chook, M. Qiao, et al. "Vitamin B-12 Supplementation Improves Arterial Function in Vegetarians with Subnormal Vitamin B-12 Status." *The Journal of Nutrition, Health & Aging* 16, no. 6 (2012): 569–573.

Lewerin, C., H. Nilsson-Ehle, S. Jacobsson, et al. "Low Holotranscobalamin and Cobalamins Predict Incident Fractures in Elderly Men: The MrOS Sweden." *Osteoporosis International* 25 (2014): 131–140.

McArthur, Jennifer O., HoMan Tang, Peter Petocz, and Samir Samman. "Biological Variability and Impact of Oral Contraceptives on Vitamins B6, B12, and Folate Status in Women of Reproductive Age." *Nutrients* 5 (2013): 3634–3645.

Miles, Lisa M., Elizabeth Allen, Kerry Mills, et al. "Vitamin B-12 Status and Neurologic Function in Older People: A Cross-Sectional Analysis of Baseline Trial Data from the

Older People and Enhanced Neurological (OPEN) Study." *American Journal of Clinical Nutrition* 104 (2016): 790–796.

Office of Dietary Supplements, National Institutes of Health. "Vitamin B12." December 30, 2017. https://ods.od.nih.gov/factsheets/VitaminB12-Consumer/.

Pawlak, R., S. E. Lester, and T. Babatunde. "The Prevalence of Cobalamin Deficiency among Vegetarians Assessed by Serum Vitamin B12: A Review of Literature." *European Journal of Clinical Nutrition* 68 (2014): 541–548.

Pfisterer, Kaylen J., Mike T. Sharratt, George G. Heckman, and Heather H. Keller. "Vitamin B12 Status in Older Adults Living in Ontario Long-Term Care Homes: Prevalence and Incidence of Deficiency with Supplementation as a Protective Factor." *Applied Physiology, Nutrition & Metabolism* 41, no. 2 (February 2016): 219–222.

Rogne, Tormod, Myrte J. Tielemans, Mary Foong-Fong Chong, et al. "Associations of Maternal Vitamin B12 Concentration in Pregnancy with the Risks of Preterm Birth and Low Birth Weight: A Systematic Review and Meta-Analysis of Individual Participant Data." *American Journal of Epidemiology* 185, no. 3 (January 20, 2017): 212–223.

University of Maryland Medical Center. "Vitamin B12 (Cobalamin)." December 30, 2017. http://www.umm.edu/health/medical/altmed/supplement/vitamin-b12-cobalamin.

van der Zwaluw, Nikita L., Rosalie A. M. Dhonukshe-Rutten, Janneke P. van Wijngaarden, et al. "Results of Two-Year Vitamin B Treatment on Cognitive Performance." *Neurology* 83 (2014): 2158–2166.

Vitamin C

Also known as ascorbic acid, vitamin C is probably one of the most highly recognized vitamins. It is water soluble, which means it is not stored by the body. New supplies of vitamin C must be taken in every day.

Vitamin C is needed for the growth and repair of tissues in the body and to absorb iron from nonheme sources. It is required for the production of collagen, a protein essential to make skin, tendons, ligaments, and blood vessels. Vitamin C is used to heal wounds and form scar tissue, and it supports bones and teeth.

Vitamin C is an antioxidant. It helps prevent damage from free radicals. Free radical damage plays a role in aging and the development of medical problems such as arthritis, heart disease, and cancer.

FOOD SOURCES AND SUPPLEMENTS

There are many excellent sources of vitamin C. These include papaya, bell peppers, broccoli, Brussels sprouts, strawberries, pineapple, oranges, kiwifruit, cantaloupe, cauliflower, kale, cabbage, bok choy, grapefruit, parsley, turnip greens, beet greens, mustard greens, collard greens, raspberries, Swiss chard, tomatoes, lemons and limes, spinach, asparagus, sea vegetables, fennel, and thyme. Very good sources of vitamin C include sweet potatoes, winter squash, green peas, blueberries, cranberries, watermelon, green beans, summer squash, carrots, plums, garlic, basil, dill, and romaine lettuce. Good sources of vitamin C include potatoes, avocados, onions, banana, apple, pears, leeks, apricot, celery, cucumber, peppermint, and cilantro.[1]

Vitamin C is generally included in multivitamins. Vitamin C may also be purchased as a single-ingredient supplement. It is sold in tablets, capsules, liquids, and chewables. There are even crystalline and effervescent alternatives. People with sensitive stomachs may wish to try buffered vitamin C. Supplements should be taken with meals.

INTAKE RECOMMENDATIONS

The National Academy of Sciences has the following Recommended Dietary Allowances for vitamin C. For infants, the academy has adequate intakes. Males who are 19 years old or older should take in 90 mg per day, while females who are 19 years or older should take in 75 mg per day. Women who are 19 years of age and older who are pregnant should take in 85 mg per day, while women who are 19 years and older who are breast-feeding should take in 115 mg per day. Individuals who smoke require 35 mg per day more vitamin C per day than nonsmokers. Male teens between the ages of 14 and 18 years should take in 75 mg per day, while female teens who are between 14 and 18 years old should take in 65 mg per day. Females between the ages of 14 and 18 years who are pregnant should take in 80 mg per day, while females between the ages of 14 and 18 years who are breast-feeding should take in 115 mg per day. Males and females between the ages of 9 and 13 years should take in 45 mg per day, while children between the ages of 4 and 8 years should take in 25 mg per day. Children between the ages of one and three should take in 15 mg per day. Infants from 7 to 12 months should take in 50 mg per day, while infants from birth to 6 months should take in 40 mg per day.

There are also tolerable upper intake levels for vitamin C. People 19 years and older should take in no more than 2,000 mg per day, while teens between the ages of 14 and 18 years should take in no more than 1,800 mg per day. Children between the ages of 9 and 13 years should take in no more than 1,200 mg per day, while children between the ages of 4 and 8 years should take in no more than 650 mg per day. Children between the ages of one and three years should take in no more than 400 mg per day, while no upper limit has been established for infants.[2]

DEFICIENCY AND EXCESS

Most people probably obtain a sufficient amount of vitamin C from their intake of various fruits and vegetables. But some people are at increased risk for deficiency. Because smoking increases the body's vitamin C requirement, smokers and those exposed to secondhand smoke have an increased risk of deficiency. People who eat a limited diet and those with malabsorption problems have an increased risk. Kidney disease requiring dialysis and some types of cancer add to the risk of deficiency. People who take in very little vitamin C for several weeks are at risk for scurvy. Symptoms of scurvy include fatigue, inflammation and/or bleeding of the gums, small red or purple spots on the skin, joint pain, poor wound healing, corkscrew hairs (kinking of individual hairs), depression, and the loosening and/or loss of teeth.

The excessive intake of vitamin C is believed to have a low toxicity. Still, a high intake of vitamin C has been associated with diarrhea, nausea, abdominal cramps, and other gastrointestinal problems.

KEY RESEARCH FINDINGS

Vitamin C Supplementation Appears to Improve Endothelial Function

In a systematic review and meta-analysis published in 2014 in the journal *Atherosclerosis*, researchers from the United Kingdom and Iraq examined the association between vitamin C supplementation and endothelial function or the functioning of the thin layers of cells that line blood vessels. Endothelial dysfunction appears in the early stages of vascular disorders and is related to the progression of clinical complications. The researchers pooled data from 44 clinical trials that included 1,129 participants. These studies found that oral doses of vitamin C supplementation greater than 500 mg per day had a significant positive effect on endothelial function. After further evaluations, the researchers learned that vitamin C supplementation improved endothelial function significantly in people with diabetes, atherosclerosis, and heart failure but not in people with high blood pressure. The researchers commented that "the effect of vitamin C supplementation appeared to be dependent on health status, with stronger effects in those at higher cardiovascular disease risk."[3]

Vitamin C Supplementation May Be Useful for Younger Men with Marginal Vitamin C Status

In a randomized, double-blind study published in 2014 in the journal *Nutrients*, researchers from Arizona (United States) wanted to determine if vitamin C supplementation would benefit men with low-to-average vitamin C intake. Specifically, what impact would vitamin C supplementation have on physical activity and respiratory tract infections in 28 healthy men between the ages of 18 and 35 years? For eight weeks, 15 men took 1,000 mg of vitamin C each day and 13 took a placebo. The researchers found that during the last two weeks of the trial, the men taking supplementation increased their level of physical activity by 40 percent. In addition, fewer men in the supplementation group reported becoming ill with colds and, when they did develop a cold, the duration was reduced by an average of 59 percent. The participants did not report any side effects from the supplementation. The researchers concluded that their data "suggested measurable health advantages associated with vitamin C supplementation in a population with adequate-to-low vitamin C status."[4]

Vitamin C Supplementation May Help Prevent Cognitive Decline

In a study published in 2017 in the journal *Annals of Pharmacotherapy*, researchers from Canada wanted to determine if vitamins C and E supplementation could slow cognitive decline in people 65 years old or older. The researchers used data from the Canadian Study of Health and Aging, a cohort study of dementia that had three evaluation waves at five-year intervals. The data were collected at 18 centers across Canada. This study included 5,269 participants. About 10 percent of the cohort reported taking vitamin C or E supplements. The researchers learned that the use of either supplement was associated with a decreased risk of all causes of dementia and Alzheimer's disease. In addition, the use of these supplements was "modestly" associated with a lower risk of cognitive impairment, not dementia. The researchers concluded that "the use of vitamin E and C supplements is associated with a reduced risk of cognitive decline."[5]

Vitamin C Supplementation Appears to Lower Blood Pressure

In a systematic review and meta-analysis published in 2012 in the *American Journal of Clinical Nutrition*, researchers from Baltimore, Maryland, and Madrid, Spain, investigated research studies that examined the association between vitamin C supplementation and blood pressure. The researchers located 29 trials that met their criteria. In the trials, the median dose of vitamin C was 500 mg per day, and the median duration was eight weeks. Trial sizes ranged from 10 to 120 participants; the mean age of the participants ranged from 22 to 74 years. The researchers learned that vitamin C supplementation was associated with significant reductions in both diastolic and systolic blood pressure, with the greatest reductions seen in people with high blood pressure (hypertension). Since most of the data were derived from smaller, short-term trials, the researchers advised future longer-term trials. "Before vitamin C supplementation can be recommended for the prevention of hypertension or as an adjuvant antihypertensive therapy, additional trials are needed, designed with large sample sizes, and with attention to quality of BP [blood pressure] assessment."[6]

Vitamin C Supplementation May Hinder Endurance Training

In a double-blind, randomized, controlled trial published in 2014 in *The Journal of Physiology*, researchers from Norway, Finland, and Little Rock, Arkansas, wanted to learn how supplementation with vitamins C and E would affect young men and women who participated in a 10-week strength training program. During the study, 32 participants took either a supplement containing vitamins C and E or a placebo, and they participated in four training sessions each week. The researchers found that the men and women taking the supplements experienced less improvement of muscular endurance than those on the placebo. The supplementation appeared to blunt the amount of training-induced increase of mitochondrial proteins, which are required for the improvement of muscular endurance. The researchers noted that people participating in endurance training should use this supplementation with a good deal of caution or not at all. The researchers concluded that "young, healthy individuals who exercise for improved strength and muscle growth should avoid consuming high doses of vitamins C and E close to the exercise sessions because, if anything, the effects tend to be undesirable."[7]

Foods High in Vitamin C May Help Prevent Cataracts

In a study published in 2016 in the journal *Ophthalmology*, researchers from the United Kingdom noted that the surgical removal of cataracts from the eyes is the most common operation performed in their country. (With cataracts, there is a clouding of the normally clear lens of the eyes.) Each year, in the United Kingdom, there are more than 300,000 of these procedures. And the risk of developing cataracts increases as one ages. The researchers examined the progression of cataracts in 324 pairs of female twins over the course of 10 years. Evaluations were made of the eye lenses, and a food questionnaire was used to measure vitamin C intake. The researchers found that, after 10 years, the participants with high levels of dietary vitamin C had clearer lenses and a 33 percent reduced risk of cataract progression. The intake of dietary vitamin C "significantly influenced nuclear cataract progression."[8]

There Appears to Be an Association between Vitamin C and the Risk of Stroke

In a meta-analysis published in 2013 in the *Journal of the American Heart Association*, researchers from China reviewed prospective studies on the relationship between vitamin C and the risk of stroke. Their review consisted of 12 articles on vitamin C intake and 6 articles on circulating vitamin C. The studies on vitamin C intake included a total of 217,454 participants with 3,762 stroke events and were published between 1995 and 2011. Six of these studies were conducted in Europe, three were from the United States, and three were from Asia. The studies on circulating vitamin C involved 29,648 participants and 989 stroke events. They were published between 1993 and 2008. Five of the studies were from Europe, and one was from Japan. The findings are notable. Both intake of dietary vitamin C and circulating vitamin C were significantly inversely associated with the risk of stroke—in a dose-response manner. Interestingly, supplemental vitamin C intake was not significantly associated with a reduced risk of strokes, but this analysis was based on only three studies and 770 stroke cases.[9]

Vitamin C Supplementation Reduces Inflammation in Hypertensive and/or Diabetic Obese Adults

In an open-label, parallel, controlled trial published in 2015 in the journal *Drug Design, Development and Therapy*, researchers from Malaysia and Gaza City (in the Gaza Strip) wanted to determine if supplemental vitamin C would be useful for the inflammation experienced by hypertensive and/or diabetic obese adults. The researchers recruited 64 obese patients, who were hypertensive and/or diabetic, from primary health-care centers in Gaza City. They ranged in age from 20 to 60 years; everyone had high levels of inflammation. The participants were randomly placed in an experimental group, which was treated with 500 mg of vitamin C twice daily, or a control group. Members of the control group were "kept free of supplements." After eight weeks, the researchers found that the vitamin C supplementation had a number of positive effects. For example, it reduced levels of high-sensitivity C-reactive protein (a measure of inflammation) and fasting blood glucose. The researchers concluded that supplemental vitamin C may reduce inflammation in hypertensive and/or diabetic obese people.[10]

Vitamin C May Reduce Breathing Problems after Exercise

In a meta-analysis published in 2014 in the journal *Allergy, Asthma & Immunology*, a researcher from Finland examined the effects of vitamin C on people who experience exercise-related respiratory problems. The analysis included three studies on people suffering from exercise-induced bronchoconstriction (coughing, wheezing, and shortness of breath), five studies on short-term heavy physical stress, and one study on male adolescent competitive swimmers with respiratory symptoms. On reviewing the studies on exercise-induced bronchoconstriction, the researchers learned that vitamin C reduced postexercise bronchoconstriction by 48 percent. In the other two groups of studies, vitamin C halved the incidence of respiratory problems. According to the researchers, "these nine randomized trials indicated that vitamin C has genuine biological effects on pulmonary functions and respiratory symptoms in people doing heavy exercise." The researchers added that people who have these exercise-related symptoms may wish to give vitamin C a try.[11]

Supplemental Vitamin C May Lower Lipid Levels in People with Type 2 Diabetes

In a prospective, double-blind, placebo-controlled 12-week study, researchers from India investigated the ability of supplemental vitamin C to lower lipid levels in people with type 2 diabetes. It is well known that people with type 2 diabetes have an increased risk of cardiovascular disease. The cohort consisted of 70 subjects between the ages of 30 and 60 years, who were patients at an outpatient diabetes clinic in a tertiary care hospital. They were divided into two groups of 35. One group was placed on vitamin C supplementation; the participants took 1,000 mg per day; the members of the other group took placebos. While the subjects maintained their usual dietary patterns, they were asked to limit consumption of dietary vitamin C. All of the subjects were on a diabetes medication known as metformin. By the end of the study, the subjects taking vitamin C supplementation had significant increases in serum vitamin C. More important, they had significant reductions in total cholesterol, triglyceride levels, low-density lipoprotein ("bad cholesterol"), and very low-density lipoprotein. These changes did not occur in the subjects in the placebo group. Although the researchers acknowledged that their findings should be "interpreted cautiously," they noted that vitamin C supplementation for people with type 2 diabetes may be "a particularly attractive therapeutic adjuvant in the treatment."[12]

Vitamin C Is Associated with a Reduced Risk of Heart Failure in Older Men

In a prospective study published in 2013 in the journal *Circulation: Heart Failure*, researchers from the United Kingdom examined the association between levels of plasma vitamin C and risk of heart failure in older men. The cohort consisted of 3,919 men between the ages of 60 and 79 years; most of the men were Caucasian and of European extraction. At baseline, none of the men had evidence of heart failure. During a mean follow-up of 11 years, there were 263 cases of heart failure. Dietary intake was obtained from a detailed seven-day recall food frequency questionnaire. Intake of vitamins and minerals was also recorded, and levels of plasma vitamin C were measured. The researchers learned that plasma vitamin C was inversely associated with cardiovascular risk factors, such as high blood pressure, adiposity, levels of "good" (high-density lipoprotein) cholesterol, and heart rate. And, when compared to men who had the lowest levels of plasma vitamin C, higher plasma levels of vitamin C were associated with a significant reduction in the risk of incident heart failure. The researchers commented that there is a need for primary intervention trials in older people who are at risk for heart failure. These could help "to confirm whether increasing plasma vitamin C levels through supplements or diet would reduce risk of HF [heart failure]."[13]

Levels of Vitamin C May Also Be Associated with Heart Failure in Women

In a prospective, population-based study published in 2011 in the *American Heart Journal*, researchers from Germany and the United Kingdom examined the association between vitamin C plasma concentrations and incident fatal and nonfatal heart failure events. The cohort consisted of 9,187 men and 11,112 women between the ages of 39 and 79 years. Data were obtained from the European Prospective Investigation into Cancer and Nutrition—Norfolk study. At baseline, all of the subjects were apparently healthy. During a mean follow-up of 12.8 years, there were 1,258 incident cases of heart failure. Of these, 154 were fatal. Vitamin C plasma levels were higher in women than men. Higher levels of serum vitamin C were associated with reduced cases of heart failure. And there was a strong correlation between dietary fruit and vegetable intake and levels of plasma vitamin C. The researchers concluded that high plasma concentrations of vitamin may be useful in the prevention of heart failure. "This observation should be regarded as [a] hypothesis generating further prospective trials."[14]

NOTES

1. The George Mateljan Foundation. "Vitamin C." December 30, 2017. http://whfoods.com/genpage.php?tname=nutrient&dbid=109.

2. Office of Dietary Supplements, National Institutes of Health. "Vitamin C." December 30, 2017. https://ods.od.nih.gov/factsheets/VitaminC-Consumer/.

3. Ashor, Ammar W., Jose Lara, John C. Mathers, and Mario Siervo. "Effect of Vitamin C on Endothelial Function in Health and Disease: A Systematic Review and Meta-Analysis of Randomised Controlled Trials." *Atherosclerosis* 235, no. 1 (2014): 9–20.

4. Johnston, Carol S., Gillean M. Barkyoumb, and Sara S. Schumacher. "Vitamin C Supplementation Slightly Improves Physical Activity Levels and Reduces Cold Incidence in Men with Marginal Vitamin C Status: A Randomized Controlled Trial." *Nutrients* 6, no. 7 (2014): 2572–2583.

5. Basambombo, Luta Luse, Pierre-Hugues Carmichael, Sharlène Côté, and Danielle Laurin. "Use of Vitamin E and C Supplements for the Prevention of Cognitive Decline." *Annals of Pharmacotherapy* 51, no. 2 (2017): 118–124.

6. Juraschek, Stephen P., Eliseo Guallar, Lawrence J. Appel, and Edgar R. Miller III. "Effects of Vitamin C Supplementation on Blood Pressure: A Meta-Analysis of Randomized Controlled Trials." *American Journal of Clinical Nutrition* 95 (2012): 1079–1088.

7. Paulsen, G., H. Hamarsland, K. T. Cumming, et al. "Vitamin C and E Supplementation Alters Protein Signaling after a Strength Training Session, but Not Muscle Growth during 10 Weeks of Training." *The Journal of Physiology* 592 (2014): 5391–5408.

8. Yonova-Doing, Ekaterina, Zoe A. Forkin, Pirro G. Hysi, et al. "Genetic and Dietary Factors Influencing the Progression of Nuclear Cataract." *Ophthalmology* 123 (2016): 1237–1244.

9. Chen, Guo-Chong, Da-Bing Lu, Zhi Pang, and Qing-Fang Liu. "Vitamin C Intake, Circulating Vitamin C and Risk of Stroke: A Meta-Analysis of Prospective Studies." *Journal of the American Heart Association* 2, no. 6 (December 2013): e000329.

10. Ellulu, Mohammed S., Asmah Rahmat, Ismail Patimah, et al. "Effect of Vitamin C on Inflammation and Metabolic Markers in Hypertensive and/or Diabetic Obese Adults: A Randomized Controlled Trial." *Drug Design, Development and Therapy* 9 (2015): 3405–3412.

11. Hemilä, Harri. "The Effect of Vitamin C on Bronchoconstriction and Respiratory Symptoms Caused by Exercise: A Review and Statistical Analysis." *Allergy, Asthma & Clinical Immunology* 10, no. 1 (2014): 58+.

12. Chaudhari, Harshal V., Ganesh N. Dakhale, Shashikumar Chaudhari, et al. "The Beneficial Effect of Vitamin C Supplementation on Serum Lipids in Type 2 Diabetic Patients: A Randomized Double Blind Study." *International Journal of Diabetes & Metabolism* 20, no. 2 (August 2012): 53–58.

13. Wannamethee, Sasiwarang Goya, Karl Richard Bruckdorfer, Andrew Gerald Shaper, et al. "Plasma Vitamin C, but Not Vitamin E, Is Associated with Reduced Risk of Heart Failure in Older Men." *Circulation: Heart Failure* 6, no. 4 (2013): 647–654.

14. Pfister, Roman, Stephen J. Sharp, Robert Luben, et al. "Plasma Vitamin C Predicts Incident Heart Failure in Men and Women in European Prospective Investigation into Cancer and Nutrition—Norfolk Prospective Study." *American Heart Journal* 162, no. 2 (August 2011): 246–253.

REFERENCES AND FURTHER READINGS

Ashor, Ammar W., Jose Lara, John C. Mathers, and Mario Siervo. "Effect of Vitamin C on Endothelial Function in Health and Disease: A Systematic Review and Meta-Analysis of Randomised Controlled Trials." *Atherosclerosis* 235, no. 1 (2014): 9–20.

Basambombo, Luta Luse, Pierre-Hugues Carmichael, Sharlène Côté, and Danielle Laurin. "Use of Vitamin E and C Supplements for the Prevention of Cognitive Decline." *Annals of Pharmacotherapy* 51, no. 2 (2017): 118–124.

Chaudhari, Harshal V., Ganesh N. Dakhale, Shashikumar Chaudhari, et al. "The Beneficial Effect of Vitamin C Supplementation on Serum Lipids in Type 2 Diabetic Patients: A Randomized Double Blind Study." *International Journal of Diabetes & Metabolism* 20, no. 2 (August 2012): 53–58.

Chen, Guo-Chong, Da-Bing Lu, Zhi Pang, and Qing-Fang Liu. "Vitamin C Intake, Circulating Vitamin C and Risk of Stroke: A Meta-Analysis of Prospective Studies." *Journal of the American Heart Association* 2, no. 6 (December 2013): e000329.

Ellulu, Mohammed S., Asmah Rahmat, Ismail Patimah, et al. "Effect of Vitamin C on Inflammation and Metabolic Markers in Hypertensive and/or Diabetic Obese Adults: A Randomized Controlled Trial." *Drug Design, Development and Therapy* 9 (2015): 3405–3412.

The George Mateljan Foundation. "Vitamin C." December 30, 2017. http://whfoods.com/genpage.php?tname=nutrient&dbid=109.

Hemilä, Harri. "The Effect of Vitamin C on Bronchoconstriction and Respiratory Symptoms Caused by Exercise: A Review and Statistical Analysis." *Allergy, Asthma & Clinical Immunology* 10, no. 1 (2014): 58+.

Johnston, Carol S., Gillean M. Barkyoumb, and Sara S. Schumacher. "Vitamin C Supplementation Slightly Improves Physical Activity Levels and Reduces Cold Incidence in Men with Marginal Vitamin C Status: A Randomized Controlled Trial." *Nutrients* 6, no. 7 (2014): 2572–2583.

Juraschek, Stephen P., Eliseo Guallar, Lawrence J. Appel, and Edgar R. Miller III. "Effects of Vitamin C Supplementation on Blood Pressure: A Meta-Analysis of Randomized Controlled Trials." *American Journal of Clinical Nutrition* 95 (2012): 1079–1088.

Office of Dietary Supplements, National Institutes of Health. "Vitamin C." December 30, 2017. https://ods.od.nih.gov/factsheets/VitaminC-Consumer/.

Paulsen, G., H. Hamarsland, K. T. Cumming, et al. "Vitamin C and E Supplementation Alters Protein Signaling after a Strength Training Session, but Not Muscle Growth during 10 Weeks of Training." *The Journal of Physiology* 592 (2014): 5391–5408.

Pfister, Roman, Stephen J. Sharp, Robert Luben, et al. "Plasma Vitamin C Predicts Incident Heart Failure in Men and Women in European Prospective Investigation into Cancer and Nutrition—Norfolk Prospective Study." *American Heart Journal* 162, no. 2 (August 2011): 246–253.

University of Maryland Medical Center. "Vitamin C (Ascorbic Acid)." December 31, 2017. http://www.umm.edu/health/medical/altmed/supplement/vitamin-c-ascorbic-acid.

Wannamethee, Sasiwarang Goya, Karl Richard Bruckdorfer, Andrew Gerald Shaper, et al. "Plasma Vitamin C, but Not Vitamin E, Is Associated with Reduced Risk of Heart Failure in Older Men." *Circulation: Heart Failure* 6, no. 4 (2013): 647–654.

Yonova-Doing, Ekaterina, Zoe A. Forkin, Pirro G. Hysi, et al. "Genetic and Dietary Factors Influencing the Progression of Nuclear Cataract." *Ophthalmology* 123 (2016): 1237–1244.

Vitamin D

Vitamin D is a fat-soluble vitamin that plays an integral role in many bodily functions. Vitamin D is probably best known for regulating the absorption of calcium and phosphorus in bone, thereby helping to build and maintain strong bones. In addition, vitamin D is a key component of the immune system, where it may prevent certain cancers, such as breast, colorectal, skin, pancreatic, and prostate cancer. Vitamin D has also been linked to high blood pressure, depression, and obesity.

There are two dietary forms of vitamin D: ergocalciferol is vitamin D2 and cholecalciferol is vitamin D3. Cholecalciferol is thought to be more effective at raising levels of serum vitamin D.

The liver and kidneys make vitamin D when the skin is exposed to sunlight. That is why many people, especially those who live in northern climates, produce insufficient amounts of vitamin D. The amount of vitamin D made also varies from person to person and is reduced by the use of sunscreen. People with darker skin absorb less sunlight than those with lighter skin, and it is also harder for the elderly to absorb sufficient sunlight to make vitamin D. Though indoor tanning equipment may be used to increase vitamin D production, they greatly increase the risk of skin cancer and should be avoided. In the United States, the majority of men and women have low levels of vitamin D.

FOOD SOURCES AND SUPPLEMENTS

Vitamin D is also found in some foods, primarily foods that are fortified with this vitamin. Milk is often fortified with vitamin D. Other commonly fortified foods include cereals and juices. Salmon is an excellent source of vitamin D. Very good sources include sardines, while good sources include tuna, eggs, and shiitake mushrooms.[1]

Vitamin D is contained in most multivitamins, and it may be purchased as a single supplement in soft gels, capsules, tablets, and liquids. Strengths vary from 50 to 1,000 IU. Higher doses are also sold, but they should not be taken without input from a medical provider. For people who are unable to digest fat, a medical provider may prescribe an injectable vitamin D.

INTAKE RECOMMENDATIONS

The Office of Dietary Supplements of the National Institutes of Health cites the following recommendations for vitamin D. Pregnant and breastfeeding women should take in 600 IU per day, while adults 71 years and older should take in 800 IU per day. People between the ages of 1 and 70 years should take in 600 IU per day, while infants should take in 400 IU per day. The tolerable upper limit for vitamin D is 4,000 IU for people nine years old and older. For children between the ages of one and eight years, the tolerable upper limit is 2,500 to 3,000 IU. And the tolerable upper limit for infants is 1,000 to 1,500 IU.[2]

DEFICIENCY AND EXCESS

Generally, younger people tend to have better levels of serum vitamin D than older people. Males have higher levels than females. By race, non-Hispanic blacks tend to have the lowest levels and non-Hispanic whites tend to have the highest levels. Breastfed infants have low levels and should take supplementation. Because vitamin D needs fat to be absorbed, people who have problems digesting fats, such as those with Crohn's disease, may be deficient. Vitamin D deficiency is more often seen in people who are obese. When their body fat binds with vitamin D, the vitamin D is not absorbed. In children, vitamin D deficiency may cause rickets, a medical problem in which the bones become soft and bend. In adults, vitamin D deficiency may lead to osteomalacia, which causes bone pain and muscle weakness.

The only way to have excessive serum levels of vitamin D is to take far too much supplementation; it is impossible to reach excessive levels from food or from sun exposure. People who have an extremely high level of vitamin D in their blood may develop a condition known as hypercalcemia, which means they have excess amounts of calcium. Hypercalcemia is associated with nausea, confusion, and fatigue. The symptoms improve when levels of serum vitamin D are dramatically reduced. Excess vitamin D is thought to be a rare condition.

KEY RESEARCH FINDINGS

Vitamin D May Be Useful for Fatigue

In a double-blind, placebo-controlled clinical trial published in 2016 in the journal *Medicine*, researchers from Switzerland wanted to learn if vitamin D3 supplementation would be useful for healthy people dealing with fatigue. The cohort consisted of 120 people with a mean age of 29 years; slightly more than half were women; 92 percent were Caucasian. All of the participants, who had low levels of serum vitamin D, were randomized to a single oral dose of 100,000 units of vitamin D or a placebo. Fifty-eight subjects took the supplement and 62 took the placebo. The supplement and placebo were manufactured to have identical appearance, taste, and smell. After four weeks, there were notable changes in the subjects who took the supplement. They had higher levels of serum vitamin D, and they were far less likely to be fatigued. The researchers commented that "a single dose of oral 100,000 IU vitamin D3 is an effective, well-tolerated, and economical treatment strategy for healthy adults who report fatigue."[3]

There May Be an Association between Levels of Vitamin D and Depressive Symptoms

In a study published in 2015 in the journal *Psychiatry Research,* researchers from Oregon and New York City wanted to learn more about the association between levels of serum vitamin D and depressive symptoms. The cohort consisted of 185 female undergraduates, between the ages of 18 and 25 years, who lived in the Pacific Northwest during the fall, winter, and spring academic terms. The subjects completed the Center for Epidemiologic Studies Depression scale weekly for four weeks, and blood was drawn to measure levels of serum vitamin D3. During the different evaluations, between 34 and 42 percent of the women reported clinically significant depressive symptoms. The women with lower levels of vitamin D3 had an increased risk for depressive symptoms. The researchers concluded that vitamin D "deficiency and insufficiency occur at high rates in healthy young women." In addition, lower levels of vitamin D3 are associated with "clinically significant depressive symptoms."[4]

In a systematic review and meta-analysis published in 2013 in the *British Journal of Psychiatry,* researchers from Canada also examined the relationship between vitamin D and depression. Why is this relationship important? The researchers noted that depression is incredibly common. In fact, in higher-income countries, it is the third leading cause of disability, and it affects about 840 million people worldwide. It is important to know if something as simple as vitamin D supplementation could reduce these daunting statistics. The researchers included 10 cross-sectional studies, 3 cohort studies, and 1 case-control study with a total of 31,424 participants. All of the participants were at least 18 years old. The researchers wrote that they "performed a transparent and methodically . . . review of the [relevant] literature." The researchers determined that, when compared to controls, people with depression had lower levels of vitamin D. Furthermore, according to the researchers, there is the need for more studies to determine if lower levels of vitamin D cause depression. "Given the high prevalence of both vitamin D deficiency and depression, an association between these two conditions could have significant public health implications, particularly as supplementation with vitamin D is cost-effective and without significant adverse effects."[5]

People with Irritable Bowel Syndrome Tend to Have Low Levels of Serum Vitamin D

In a randomized, double-blind pilot study published in 2015 in the journal *BMJ Open Gastroenterology*, researchers from the United Kingdom investigated the use of vitamin D supplementation for irritable bowel syndrome (IBS). The initial cohort consisted of 51 patients with IBS. The subjects, with mean ages in their mid-30s, provided blood samples and completed a food frequency questionnaire. Another questionnaire obtained information on IBS symptoms—IBS with diarrhea, IBS with constipation, or IBS with mixed bowel habits. At baseline, between 70 and 81.8 percent of the subjects were deficient in vitamin D. For 12 weeks, the subjects took either a placebo or vitamin D supplementation or a probiotic and vitamin D supplement. By the end of the study, all of the subjects experienced increases in serum vitamin D. The group that took only vitamin D had the highest increases. The researchers acknowledged that their findings were limited by the small sample size and relatively short duration of the study. And nine of the participants failed to complete all the required paperwork. Studies with more subjects that continue for longer periods of time are needed. "As a pilot study the current trial is inherently underpowered."[6]

Adolescents Need a Regular Intake of Vitamin D

In a study published in 2016 in the *American Journal of Clinical Nutrition*, researchers from the United Kingdom wanted to learn more about the vitamin D requirements of teenagers. In the past, researchers have observed high levels of vitamin D inadequacy in adolescents. Adolescence is a period of rapid skeletal growth; having adequate amounts of vitamin D is essential for this growth to occur. During this trial, which took place in the winter, 110 male and female teens, between the ages of 14 and 18 years, were randomly assigned to take a placebo or 10 mcg or 20 mcg of vitamin D3 every day for 20 weeks. One hundred and five subjects completed the entire trial. The researchers found that in order to maintain adequate levels of serum vitamin D, teens must take in between 10 and about 30 mcg of vitamin D each day. The researchers added that their study "was conducted with healthy white subjects and should be repeated in other ethnic population groups for whom Vitamin D requirements may be higher."[7]

Bones of Healthy Children and Adolescents with Normal Vitamin D Levels May Not Benefit from Supplementation

In a systematic review and meta-analysis published in 2011 in the journal *BMJ*, researchers from Australia examined the effectiveness of vitamin D supplementation for improving bone mineral density in healthy children and adolescents. The cohort consisted of six studies with a total of 343 participants taking placebos and 541 participants taking vitamin D supplementation. All of the studies were conducted for at least three months in healthy children and teens between the ages of 8 and 17 years. The studies administered vitamin D3 with doses ranging from 132 IU daily to 14,000 IU per week. While the supplementation appeared to be well tolerated, the overall findings were that the supplementation did not have a statistically significant effect on the percentage change in total bone mineral content or bone mineral density of the hip or forearm. The researchers concluded that "targeting children and adolescents with low serum vitamin D concentrations could result in clinically important improvements in bone density but that vitamin D supplementation in healthy children and adolescents generally to improve bone density is not justified."[8]

There Is a Strong Association between Vitamin D Deficiency and Severe Obesity, and Low Socioeconomic Status Appears to Be a Risk Factor for Vitamin D Deficiency in Severely Obese Adults

In a retrospective study published in 2017 in the *Journal of Human Nutrition and Dietetics*, researchers from France wanted to learn more about the association between vitamin D and obesity. Their cohort consisted of 564 patients with severe or morbid obesity. The subjects recorded their dietary intake for five days. They also met with dietitians for face-to-face interviews. The researchers determined that almost all of the patients were deficient in vitamin D. In fact, 543 subjects had vitamin D deficiency; 35 percent of the subjects had severe vitamin deficiency. Only 21 people (4%) had a normal vitamin D status. Moreover, there was an inverse relationship between vitamin D status, body mass index, and fat mass. The researchers also learned that low socioeconomic status independently increased the risk of severe vitamin D deficiency. "These new findings highlight the need to pay particular attention to the health impact of vitamin D deficiency in socio-economically disadvantaged populations."[9]

Vitamin D Deficiency Is Common in Psychogeriatric Patients

In a study published in 2014 in the journal *BMC Psychiatry*, researchers from Norway examined the vitamin D status of psychogeriatric patients. Between March 2010 and December 2011, the researchers created a psychogeriatric patient group of 95 people (90 inpatients and 5 outpatients) and a matching control group of 104. All of the participants were older than 64 years and lived in northern Norway. Blood tests determined that 19.2 percent of the people in the control group were vitamin D deficient; at the same time, 71.6 percent of the elderly psychiatric patients were vitamin D deficient. The researchers noted that there is a possibility that vitamin D deficiency actually contributes to the development of at least some psychiatric disorders. And they suggested that "increased attention should be given to vitamin D deficiency in elderly patients with psychiatric disorders."[10]

There Appears to Be an Association between Serum Vitamin D Concentrations and Cognitive Function in Older Adults

In a population-based study published in 2015 in the *Journal of Alzheimer's Disease*, researchers from Germany examined the association between serum levels of vitamin D and cognitive functioning, specifically dementia, among community-dwelling older adults from southern Germany. The researchers collected data on 1,373 subjects (56.2% men) who were 65 years or older; they had a mean age of 75.6 years. The researchers determined that 75 subjects had mild dementia. And the subjects with dementia had significantly lower levels of serum vitamin D. The researchers noted that other studies have found similar results. Still, according to these researchers, additional studies are needed to confirm that vitamin D offers protection against cognitive decline. "Whether higher serum levels may offer protection against dementia in elderly should be clarified by randomized interventional trials."[11]

Higher Doses of Vitamin D Supplementation May Benefit Cognition

In a study published in 2017 in the journal *Experimental Gerontology*, a researcher from Canada wanted to learn if higher doses of vitamin D supplementation would improve human cognition. The cohort consisted of 82 healthy adults from northern British Columbia, Canada. Everyone was enrolled during the winter and early spring months. For 18 weeks, they were randomly placed on 400 IU per day (low dose) or 4,000 IU per day (high dose) of vitamin D. At baseline, there were no significant cognitive differences between the low-dose (n = 40) and high-dose (n = 42) groups. By the end of the trial, assessment testing determined that the members of the high-dose group had significantly higher levels of serum vitamin D. In addition, they experienced improvements in nonverbal (visual) memory. Verbal memory appeared to improve only with low-dose vitamin D. The researchers noted that their findings "should be viewed as being preliminary, and possibly due to chance effects, requiring confirmation in larger follow-up studies."[12]

Low Levels of Serum Vitamin D Appear to Be Associated with Metabolic Syndrome

In a prospective study published in 2012 in the *Journal of Clinical Endocrinology & Metabolism*, researchers from Canada and Australia investigated the association between low levels of serum vitamin D and metabolic syndrome, a clustering of metabolic traits including abdominal obesity, glucose intolerance, hypertension, and elevated cholesterol. The baseline data, which were derived from the Australian Diabetes, Obesity, and Lifestyle Study (AusDiab), included 4,164 people, with a mean age of 50 years, who did not have metabolic syndrome. Over a five-year period, there were 528 incident cases of metabolic syndrome (12.7%). The subjects who developed metabolic syndrome had lower levels of serum vitamin D. Moreover, when compared to subjects with higher levels of serum vitamin D, the subjects with low levels were associated "with up to a significant 74 percent" increased rate of developing metabolic syndrome. The researchers concluded that low levels of serum vitamin D should be considered "an independent risk factor for the development of MetS [metabolic syndrome]."[13]

Vitamin D Deficiency Is Highly Prevalent among Overweight and Obese U.S. Children

In a study published in 2013 in the journal *Pediatrics*, researchers from Dallas, Texas, noted that adequate vitamin D is essential for skeletal health in growing children. They wanted to learn if overweight and obese children had adequate amounts of vitamin D. The researchers used data on 6- to 18-year-old children who were enrolled in a cross-sectional study (2003–2006 National Health and Nutrition Examination Survey). Body weight and height were measured, and children were classified as healthy-weight, overweight, obese, or severely obese. Of the 12,292 children in the sample, the prevalence of vitamin D deficiency among healthy-weight, overweight, obese, and severely obese children was 21, 29, 34, and 49 percent, respectively. Vitamin D deficiency was more often seen among minority, older, and female children. In addition, there were significant racial and ethnic disparities. While severe vitamin D deficiency was found in 27 percent of white children, Latino children exceeded 50 percent, and African American children approached 90 percent. The researchers noted that there is a "need for vigilance in vitamin D deficiency screening and treatment of obese and minority children."[14]

Vitamin D Deficiency Is Common among Younger Children

In a study published in 2016 in the *British Journal of Nutrition*, researchers from Norway examined rates of vitamin D deficiency among children between the ages of six and eight years. Data were obtained from the Physical Activity and Nutrition in Children (PANIC) study. The cohort consisted of 184 females and 190 males. Dietary intake of vitamin D was assessed using food records for four consecutive days. There were also questions about the intake of vitamin and mineral supplements. Blood samples were collected after a 12-hour overnight fast. The researchers learned that almost all of the children took in insufficient amounts of vitamin D; less than half took vitamin D supplementation. The girls had lower intakes of vitamin D than the boys. The primary dietary sources of vitamin D were vitamin D–fortified milk, which is commonly used in Finland.

Other dietary sources of vitamin D included milk products, fat, and fish products. Only 20 percent of the vitamin D was obtained from natural dietary sources. The researchers concluded that "more attention should be paid to the sufficient intake of vitamin D from food and supplements, especially among children who do not use fortified milk products."[15]

Increased Levels of Vitamin D May Improve Treatment for Inflammatory Bowel Diseases

In a single-center, retrospective study published in 2017 in the journal *Alimentary Pharmacology & Therapeutics*, researchers based in Boston analyzed the association between levels of serum vitamin D and the effectiveness of treatment for inflammatory bowel diseases (IBD). The cohort consisted of 173 IBD patients at the Brigham and Women's Hospital in Boston; the collected data contained information on levels of serum vitamin D and the effectiveness of their three months of IBD treatments (with antitumor necrosis factor-α). The researchers learned that patients with low levels of vitamin D at the beginning of treatment had decreased odds of being in remission by the end of the treatment. According to the researchers, there appears to be a significant association between vitamin D status and remission of IBD with antitumor necrosis factor-α medication. And they concluded that larger studies on this association are needed. In time, it may be determined that vitamin D may play a supporting role in the treatment of IBD.[16]

Children with Vitamin D Deficiency Are More Likely to Develop Asthma, Allergies, and Eczema

In a study published in 2017 in the *Journal of Allergy and Clinical Immunology*, researchers from Australia wanted to learn more about the association between serum levels of vitamin D and the development of asthma, hay fever, and eczema in children. The initial cohort consisted of 263 children with a doctor-diagnosed history of asthma, hay fever, or eczema. The children were assessed at birth and at numerous follow-ups until the age of 10. The researchers learned that repeated bouts of vitamin D deficiency during early childhood heightened the risk for allergic sensitization and severe respiratory tract infections, which, in turn, increased the risk of asthma, hay fever, and eczema at the age of 10. The researchers commented that their findings "suggest that vitamin D deficiency during the first few years after birth might be one of the determinants of risk for the expression of current wheeze, asthma, or both in conjunction with atopy at 10 years."[17]

Vitamin D Deficiency in Childhood May Be Linked to Subclinical Atherosclerosis Later in Life

In a study published in 2015 in the *Journal of Clinical Endocrinology & Metabolism*, researchers from Finland and Australia wanted to learn more about the relationship between vitamin D deficiency and subclinical atherosclerosis later in life. (Subclinical means that there no symptoms.) The researchers measured the serum vitamin D levels of 2,148 Finnish children (1,187 females and 961 males) between the ages of 3 and 18 years. The subjects were reexamined 27 years later at the age of 30 to 45 years. During the adult examination, an ultrasound was used to measure carotid intima-thickness, an indicator of structural atherosclerosis (hardening and narrowing of the arteries). The researchers learned that the subjects in the lowest vitamin D quartile during childhood were at significantly higher risk for carotid intima-thickness in adulthood. The association was independent of conventional cardiovascular risk factors such as serum lipids, blood pressure, and smoking. On the other hand, low levels of vitamin D in adults were not associated with subclinical atherosclerosis. The researchers commented that their findings "suggested that subclinical vitamin D levels in childhood should be considered a possible risk factor for cardiovascular disease, although the therapeutic implications are unknown."[18]

There May Be an Association between Gestational Vitamin D Deficiency and Autism-Spectrum Disorders

In a study published online in 2016 in the journal *Molecular Psychiatry*, researchers from Australia, the Netherlands, and Denmark commented that there has been "intense interest" in identifying metabolic factors that may be associated with autism-spectrum disorders. The researchers used data on 4,229 mothers and children from the Generation R study, a population-based prospective cohort from fetal life onward, based in Rotterdam, the Netherlands. Maternal mid-gestation and neonatal blood tests revealed which women had low vitamin D levels, and a questionnaire completed by parents enabled researchers to learn which children had autistic traits by the age of six years. The researchers found that the women who were vitamin D deficient during pregnancy were significantly more likely to have children with autism-spectrum disorders. And the researchers concluded that "because gestational vitamin D deficiency is readily preventable with safe, cheap and accessible supplements, this candidate risk factor warrants closer scrutiny."[19]

NOTES

1. The George Mateljan Foundation. "Vitamin D." December 31, 2017. http://whfoods.com/genpage.php?tname=nutrient&dbid=110.

2. Office of Dietary Supplements, National Institutes of Health. "Vitamin D." December 31, 2017. https://ods.od.nih.gov/factsheets/VitaminD-Consumer/.

3. Nowak, Albina, Lukas Boesch, Erik Andres, et al. "Effect of Vitamin D3 on Self-Perceived Fatigue: A Double-Blind Randomized Placebo-Controlled Trial." *Medicine* 95, no. 52 (2016): e5353.

4. Kerr, David C. R., David T. Zava, Walter T. Piper, et al. "Associations between Vitamin D Levels and Depressive Symptoms in Healthy Young Adult Women." *Psychiatry Research* 227 (2015): 46–51.

5. Anglin, Rebecca E. S., Zainab Samaan, Stephen D. Walter, and Sarah D. McDonald. "Vitamin D Deficiency and Depression in Adults: Systematic Review and Meta-Analysis." *British Journal of Psychiatry* 202 (2013): 100–107.

6. Tazzyman, Simon, Nicholas Richards, Andrew R. Trueman, et al. "Vitamin D Associates with Improved Quality of Life in Participants with Irritable Bowel Syndrome: Outcomes from a Pilot Trial." *BMJ Open Gastroenterology* 2 (2015): e000052.

7. Smith, Taryn J., Laura Tripkovic, Camilla T. Damsgaard, et al. "Estimation of the Dietary Requirement for Vitamin D in Adolescents Ages 14–18 Years: A Dose-Response, Double-Blind, Randomized Placebo-Controlled Trial." *American Journal of Clinical Nutrition* 104 (2016): 1301–1309.

8. Winzenberg, Tania, Sandi Powell, Kelly Anne Shaw, and Graeme Jones. "Effects of Vitamin D Supplementation on Bone Density in Healthy Children: Systematic Review and Meta-Analysis." *BMJ* 342 (2011): c7254.

9. Léger-Guist'hau, J., C. Domingues-Faria, M. Miolanne, et al. "Low Socio-Economic Status Is a Newly Identified Independent Risk Factor for Poor Vitamin D Status in Severely Obese Adults." *Journal of Human Nutrition and Dietetics* 30, no. 2 (April 2017): 203–215.

10. Grønli, Ole, Jan Magnus Kvamme, Rolf Jorde, and Rolf Wynn. "Vitamin D Deficiency Is Common in Psychogeriatric Patients, Independent of Diagnosis." *BMC Psychiatry* 14 (2014): 134+.

11. Nagel, Gabriele, Florian Herbolsheimer, Matthias Riepe, et al. "Serum Vitamin D Concentrations and Cognitive Function in a Population-Based Study among Older Adults in South Germany." *Journal of Alzheimer's Disease* 45 (2015): 1119–1126.

12. Pettersen, Jacqueline A. "Does High Dose Vitamin D Supplementation Enhance Cognition?: A Randomized Trial in Healthy Adults." *Experimental Gerontology* 90 (April 2017): 90–97.

13. Gagnon, Claudia, Zhong X. Lu, Dianna J. Magliano, et al. "Low Serum 25-Hydroxyvitamin D Is Associated with Increased Risk of the Development of the Metabolic Syndrome at Five Years: Results from a National Population-Based Prospective Study (the Australian Diabetes, Obesity and Lifestyle Study: AusDiab)." *Journal of Clinical Endocrinology & Metabolism* 97, no. 6 (June 2012): 1953–1961.

14. Turer, Christy, Hua Lin, and Glenn Flores. "Prevalence of Vitamin D Deficiency among Overweight and Obese US Children." *Pediatrics* 131, no. 1 (January 2013): e152–e161.

15. Soininen, Sonja, Aino-Maija Eloranta, Virpi Lindi, et al. "Determinants of Serum 25-Hydroxyvitamin D Concentration in Finnish Children: The Physical Activity and Nutrition in Children (PANIC) Study." *British Journal of Nutrition* 115 (2016): 1080–1091.

16. Winter, R. W., E. Collins, B. Cao, et al. "Higher 25-Hydroxyvitamin D Levels Are Associated with Greater Odds of Remission with Anti-Tumour Necrosis Factor-α Medications among Patients with Inflammatory Bowel Diseases." *Alimentary Pharmacology & Therapeutics* 45 (2017): 653–659.

17. Hollams, Elysia M., Shu Mei Teo, Merci Kusel, et al. "Vitamin D over the First Decade and Susceptibility to Childhood Allergy and Asthma." *Journal of Allergy and Clinical Immunology* 139 (2017): 472–481.

18. Juonala, Markus, Atte Voipio, Katja Pahkala, et al. "Childhood 25-OH Vitamin D Levels and Carotid Intima-Media Thickness in Adulthood: The Cardiovascular Risk in Young Finns Study." *Journal of Clinical Endocrinology & Metabolism* 100, no. 4 (April 2015): 1469–1476.

19. Vinkhuyzen, A. A. E., D. W. Eyles, T. H. J. Burne, et al. "Gestational Vitamin D Deficiency and Autism-Related Traits: The Generation R Study." *Molecular Psychiatry.* Online, 2016.

REFERENCES AND FURTHER READINGS

Anglin, Rebecca E. S., Zainab Samaan, Stephen D. Walter, and Sarah D. McDonald. "Vitamin D Deficiency and Depression in Adults: Systematic Review and Meta-Analysis." *British Journal of Psychiatry* 202 (2013): 100–107.

Gagnon, Claudia, Zhong X. Lu, Dianna J. Magliano, et al. "Low Serum 25-Hydroxyvitamin D Is Associated with Increased Risk of the Development of the Metabolic Syndrome at Five Years: Results from a National, Population-Based Prospective Study (The Australian Diabetes, Obesity and Lifestyle Study: AusDiab)." *Journal of Clinical Endocrinology & Metabolism* 97, no. 6 (June 2012): 1953–1961.

The George Mateljan Foundation. "Vitamin D." December 31, 2017. http://whfoods.com/genpage.php?tname=nutrient&dbid=110.

Grønli, Ole, Jan Magnus Kvamme, Rolf Jorde, and Rolf Wynn. "Vitamin D Deficiency Is Common in Psychogeriatric Patients, Independent of Diagnosis." *BMC Psychiatry* 14 (2014): 134+.

Hollams, Elysia M., Shu Mei Teo, Merci Kusel, et al. "Vitamin D over the First Decade and Susceptibility to Childhood Allergy and Asthma." *Journal of Allergy and Clinical Immunology* 139 (2017): 472–481.

Juonala, Markus, Atte Voipio, Katja Pahkala, et al. "Childhood 25-OH Vitamin D Levels and Carotid Intima-Media Thickness in Adulthood: The Cardiovascular Risk in Young Finns Study." *Journal of Clinical Endocrinology & Metabolism* 100, no. 4 (April 2015): 1469–1476.

Kerr, David C. R., David T. Zava, Walter T. Piper, et al. "Associations between Vitamin D Levels and Depressive Symptoms in Healthy Young Adult Women." *Psychiatry Research* 227 (2015): 46–51.

Léger-Guist'hau, J., C. Domingues-Faria, M. Miolanne, et al. "Low Socio-Economic Status Is a Newly Identified Independent Risk Factor for Poor Vitamin D Status in Severely Obese Adults." *Journal of Human Nutrition and Dietetics* 30, no. 2 (April 2017): 203–215.

Nagel, Gabriele, Florian Herbolsheimer, Matthias Riepe, et al. "Serum Vitamin D Concentrations and Cognitive Function in a Population-Based Study among Older Adults in South Germany." *Journal of Alzheimer's Disease* 45 (2015): 1119–1126.

Nowak, Albina, Lukas Boesch, Erik Andres, et al. "Effect of Vitamin D3 on Self-Perceived Fatigue: A Double-Blind Randomized Placebo-Controlled Trial." *Medicine* 95, no. 52 (2016): e5353.

Office of Dietary Supplements, National Institutes of Health. "Vitamin D." December 31, 2017. https://ods.od.nih.gov/factsheets/VitaminD-Consumer/.

Pettersen, Jacqueline A. "Does High Dose Vitamin D Supplementation Enhance Cognition?: A Randomized Trial in Healthy Adults." *Experimental Gerontology* 90 (April 2017): 90–97.

Smith, Taryn J., Laura Tripkovic, Camilla T. Damsgaard, et al. "Estimation of the Dietary Requirement for Vitamin D in Adolescents Ages 14–18 Years: A Dose-Response, Double-Blind, Randomized Placebo-Controlled Trial." *American Journal of Clinical Nutrition* 104 (2016): 1301–1309.

Soininen, Sonja, Aino-Maija Eloranta, Virpi Lindi, et al. "Determinants of Serum 25-Hydroxyvitamin D Concentration in Finnish Children: The Physical Activity and Nutrition in Children (PANIC) Study." *British Journal of Nutrition* 115 (2016): 1080–1091.

Tazzyman, Simon, Nicholas Richards, Andrew R. Trueman, et al. "Vitamin D Associates with Improved Quality of Life in Participants with Irritable Bowel Syndrome: Outcomes from a Pilot Trial." *BMJ Open Gastroenterology* 2 (2015): e000052.

Turer, Christy, Hua Lin, and Glenn Flores. "Prevalence of Vitamin D Deficiency among Overweight and Obese US Children." *Pediatrics* 131, no. 1 (January 2013): e152–e161.

Vinkhuyzen, A. A. E., D. W. Eyles, T. H. J. Burne, et al. "Gestational Vitamin D Deficiency and Autism-Related Traits: The Generation R Study." *Molecular Psychiatry*. Online, 2016.

Winter, R. W., E. Collins, B. Cao, et al. "Higher 25-Hydroxyvitamin D Levels Are Associated with Greater Odds of Remission with Anti-Tumour Necrosis Factor-α Medications among Patients with Inflammatory Bowel Diseases." *Alimentary Pharmacology & Therapeutics* 45 (2017): 653–659.

Winzenberg, Tania, Sandi Powell, Kelly Anne Shaw, and Graeme Jones. "Effects of Vitamin D Supplementation on Bone Density in Healthy Children: Systematic Review and Meta-Analysis." *BMJ* 342 (2011): c7254.

Vitamin E

"Vitamin E" is a term used to describe eight different naturally occurring nutrients; these consist of four different tocopherols (alpha, beta, gamma, delta) and four different tocotrienols (alpha, beta, gamma, delta). Found in varying amounts in the diet, each of these is a fat-soluble antioxidant. Therefore, they offer protection from free radicals. Sometimes, the eight types are collectively said to be "tocochromanols."

Of the eight nutrients, the best known and most studied is alpha-tocopherol. That is why recommendations for vitamin E intake are usually measured in milligram equivalents or alpha-tocopherol or mg ATE.[1]

The body needs vitamin E to boost the immune system. It helps the body fight off bacteria and viruses, and it widens blood vessels and prevents clotting within the vessels.

FOOD SOURCES AND SUPPLEMENTS

Excellent sources of vitamin E include sunflower seeds, spinach, Swiss chard, turnip greens, asparagus, beet greens, mustard greens, and chili peppers. Very good sources of vitamin E include almonds, broccoli, bell peppers, kale, and tomatoes. Good sources of vitamin E include avocado, peanuts, shrimp, olives, olive oil, collard greens, cranberries, raspberries, kiwifruit, carrots, green beans, and leeks.[2] Small amounts of vitamin E are generally found in multivitamins. Vitamin E supplementation is sold in softgels, tablets, capsules, and topical oils. Health-care providers tend to recommend alpha-tocopherol or natural mixed tocopherols. But the doses in vitamin E supplements may be higher than most health professionals recommend. In addition, vitamin E supplementation may be made from food or synthetic sources. The vitamin E food supplementation, also known as natural vitamin E, is more potent than the synthetic form.

INTAKE RECOMMENDATIONS

The National Academy of Sciences established Dietary Reference Intakes for vitamin E. These include adequate intake levels for infants and Recommended Dietary Allowances for everyone over the age of one year. These amounts represent alpha-tocopherol equivalents. Adults, pregnant teens and women, and teens between the ages of 14 and 18 years should take in 15 mg or 22.4 IU per day, while breastfeeding teens and women should take in 19 mg or 28.4 IU per day. Children between the ages of 9 and 13 years should take in 11 mg or 16.4 IU per day, while children between the ages of 4 and 8 years should take in 7 mg or 10.4 IU per day. Children between the ages of one and three years should take in 6 mg or 9 IU per day. Infants over the age of six months should take in 5 mg (7.5 IU) per day, while infants up to six months should take in 4 mg (6 IU) per day. The tolerable upper limit of vitamin E for adults is 1,500 IU per day for supplements made from the natural form of vitamin E and 1,100 IU per day for supplements made from synthetic vitamin E. The upper limit for children should be lower.[3]

DEFICIENCY AND EXCESS

Most Americans consume less than the recommended amounts of vitamin E. Still, healthy Americans rarely experience any related symptoms. Vitamin E deficiency in more common in people who have problems digesting and/or absorbing fats, such as in those with Crohn's disease and cystic fibrosis. Diets that highly restrict fat may also increase the risk of deficiency. Long-term deficiency may cause liver and kidney problems. Symptoms of vitamin E deficiency include the loss of feeling in the arms and legs caused by nerve and muscle damage, the loss of body movement control, muscle weakness, vision problems, and a weakened immune system.

It appears to be impossible to consume too much vitamin E in foods. Taking in excessive amounts of vitamin E supplementation may increase the risk of bleeding, especially in the brain, which may cause a stroke.

KEY RESEARCH FINDINGS

Vitamin E Supplementation Does Not Appear to Affect All-Cause Mortality

In a meta-analysis published in 2011 in the journal *Current Aging Science*, researchers from Kentucky (United States) investigated randomized, controlled studies on the association between vitamin E supplementation and all causes of mortality. The 57 trials that were included in the analysis were published between 1988 and 2009. In all but 11 of the trials, vitamin E was used in combination with other supplements. Sample sizes ranged from 28 to 39,876, with a median sample size of 423. In total, there were 246,371 subjects and 29,295 deaths, and the trials continued for 1 to 10.1 years, with a mean time period of 2.6 years. The researchers learned that vitamin E supplementation was not associated with any increases or reductions in all causes of mortality. And the researchers concluded that "supplementation with vitamin E appears neither beneficial nor harmful in terms of mortality." That is why "vitamin E supplementation should not be recommended as a means of improving longevity."[4]

Many People May Have Low Levels of Serum Vitamin E

In a systematic review published online in 2016 in the *International Journal for Vitamin and Nutrition Research*, researchers from Switzerland and Germany wanted to learn more about the global intake of vitamin E. The researchers reviewed studies published between 2000 and 2012; a total of 176 articles referring to 132 single studies were included. There were 249,637 participants from 46 countries. Ranging in age from newborn to 106 years, the participants had a mean age of 49.8 years. Almost half of the studies were conducted in Europe. The findings were alarming. Only about one-fifth of the global population met recommended levels of vitamin E. The highest levels of deficiencies were found in populations in the Middle East and Africa (27%). But Asia Pacific had a deficiency rate of 16 percent, and Europe had a deficiency rate of 8 percent. Newborns and children were the most affected age groups. They tend to have lower levels of serum vitamin E than adults. According to these researchers, their findings suggest that much of the world takes in too little vitamin E. "Possible measures include encouragement of consumptions of vitamin E-rich food sources (e.g. vegetables, dairy products, eggs), adequate fortification of food products (e.g. vegetable oils), and supplementation."[5]

In a study published in 2015 in the online journal *PLoS ONE*, researchers from New Jersey, New York, the Netherlands, and Switzerland wanted to learn if young adults in the United States had sufficient levels of serum vitamin E. Data were obtained from the National Health and Nutrition Examination Survey (NHANES 2003–2006). For this survey, the data collection process included blood samples and interviews. The cohort included 7,922 subjects. The researchers learned that the subjects who obtained vitamin E only from food tended to be vitamin E deficient. In fact, nearly 9 in 10 of the subjects who were 20 to 30 years old were deficient; 7 in 10 of those between the ages of 31 and 50 years had low levels, as did 4 in 10 in those 51 years and older. Low levels of vitamin E were more often seen in African Americans and Mexican Americans than in non-Hispanic Whites. "Clearly, there is an opportunity for increased consumption of vitamin E rich foods such as nuts, oils, and whole grains or dietary supplement use." In addition, the findings underscore the importance "to continue monitoring vitamin E status in Americans."[6]

Vitamin E May Not Prevent Cardiovascular Disease

In a meta-analysis of randomized, controlled trials published in 2013 in the journal *BMJ*, researchers from Korea assessed the efficacy of vitamin and antioxidant supplements, including vitamin E, to prevent cardiovascular diseases, "the leading causes of deaths and disability worldwide." The cohort consisted of 50 trials with 294,478 participants (156,663 in intervention groups and 137,815 in control groups). The number of participants ranged from 61 to 39,876. When analyzing the data, the researchers considered a number of factors, such as types of vitamins and antioxidants, supplement doses, cardiovascular outcomes, methodological quality, duration of treatment, number of participants, type of control (placebo vs. no placebo), funding source, and provider of supplements. The data included all types of cardiovascular conditions. In the trials that reported age, the mean ages ranged from 49 to 82 years. The trials were published from 1989 to 2012. The researchers noted that they found "no evidence to support the use of vitamin or antioxidant supplements" to prevent cardiovascular problems. While some vitamin E trials demonstrated lower rates of heart attacks, "these beneficial effects were shown only in trials with supplements provided by the pharmaceutical industry."[7]

However, in Some Instances, Supplementation with Vitamin E May Be Associated with Reduced Risk of a Heart Attack

In a meta-analysis published in 2015 in the journal *Nutrition, Metabolism & Cardiovascular Diseases*, researchers from Italy wanted to learn if supplemental vitamin E would reduce the risk of cardiovascular events, such as heart attacks. They hoped to compare the effect of vitamin E alone or in combination with other antioxidants. The researchers pooled data from 16 randomized, controlled trials. The doses of vitamin E ranged from 33 to 800 IU, and the follow-ups ranged from 6 months to 9.4 years. The studies included between 100 and 39,876 participants. Researchers learned that when vitamin E was given alone, the risk of heart attack was significantly reduced. However, when combined with other antioxidants, no effects were observed. "It appears ineffective when associated with other antioxidants." The researchers commented that their findings provided "evidence that vitamin E supplementation in a range of 400–800 IU/daily is able to decrease myocardial infarction."[8]

Vitamin E Supplementation May Benefit People with Metabolic Syndrome

In a randomized, double-blind crossover trial published in 2017 in the *American Journal of Clinical Nutrition*, researchers from Oregon and Ohio (United States) examined the association between the ingestion of vitamin E and people with and without metabolic syndrome, a disorder characterized by a clustering of metabolic traits, including abdominal obesity, glucose intolerance, hypertension, and elevated cholesterol. The researchers recruited 20 participants: 10 were healthy and 10 had metabolic syndrome. During four 72-hour interventions, the participants ingested vitamin E with either nonfat milk, reduced-fat milk, whole milk, or soymilk. To determine levels of vitamin E, researchers assessed specific biomarkers in the urine and blood. The researchers learned that the subjects with metabolic syndrome excreted significantly less vitamin E than the healthy subjects. In fact, they retained between 30 and 50 percent more vitamin E than the healthy subjects. The researchers concluded that the subjects with metabolic syndrome had an increased need for vitamin E. The "participants with MetS [metabolic syndrome] had decreased vitamin E catabolism."[9] (Catabolism is the breakdown of complex molecules into simpler ones.)

Vitamin E Supplementation May Be Useful in the Prevention of Cognitive Decline

In a study published in 2017 in the journal *Annals of Pharmacotherapy*, researchers from Canada investigated the use of vitamins E and C for the prevention of cognitive decline in older people. Data on 5,269 subjects were obtained from the Canadian Study of Health and Aging (1991–2002), a cohort study of dementia that included three evaluation waves at five-yearly intervals. The fieldwork for this survey was conducted in 18 centers across Canada; all of the participants were 65 years or older. About 10 percent of the participants reported taking vitamin E or C supplements, the majority taking either vitamin supplement alone. When the researchers compared the participants taking the vitamin supplements to those who did not, the use of vitamin E and/or vitamin C supplements was significantly associated with dramatic reductions in dementia and Alzheimer's disease. When adjustments were made for confounders, all of the results remained significant. Supplementation with vitamins E and C was "modestly" associated with a lower risk of cognitive impairment, not dementia. According to these researchers, "These findings indicate additional support for the use of antioxidants as a preventive strategy against cognitive decline."[10]

In a population-based study published in 2013 in the journal *Experimental Gerontology*, researchers from Sweden, Italy, and Finland investigated the relationship between vitamin E and cognitive impairment. The cohort consisted of 140 non-cognitively impaired elderly subjects obtained from the Cardiovascular Risk Factors, Aging, and Dementia study in Finland. At baseline, all of the subjects were 65 years old or older. To detect cognitive impairment, the subjects were followed for a mean of eight years. None of the subjects reported using vitamin E supplements. The researchers determined that the subjects with higher levels of serum vitamin E had a reduced risk of cognitive impairment. They concluded that "various vitamin E forms might play a role in cognitive impairment."[11]

On the Other Hand, Vitamin E May Not Prevent Dementia

In a study published in 2017 in the journal *JAMA Neurology*, researchers from several locations in Kentucky and Seattle, Washington, examined the association between vitamin E, selenium, and dementia. The study initially began in 2002 as an investigation into the relationship between vitamin E and/or selenium in the prevention of prostate cancer in older men. In 2009, when it was evident that neither vitamin was useful against prostate cancer, the trial was stopped. About 3,790 of the participants agreed to remain in the cohort to test the usefulness of the supplements for the prevention of dementia. At baseline, none of the participants had dementia or any neuropsychiatric disorder that might affect cognition. The participants, who were all at least 60 years old, were placed on vitamin E, selenium, both, or a placebo until the study ended in May 2015. The researchers determined that the incidence of dementia was between 4 and 5 percent in each of the four groups. As a result, there was no statistical difference between the groups. Neither supplement appeared to prevent dementia. The researchers concluded that "supplemental use of vitamin E and selenium did not forestall dementia and are not recommended as preventive agents."[12]

Vitamin E Supplementation May Not Protect against Cancer

In a study published in 2014 in the *American Journal of Clinical Nutrition*, researchers from different locations in Boston investigated the use of vitamins E and C for the prevention of cancer in men. Beginning in 1997, 14,641 male physicians in the United States, who were 50 years or older, were randomly assigned to take 400 IU of vitamin E every other day, 500 mg of vitamin C every day, or a placebo. Though the vitamin treatment ended in 2007, observational follow-up continued through 2011. During the course of the trial, there were a total of 1,373 incident cases of prostate cancer and a total of 2,669 cases of documented cancers. There was no significant difference in the incidence of cancers between the subjects taking vitamin E and the subjects taking a placebo. The supplementation appeared to have "no effect." The use of vitamin E supplementation "has no immediate or long-term effect on cancer risk."[13]

Vitamin E Supplementation May Increase the Risk of Prostate Cancer in Healthy Men

In a study published in 2011 in *JAMA*, researchers from multiple locations in the United States and Canada wanted to determine the long-term effect of vitamin E and selenium supplementation on the risk of prostate cancer in relatively healthy men. The researchers randomized around 35,000 men from 427 study sites in the United States, Canada, and Puerto Rico; their data were known as the "Selenium and Vitamin E Cancer Prevention Trial" or SELECT. The men were randomly assigned to take vitamin E or selenium or both vitamin E and selenium or a placebo. When the original study ended in 2008, the researchers learned that vitamin E did not reduce the rates of prostate cancer. However, there was a slight "statistically nonsignificant" increase in prostate cancer. Three years later, almost 150 men in the vitamin E group were diagnosed with prostate cancer. That number stands in contrast to the 113 men in the placebo group diagnosed with prostate cancer. As a result, the men taking vitamin E had a 17 percent higher risk for prostate cancer than those taking the placebo. According to the researchers, "The findings show that vitamin E supplementation in the general population of healthy men significantly increases the risk of being diagnosed with prostate cancer." Likewise, "the observed 17% increase in prostate cancer incidence demonstrates the potential for seemingly innocuous yet biologically active substances such as vitamins to cause harm."[14]

Vitamin E Supplementation Does Not Appear to Affect the Overall Risk of Heart Failure

In a randomized, double-blind, placebo-controlled trial published in 2012 in the journal *Circulation: Heart Failure*, researchers from Boston wanted to learn more about the association between vitamin E and the risk of heart failure. The data, which were obtained from the Women's Health Study, included 39,815 initially healthy women, who were at least 45 years at baseline. The women were randomly assigned to take a vitamin E supplement every other day or a placebo. Over a median follow-up of 10.2 years, there were 220 incident cases of heart failure. There were 106 incident cases of heart failure in the vitamin E group and 114 cases in the placebo group. The small difference between the groups was not statistically significant. Still, the researchers cautioned that because their sample consisted primarily of healthy, middle-aged, Caucasian women, their findings "may not be generalized to other populations." And they underscored the need to focus on other primary prevention measures such as controlling blood pressure.[15]

NOTES

1. The George Mateljan Foundation. "Vitamin E." January 1, 2018. http://whfoods.com/genpage.php?tname=nutrient&dbid=111.

2. Ibid.

3. Office of Dietary Supplements, National Institutes of Health. "Vitamin E." January 1, 2018. https://ods.od.nih.gov/factsheets/VitaminE-Consumer/.

4. Abner, Erin L., Frederick A. Schmitt, Marta S. Mendiondo, et al. "Vitamin E and All-Cause Mortality: A Meta-Analysis." *Current Aging Science* 4, no. 2 (July 2011): 158–170.

5. Péter, Szabolcs, Angelika Friedel, Franz F. Roos, et al. "A Systematic Review of Global Alpha-Tocopherol Status as Assessed By Nutritional Intake Levels and Blood Serum Concentrations." *International Journal for Vitamin and Nutrition Research*. Online, July 14, 2016.

6. McBurney, M. I., E. A. Yu, E. D. Ciappio, et al. "Suboptimal Serum α-Tocopherol Concentrations Observed among Younger Adults and Those Depending Exclusively upon Food Sources, NHANES 2003–2006." *PLoS ONE* 10, no. 8 (August 19, 2015): e0135510.

7. Myung, S. K., W. Ju, B. Cho, et al. "Efficacy of Vitamin and Antioxidant Supplements in Prevention of Cardiovascular Disease: Systematic Review and Meta-Analysis of Randomised Controlled Trials." *BMJ* 346 (2013): f10.

8. Loffredo, L., L. Perri, A. Di Castelnuovo, et al. "Supplementation with Vitamin E Alone Is Associated with Reduced Myocardial Infarction: A Meta-Analysis." *Nutrition, Metabolism & Cardiovascular Diseases* 25 (2015): 354–363.

9. Traber, Maret G., Eunice Mah, Scott W. Leonard, et al. "Metabolic Syndrome Increases Dietary α-Tocopherol Requirements as Assessed Using Urinary and Plasma Vitamin E Catabolites: A Double-Blind, Crossover Clinical Trial." *American Journal of Clinical Nutrition* 105, no. 3 (March 2017): 571–579.

10. Basambombo, Luta Luse, Pierre-Hugues Carmichael, Sharlène Côté, and Danielle Laurin. "Use of Vitamin E and C Supplements for the Prevention of Cognitive Decline." *Annals of Pharmacotherapy* 51, no. 2 (February 2017): 118–124.

11. Mangialasche, Francesca, Alina Solomon, Ingemar Kåreholt, et al. "Serum Levels of Vitamin E Forms and Risk of Cognitive Impairment in a Finnish Cohort of Older Adults." *Experimental Gerontology* 48 (2013): 1428–1435.

12. Kryscio, Richard J., Erin L. Abner, Allison Caban-Holt, et al. "Association of Antioxidant Supplement Use and Dementia in the Prevention of Alzheimer's Disease by Vitamin E and Selenium Trial (PREADViSE)." *JAMA Neurology* 74, no. 5 (2017): 567–573.

13. Wang, L., H. D. Sesso, R. J. Glynn, et al. "Vitamin E and C Supplementation and Risk of Cancer in Men: Post-Trial Follow-Up in the Physicians' Health Study II Randomized Trial." *American Journal of Clinical Nutrition* 100, no. 3 (September 2014): 915–923.

14. Klein, Eric A., Ian M. Thompson Jr., Catherine M. Tangen, et al. "Vitamin E and the Risk of Prostate Cancer: Updated Results of the Selenium and Vitamin E Cancer Prevention Trial (SELECT)." *JAMA* 306, no. 14 (October 12, 2011): 1549–1556.

15. Chae, Claudia U., Christine M. Albert, M. V. Moorthy, et al. "Vitamin E Supplementation and the Risk of Heart Failure in Women." *Circulation: Heart Failure* 5 (2012): 176–182.

REFERENCES AND FURTHER READINGS

Abner, Erin L., Frederick A. Schmitt, Marta S. Mendiondo, et al. "Vitamin E and All-Cause Mortality: A Meta-Analysis." *Current Aging Science* 4, no. 2 (July 2011): 158–170.

Basambombo, Luta Luse, Pierre-Hugues Carmichael, Sharlène Côté, and Danielle Laurin. "Use of Vitamin E and C Supplements for the Prevention of Cognitive Decline." *Annals of Pharmacotherapy* 51, no. 2 (February 2017): 118–124.

Chae, Claudia U., Christine M. Albert, M. V. Moorthy, et al. "Vitamin E Supplementation and the Risk of Heart Failure in Women." *Circulation: Heart Failure* 5 (2012): 176–182.

The George Mateljan Foundation. "Vitamin E." January 1, 2018. http://whfoods.com/genpage.php?tname=nutrient&dbid=111.

Klein, Eric A., Ian M. Thompson Jr., Catherine M. Tangen, et al. "Vitamin E and the Risk of Prostate Cancer: Updated Results of the Selenium and Vitamin E Cancer Prevention Trial (SELECT)." *JAMA* 306, no. 14 (October 12, 2011): 1549–1556.

Kryscio, Richard J., Erin L. Abner, Allison Caban-Holt, et al. "Association of Antioxidant Supplement Use and Dementia in the Prevention of Alzheimer's Disease by Vitamin E and Selenium Trial (PREADViSE)." *JAMA Neurology* 74, no. 5 (2017): 567–573.

Loffredo, L., L. Perri, A. Di Castelnuovo, et al. "Supplementation with Vitamin E Alone Is Associated with Reduced Myocardial Infarction: A Meta-Analysis." *Nutrition, Metabolism & Cardiovascular Diseases* 25 (2015): 354–363.

Mangialasche, Francesca, Alina Solomon, Ingemar Kåreholt, et al. "Serum Levels of Vitamin E Forms and Risk of Cognitive Impairment in a Finnish Cohort of Older Adults." *Experimental Gerontology* 48 (2013): 1428–1435.

McBurney, M. I., E. A. Yu, E. D. Ciappio, et al. "Suboptimal Serum α-Tocopherol Concentrations Observed among Younger Adults and Those Depending Exclusively upon Food Sources, NHANES 2003–2006." *PLoS ONE* 10, no. 8 (August 19, 2015): e0135510.

Myung, S. K., W. Ju, B. Cho, et al. "Efficacy of Vitamin and Antioxidant Supplements in Prevention of Cardiovascular Disease: Systematic Review and Meta-Analysis of Randomised Controlled Trials." *BMJ* 346 (2013): f10.

Office of Dietary Supplements, National Institutes of Health. "Vitamin E." January 1, 2018. https://ods.od.nih.gov/factsheets/VitaminE-Consumer/.

Péter, Szabolcs, Angelika Friedel, Franz F. Roos, et al. "A Systematic Review of Global Alpha-Tocopherol Status as Assessed by Nutritional Intake Levels and Blood Serum Concentrations." *International Journal for Vitamin and Nutrition Research*. Online, July 14, 2016.

Traber, Maret G., Eunice Mah, Scott W. Leonard, et al. "Metabolic Syndrome Increases Dietary α-Tocopherol Requirements as Assessed Using Urinary and Plasma Vitamin E Catabolites: A Double-Blind, Crossover Clinical Trial." *American Journal of Clinical Nutrition* 105, no. 3 (March 2017): 571–579.

University of Maryland Medical Center. "Vitamin E." January 1, 2018. http://www.umm.edu/health/medical/altmed/supplement/vitamin-e.

Wang, L., H. D. Sesso, R. J. Glynn, et al. "Vitamin E and C Supplementation and Risk of Cancer in Men: Post-Trial Follow-Up in the Physicians' Health Study II Randomized Trial." *American Journal of Clinical Nutrition* 100, no. 3 (September 2014): 915–923.

Vitamin K

Named after the German word for blood clotting (*koagulation*), vitamin K is a fat-soluble vitamin, which is stored in fat tissue and the liver, that helps the body make proteins needed for normal blood clotting. Vitamin K is also required to make important bone proteins. Though there are actually three types of vitamin K (K1, K2, and K3), the vast majority of information and research on vitamin K focuses on K1. Therefore, this entry addresses vitamin K1, the natural form of the vitamin, which is the primary source of vitamin K that humans obtain from food.

Information on vitamin K frequently addresses its blood clotting properties. Why is that important? People who have low levels of vitamin K increase their risk for excessive bleeding, which may begin as oozing from the gums or nose. In addition, vitamin K is used to counteract an overdose of the blood thinner Coumadin. It has also been repeatedly shown that vitamin K supports bone health. People with deficient levels of vitamin K are at increased risk for bone fractures. There is limited evidence that vitamin K may be useful for postmenopausal women who are at increased risk for fractures.

FOOD SOURCES AND SUPPLEMENTS

Many vegetables contain excellent amounts of vitamin K. These include kale, spinach, mustard greens, collard greens, parsley, broccoli, Brussels sprouts, asparagus, cabbage, bok choy, green beans, and cauliflower. Top fruit sources of vitamin K are kiwifruit, blueberries, prunes, and grapes. Soybeans and miso are two good legume sources. Fish, liver, meat, eggs, and cereals contain small amounts.

Vitamin K may be included in a multivitamin, and vitamin K supplementation may be readily purchased online in pill and liquid forms. In some instances, medical providers give a shot of vitamin K. Still, before beginning a vitamin K regime, it is a good idea to discuss the issue with a medical provider.

INTAKE RECOMMENDATIONS

The Food and Nutrition Board at the Institute of Medicine recommends the following adequate intakes for vitamin K: Males age 19 years and older should have 120 mcg per day, while females aged 19 years and older need at least 90 mcg per day. Males and females aged 14 to 18 years should have 75 mcg per day, while children 9 to 13 years need 60 mcg per day. Children four to eight years need 55 mcg per day, and children one to three years require 30 mcg per day. Infants 7 to 12 months need 2.5 mcg per day, and infants 0 to 6 months need 2 mcg per day.[1]

DEFICIENCY AND EXCESS

Vitamin K deficiencies appear to be uncommon. Green vegetables tend to have excellent amounts of vitamin K. A single one-cup serving of broccoli provides more vitamin K than people need. Yet some people are at increased risk for vitamin K deficiency. People who have a medical problem that affects absorption in the digestive tract, such as Crohn's disease, may not absorb sufficient amounts of vitamin K. That may also be true for people who have taken certain medication, such as antibiotics, for long periods of time. People who are malnourished or drink alcohol in excess may have insufficient vitamin K. For these people, a health provider may recommend vitamin K supplementation. People with low levels of vitamin K are at increased risk for bleeding problems and osteoporosis, a condition in which the body's bones become increasingly more porous. Symptoms of vitamin K deficiency include bruising, gastrointestinal bleeding, excessive menstrual bleeding, and blood in the urine.

Though vitamin K deficiencies are thought to be rare in adults, vitamin K deficiencies are very common is newborn infants. Vitamin K does not cross the placenta to the fetus in sufficient amounts, and it may require several weeks for a newborn to develop enough vitamin K. That is why newborns are generally given a single injection of vitamin K.

There is no evidence that consuming vitamin K in food may lead to toxicity. On the other hand, high levels of vitamin K supplementation have the potential to be toxic. It may cause numbness or tingling in extremities. In general, people who take anticoagulant medications or blood thinners should check with their health-care provider before taking any vitamin K supplementation. Vitamin K supplements may interfere with the medication.

KEY RESEARCH FINDINGS

Dietary Intake of Vitamin K Appears to Be Inversely Associated with Mortality Risk

In a prospective study published in 2014 in *The Journal of Nutrition*, researchers from Spain wanted to learn more about the association between dietary intake of vitamin K and mortality in a Mediterranean population at high risk for cardiovascular disease. The cohort consisted of 7,216 participants in the PREDIMED study which had a median follow-up of 4.8 years. (The PREDIMED study was a large, parallel-group, multicenter, controlled, randomized clinical trial trying to assess the effect of the Mediterranean diet on the primary prevention of cardiovascular disease in elderly people at high risk for cardiovascular disease.) The participants were all community-dwelling men and women between the ages of 55 and 80 years. The intake of energy and nutrients were evaluated with the assistance of a 137-item food frequency questionnaire. The researchers determined that the participants with higher levels of dietary vitamin K had lower body mass index measurements and smaller waist circumference values. They were more physically active and less likely to smoke. The participants in the upper quartile of vitamin K dietary intake consumed nearly twice as many vegetables, especially leafy green vegetables, as those in the lower quartile. During the follow-up years, 81 of the participants died from cardiovascular events and 130 died from cancer. A total of 323 died from all causes. The researchers determined an inverse association between an increased dietary intake of vitamin K and all causes of mortality. The researchers concluded that dietary intake of vitamin K, which was relatively high in this cohort, played a "protective role in cardiovascular mortality, cancer mortality, and all-cause mortality."[2]

There May Be an Association between Low Levels of Vitamin K and Morbid Obesity

In a study published in 2015 in *International Journal of Clinical Practice*, the researchers from the United Kingdom wanted to assess vitamin K deficiencies in morbidly obese people prior to their bariatric surgery. The cohort consisted of 118 people who were referred to an obesity clinic between January 2010 and February 2011. They were all evaluated for potential bariatric surgery, or surgery that helps to facilitate weight loss. The cohort was predominately female and middle aged. Almost half of the subjects had hypertension or high blood pressure, and about one-third had type 2 diabetes. Forty percent of the subjects had low levels of vitamin K. Therefore, while these subjects consumed too many calories, they had "vitamin insufficiency." Vitamin K levels appeared to be inversely associated with body mass index. Subjects with lower levels of vitamin K had higher levels of body mass index. The researchers concluded that "vitamin K supplementation should be considered prebariatric surgery in patients with diabetes or severe insulin resistance."[3]

Vitamin K Supplementation Seems to Help Blood Sugar Levels in Premenopausal Women with Prediabetes

In a double-blind, placebo-controlled study published in 2015 in the *Journal of Diabetes & Metabolic Disorders*, researchers from Iran wanted to learn if vitamin K would be useful for premenopausal women with prediabetes. For four weeks, 82 women were randomized to consume vitamin K supplement (n = 39) or a placebo (n = 43). Their average age was 40.17 years, and their average weight was 156.2 pounds. As a result, most of the women were overweight. Blood samples were taken at baseline and after four weeks, and body mass index and body fat were measured before and after the intervention. At the end of the study, the researchers found that the vitamin K significantly decreased insulin and glucose levels. Vitamin K supplementation "improved glycemic status in premenopausal prediabetic women."

Dietary Intake of Vitamin K Seems to Support Better Bone Mineral Density

In a study published in 2015 in the *Journal of Clinical Biochemistry and Nutrition*, researchers from Korea examined the association between dietary intake of vitamin K and levels of bone mineral density in Korean adults. The cohort consisted of 2,785 men and 4,307 women, aged 19 years or older, from the fifth Korea National Health and Nutrition Examination Survey. The researchers found only a positive association between vitamin K intake and femur bone mineral density in men. In women, high levels of vitamin K intake were associated with significantly higher femur and lumber bone mineral density. It initially appeared that as vitamin K intake increased in women, the risk for osteoporosis decreased. But after adjusting for several factors, the effect was not sustained. But the researchers did learn that low dietary vitamin K intake was associated with low bone mineral density. The researchers concluded that "vitamin K is indeed a factor that influences bone density."[4]

Low Levels of Vitamins K1 and D Appear to Be Associated with Increased Risk for Hip Fractures in the Elderly

In a study published in 2016 in *Osteoporosis International*, researchers from Norway investigated the association between serum concentrations of vitamins K1 and D and the risk of hip fractures in elderly Norwegians. The cohort consisted of 21,774 community-residing men and women between the ages of 65 and 79 years from four population-based studies in Norway. Hip fracture data were obtained from hospitals during a follow-up period of 8.2 years. The researchers determined that low serum concentrations of K1 were associated with an increased risk for hip fractures. Moreover, when compared to the subjects with high serum concentrations of both vitamins, the subjects who had low levels of vitamins K1 and D had an even higher statistically significant risk of hip fractures. Elderly people with low levels of serum vitamins K1 and D are at increased risk for hip fractures.[5]

NOTES

1. Medlineplus. "Vitamin K." January 1, 2018. U.S. National Library of Medicine, National Institutes of Health. https://medlineplus.gov/vitamink.html.

2. Juanola-Falgarona, Martí, Jordi Salas-Salvadó, Miguel Ángel Martínez-González. "Dietary Intake of Vitamin K Is Inversely Associated with Mortality Risk." *The Journal of Nutrition* 144 (2014): 743–750.

3. Ewang-Emukowhate, M., D. J. Harrington, A. Botha, et al. "Vitamin K and Other Markers of Micronutrient Status in Morbidly Obese Patients before Bariatric Surgery." *International Journal of Clinical Practice* 69, no. 6 (June 2015): 638–642.

4. Kim, Mi-Sung, Eun-Soo Kim, and Cheong-Min Sohn. "Dietary Intake of Vitamin K in Relation to Bone Mineral Density in Korea Adults: The Korea National Health and Nutrition Examination Survey (2010–2011)." *Journal of Clinical Biochemistry and Nutrition* 57, no. 3 (November 2015): 223–227.

5. Finnes, T. E., C. M. Lofthus, H. E. Meyer, et al. "A Combination of Low Serum Concentrations of Vitamins K1 and D Is Associated with Increased Risk of Hip Fractures in Elderly Norwegians: A NOREPOS Study." *Osteoporosis International* 27, no. 4 (April 2016): 1645–1652.

REFERENCES AND FURTHER READINGS

Ewang-Emukowhate, M., D. J. Harrington, A. Botha, et al. "Vitamin K and Other Markers of Micronutrient Status in Morbidly Obese Patients before Bariatric Surgery." *International Journal of Clinical Practice* 69, no. 6 (June 2015): 638–642.

Finnes, T. E., C. M. Lofthus, H. E. Meyer, et al. "A Combination of Low Serum Concentrations of Vitamins K1 and D Is Associated with Increased Risk of Hip Fractures in Elderly Norwegians: A NOREPOS Study." *Osteoporosis International* 27, no. 4 (April 2016): 1645–1652.

Juanola-Falgarona, Martí, Jordi Salas-Salvadó, Miguel Ángel Martínez-González, et al. "Dietary Intake of Vitamin K Is Inversely Associated with Mortality Risk." *The Journal of Nutrition* 144 (2014): 743–750.

Kim, Mi-Sung, Eun-Soo Kim, and Cheong-Min Sohn. "Dietary Intake of Vitamin K in Relation to Bone Mineral Density in Korea Adults: The Korea National Health and Nutrition Examination Survey (2010–2011)." *Journal of Clinical Biochemistry and Nutrition* 57, no. 3 (November 2015): 223–227.

Medlineplus. "Vitamin K." January 1, 2018. U.S. National Library of Medicine, National Institutes of Health. https://medlineplus.gov/vitamink.html.

Rasekhi, Hamid, Majid Karandish, Mohammad Taha Jalali, et al. "Phylloquinone Supplementation Improves Glycemic Status Independent of the Effects of Adiponectin Levels in Premenopause Women with Prediabetes: A Double-Blind Randomized Controlled Clinical Trials." *Journal of Diabetes & Metabolic Disorders* 14, no. 1 (2015): 1.

Zinc

Zinc is an essential trace mineral found in every cell of the human body. Zinc is known to help heal wounds, and it plays a role in the immune system, reproduction, growth, taste, vision, smell, blood clotting, insulin regulation, and thyroid function. Interestingly, many people know about zinc from its alleged ability to reduce the symptoms of the common cold. While there are several over-the-counter zinc products to fight colds, researchers have been unable to explain how this works. It has also been suggested that zinc may be useful against the herpes virus.

In addition, zinc has antioxidant properties, which prevents damage to the cells from free radicals. Free radicals accelerate aging and support the development of cancer and heart disease.[1]

FOOD SOURCES AND SUPPLEMENTS

Oysters contain more zinc per serving than any other food. But people who eat more than a few oysters may be taking in excess amounts of zinc. Very good sources of zinc include beef, spinach, asparagus, shiitake mushrooms, and crimini mushrooms. Good sources include lamb, sesame seeds, pumpkin seeds, garbanzo beans, lentils, cashews, quinoa, turkey, shrimp, tofu, scallops, green peas, oats, yogurt, beet greens, summer squash, broccoli, Swiss chard, Brussels sprouts, miso, parsley, sea vegetables, tomatoes, and bok choy.[2] Almost all multivitamins contain zinc. Zinc is also available alone or combined with calcium, magnesium, or other ingredients in supplements. Zinc may be found in nasal sprays and gels; it may be sold as zinc gluconate, zinc sulfate, and zinc acetate. In addition, zinc may be found in over-the-counter products for colds, wounds, and denture adhesive creams.

INTAKE RECOMMENDATIONS

The Food and Nutrition Board of the Institute of Medicine has established Recommended Dietary Allowance quantities for zinc. Breastfeeding women 19 years or older should take in 12 mg per day, while teens between the ages of 14 and 18 years who are breast-feeding should take in 13 mg per day. Pregnant women 19 years or older should take in 11 mg per day, while pregnant teens between the ages of 14 and 18 years should take in 12 mg per day. Males who are 19 years or older should take in 11 mg per day, while females who are 19 years or older should take in 8 mg per day. Male teens between the ages of 14 and 18 years should take in 11 mg per day, while females between the ages of 14 and 18 years should take in 9 mg per day. Children between the ages of 9 and 13 years should take in 8 mg per day, while children between the ages of 4 and 8 years should take in 5 mg per day. Children between the ages of six months and three years should take in 3 mg per day. The adequate intake levels for zinc for infants from birth to six months is 2 mg per day. The tolerable upper intake level for zinc is 40 mg per day.[3]

DEFICIENCY AND EXCESS

Although zinc deficiency is more common in other parts of the world, in North America, most people take in adequate amounts of zinc. However, certain people are at increased risk for a zinc deficiency. These include people who have had gastrointestinal surgery or dealing with chronic digestive disorders, such as ulcerative colitis and Crohn's disease. Because beef contains very good amounts of zinc, vegetarians may be at increased risk for deficiency. Infants over the age of six months who are breastfed may need supplementation. People who consume larger amounts of alcohol and people with sickle cell disease may be deficient.

Zinc deficiency slows the growth of infants and children and delays sexual development in teens. It causes impotence in men and hair loss, diarrhea, eye and skin sores, and the loss of appetite. Other problems associated with zinc deficiency include weight loss, slowed wound healing, decreased ability to taste foods, and lower levels of alertness.

With the possible exception of oysters, it appears unlikely that the intake of zinc from food may be toxic. Toxicity seems to be caused by zinc supplementation or a nondietary exposure, such as from the ongoing use of denture creams that contain zinc. High intake of zinc is known to impair the absorption of copper, which may cause anemia and fatigue. Other side effects of the excessive amounts of zinc include nausea, vomiting, loss of appetite, stomach cramps, diarrhea, headaches, reduced immunity, and low levels of HDL or "good cholesterol."

KEY RESEARCH FINDINGS

Zinc and Multivitamin Supplementation Appears to Benefit Schoolchildren

In a randomized, controlled trial published in 2016 in the journal *Pediatrics International*, researchers from Thailand wanted to learn if zinc and multivitamin supplementation would improve the growth of healthy Thai schoolchildren. The cohort consisted of 140 children between the ages of 4 and 13 years (kindergarten to sixth grade). The children were divided into two groups of 70. For six months, during schooldays, the children received either zinc and multivitamins or a placebo. After two months, the children who received the zinc and multivitamins had a significantly higher gain in height. This was especially apparent in the preadolescents. Over the course of six months, the children in the supplementation group grew an average of 4.9 cm, compared to 3.6 cm in the placebo group. The supplements also improved the weight of children who were lighter than average. No significant adverse effects were reported. "Supplementation of chelated zinc plus multivitamins for 6 months significantly increased height gain in Thai schoolchildren and was well tolerated."[4]

As People Age, They May Have a Reduced Ability to Absorb Zinc

In a study published in 2013 in the *Journal of Nutritional Biochemistry*, researchers from Oregon wanted to learn more about the ability of aged mice to absorb zinc. As a result, they compared zinc levels in young and old mice. The researchers determined that the older mice had lower levels of zinc and increased chronic inflammation. And they commented that the current recommended intakes for zinc do not advise older people to take in higher levels. In fact, older people are told to take in the same amount as younger and middle-aged adults. Those recommendations may need to be adjusted. In many instances, zinc supplementation may be advised; in order to maintain their zinc requirement, older people may need to take in larger amounts of this mineral. "Improving zinc status in the aged mice via dietary zinc supplementation can overcome age-related chronic inflammation."[5]

Vegetarian Diets May Be Low in Zinc

In a meta-analysis and systematic review published in 2013 in the *Journal of the Science of Food and Agriculture*, researchers from Australia examined 34 observational studies on the association between vegetarian diets and levels of zinc. When compared to nonvegetarians, the researchers determined that vegetarians consumed less dietary zinc. "Populations who habitually consume strict vegetarian diets have lower zinc intakes and status." This difference in values between vegetarians and nonvegetarians was higher in females than males and greater in developing countries than developed countries. The researchers suggested that vegetarians on the low-zinc spectrum line should consider "dietary practices that increase zinc bioavailability . . . [and] the consumption of foods fortified with zinc or low-dose supplementation."[6]

Zinc Supplementation May Impact Pregnancy Outcomes

In a double-blind, placebo-controlled study published in 2015 in the *British Journal of Nutrition*, researchers from Egypt examined the association between levels of zinc supplementation and pregnancy outcomes. Their initial cohort consisted of 675 healthy pregnant women between the ages of 20 and 45 years; all of the participants had low levels of serum zinc. The women were then divided into three groups. One group took a daily zinc supplement; another group took a daily zinc supplement and multivitamins; and another group (control) took a placebo. The women were monitored from recruitment until one week after delivery. Five hundred and ninety-seven women completed the study. The researchers determined that the women in both supplement groups had significantly lower rates of stillbirth, preterm delivery, and early neonatal morbidity. In addition, both supplement regimens were almost equally effective in reducing second- and third-trimester pregnancy complications. The researchers noted that in Egypt pregnant women are routinely given iron and folic acid supplementation. It may well be advantageous to add zinc supplementation, which "was effective in reducing pregnancy complications and early neonatal infection among the Zn [zinc]–deficient women of the present trial."[7]

Zinc Supplementation May Increase Immunity Markers in the Elderly

In a randomized, double-blind, placebo-controlled study published in 2016 in the *American Journal of Clinical Nutrition*, researchers from the Boston area wanted to determine if zinc supplementation would improve markers of immunity for an elderly, nursing home population. The researchers recruited 31 residents of a nursing facility; all of the participants had low levels of serum zinc. For three months, 16 residents took zinc supplementation and 15 residents took a placebo. A total of 25 people completed the entire study, with 13 and 12 receiving the placebo and zinc capsules, respectively. The researchers learned that the zinc serum levels of the supplementation group increased by 16 percent over the placebo group. The researchers commented that their main finding was "that it is feasible to increase serum zinc concentration in nursing home residents with a low serum zinc concentration through supplementation with zinc." Some of the participants with low initial levels of zinc failed to reach recommended levels. They may require higher doses of zinc or may need to remain on supplementation for longer periods of time. Since high levels of zinc are associated with better T cell function and improved immunity, "the potential for reduction in infections and other chronic disease is high."[8]

Two Different Types of Zinc Lozenges Appear to Be Similarly Effective against the Common Cold

In a meta-analysis published in 2017 in the *Journal of the Royal Society of Medicine Open*, a researcher from Finland compared the efficacy of zinc acetate lozenges to zinc gluconate lozenges in treating the symptoms of a common cold. The analysis included seven randomized trials with 575 participants with "naturally acquired" common colds. The zinc doses ranged from 80 to 207 mg per day; three of the trials used zinc acetate, and four used zinc gluconate. All of the trials were randomized, placebo-controlled, and double-blind. The researchers determined that the zinc supplementation reduced the cold symptoms by 33 percent. Yet doses higher than 80 to 92 mg per day had no additional impact. According to the researchers, "The current evidence of efficacy for zinc lozenges . . . is so strong that common cold patients may be encouraged to try them for treating their colds."[9]

Low Levels of Zinc May Be Associated with Depressive Symptoms in Women

In a study published in 2012 in the *Journal of Affective Disorders*, researchers from Watertown, Massachusetts, investigated the association between zinc and depressive symptoms. The researchers analyzed cross-sectional, observational epidemiological data from the Boston Area Community Health (BACH) Survey. BACH included 2,301 men and 3,201 women between the ages of 30 and 79 years. Data were obtained during two-hour, in-person home interviews by a trained phlebotomist-interviewer. The final sample size was 3,708, with 2,163 women and 1,545 men. The researchers learned that depressive symptoms were seen in 15.9 percent of the men and 23.5 percent of the women. While an association was not seen in men, among women, dietary, supplemental and total zinc were significantly associated with the presence of depressive symptoms. Women in the lowest dietary zinc quartile were about 80 percent more likely to have depressive symptoms than those in the highest quartile. The risk for depression increased as the intake of zinc decreased. The association was strongest among women taking antidepressant (selective serotonin reuptake inhibitor) medications. The researchers commented that the "pronounced gender difference" that they observed "warrants further attention."[10]

In Spain, Large Percentages of the Population Are Not Meeting Their Zinc Requirements. This May Well Be Happening in Other Populations

In a study published in 2017 in the journal *Nutrients*, researchers from Spain examined the intake levels of six nutrients, including zinc, in the population of Spain. Data were obtained from the Spanish "Anthropometry, Intake and Energy Balance in Spain" (ANIBES) study, which included 2,009 participants between the ages of 9 and 75 years. The data were collected using a validated, photo-based, three-day food record. The fieldwork was performed at 128 sampling points across Spain from mid-September 2013 to mid-November 2013. The primary sources of zinc were meat, meat products, cereals, grains, and milk and dairy products. The researchers determined that a notable 83 percent of the population did not fulfill their zinc requirements. Elderly people were the most likely to have a lower reported intake of zinc. The researchers concluded that "a significant percentage of the Spanish ANIBES population does not meet the recommended intakes for zinc."[11]

Adolescents Who Consume a Mediterranean Diet Tend to Consume Sufficient Amounts of Zinc

In a study published in 2012 in the journal *Public Health Nutrition*, researchers from Spain examined the ability of the Mediterranean diet to provide sufficient zinc for adolescents. The Mediterranean diet is one that consists of higher amounts of vegetables, fish, legumes, and grains, and lower amounts of meats and dairy products. The cohort consisted of 20 healthy male adolescents between the ages of 11 and 14 years. The teens ate a Mediterranean diet—mostly supplied by a caterer hired by the researchers—for 28 days. Levels of zinc were assessed. When tested for zinc biomarkers, all of the teens had normal levels. Acknowledging that their findings may be limited by the small sample size and relatively brief duration of the study, the researchers recommended studies that last for longer periods of time. "Due to the importance of Zn [zinc] in preventing growth and behavioural disorders among adolescents, long-term trials to investigate the suitability of the Mediterranean diet with respect to Zn requirements at this time of life are needed."[12]

Zinc in Dental Fixtures May Cause Copper Deficiency Myelopathy

In an article published online in 2017 in the journal *BMJ Case Reports*, researchers from the United Kingdom described a 62-year-old patient who was referred to their neurology clinic after he developed numbness, pain, and weakness in his legs that continued for six months. After a number of tests, including magnetic resonance imaging, he was diagnosed with copper deficiency myelopathy.

The man, who had dentures that did not fit properly, had been using two to four tubes of denture fixative every week for 15 years. The man was told to discontinue the use of the fixative and begin taking copper supplementation. However, while the treatment did stop the progression of the illness, the man had a degree of irreversible nerve damage and was unable to achieve a complete recovery. Earlier treatment may have resulted in a better outcome. "Prompt recognition and treatment . . . may have prevented any irreversible neurological deficit."[13]

NOTES

1. Office of Dietary Supplements, National Institutes of Health. "Zinc." January 1, 2018. https://ods.od.nih.gov/factsheets/Zinc-Consumer/.

2. The George Mateljan Foundation. "Zinc." January 1, 2018. http://whfoods.com/genpage.php?tname=nutrient&dbid=115.

3. Office of Dietary Supplements, National Institutes of Health. "Zinc." January 1, 2018. https://ods.od.nih.gov/factsheets/Zinc-Consumer/.

4. Rerksuppaphol, Sanguansak and Lakkana Rerksuppaphol. "Effect of Zinc plus Multivitamin Supplementation on Growth in School Children." *Pediatrics International* 58 (2016): 1193–1199.

5. Wong, Carmen P., Kathy R. Magnusson, and Emily Ho. "Increased Inflammatory Response in Aged Mice Is Associated with Age-related Zinc Deficiency and Zinc Transporter Dysregulation." *Journal of Nutritional Biochemistry* 24 (2013): 353–359.

6. Foster, Meika, Anna Chu, Peter Petocz, and Samir Samman. "Effect of Vegetarian Diets on Zinc Status: A Systematic Review and Meta-Analysis of Studies in Humans." *Journal of the Science of Food and Agriculture* 93 (2013): 2362–2371.

7. Nossier, S. A., N. E. Naeim, N. A. El-Sayed, and A. A. Abu Zeid. "The Effect of Zinc Supplementation on Pregnancy Outcomes: A Double-Blind, Randomised Controlled Trial, Egypt." *British Journal of Nutrition* 114, no. 2 (July 2015): 274–285.

8. Barnett, Junaidah B., Maria C. Dao, Davidson H. Hamer, et al. "Effect of Zinc Supplementation on Serum Zinc Concentration and T Cell Proliferation in Nursing Home Elderly: A Randomized, Double-Blind, Placebo-Controlled Trial." *American Journal of Clinical Nutrition* 103 (2016): 942–951.

9. Hemilä, Harri. "Zinc Lozenges and the Common Cold: A Meta-Analysis Comparing Zinc Acetate and Zinc Gluconate, and the Role of Zinc Dosage." *Journal of the Royal Society of Medicine Open* 8, no. 5 (May 2017): 2054270417694291.

10. Maserejian, Nancy N., Susan A. Hall, and John B. McKinlay. "Low Dietary or Supplemental Zinc Is Associated with Depression Symptoms among Women, but Not Men, in a Population-Based Epidemiological Survey." *Journal of Affective Disorders* 136 (2012): 781–788.

11. Olza, Josune, Javier Aranceta-Bartrina, Marcela González-Gross, et al. "Reported Dietary Intake and Food Sources of Zinc, Selenium, and Vitamins A, E and C in the Spanish Population: Findings from the ANIBES Study." *Nutrients* 9, no. 7 (July 2017): 697.

12. Mesias, Marta, Isabel Seiquer, and M. Pilar Navarro. "Is the Mediterranean Diet Adequate to Satisfy Zinc Requirements during Adolescence?" *Public Health Nutrition* 15, no. 8 (2012): 1429–1436.

13. Carroll, L. S., A. H. Abdul-Rahim, and R. Murray. "Zinc Containing Dental Fixative Causing Copper Deficiency Myelopathy." *BMJ Case Reports*. Online, August 8, 2017. doi:10.1136/bcr-2017-219802.

REFERENCES AND FURTHER READINGS

Barnett, Junaidah B., Maria C. Dao, Davidson H. Hamer, et al. "Effect of Zinc Supplementation on Serum Zinc Concentration and T Cell Proliferation in Nursing Home Elderly: A Randomized, Double-Blind, Placebo-Controlled Trial." *American Journal of Clinical Nutrition* 103 (2016): 942–951.

Carroll, L. S., A. H. Abdul-Rahim, and R. Murray. "Zinc Containing Dental Fixative Causing Copper Deficiency Myelopathy." *BMJ Case Reports*. Online, August 8, 2017. doi:10.1136/bcr-2017-219802.

Foster, Meika, Anna Chu, Peter Petocz, and Samir Samman. "Effect of Vegetarian Diets on Zinc Status: A Systematic Review and Meta-Analysis of Studies in Humans." *Journal of the Science of Food and Agriculture* 93 (2013): 2362–2371.

The George Mateljan Foundation. "Zinc." January 1, 2018. http://whfoods.com/genpage.php?tname=nutrient&dbid=115.

Hemilä, Harri. "Zinc Lozenges and the Common Cold: A Meta-Analysis Comparing Zinc Acetate and Zinc Gluconate, and the Role of Zinc Dosage." *Journal of the Royal Society of Medicine Open* 8, no. 5 (May 2017): 2054270417694291.

Maserejian, Nancy N., Susan A. Hall, and John B. McKinlay. "Low Dietary or Supplemental Zinc Is Associated with Depression Symptoms among Women, but Not Men, in a Population-Based Epidemiological Survey." *Journal of Affective Disorders* 136 (2012): 781–788.

Medlineplus. "Zinc." January 1, 2018. https://ods.od.nih.gov/factsheets/Zinc-Consumer/.

Mesias, Marta, Isabel Seiquer, and M. Pilar Navarro. "Is the Mediterranean Diet Adequate to Satisfy Zinc Requirements during Adolescence?" *Public Health Nutrition* 15, no. 8 (2012): 1429–1436.

Nossier, S. A., N. E. Naeim, N. A. El-Sayed, and A. A. Abu Zeid. "The Effect of Zinc Supplementation on Pregnancy Outcomes: A Double-Blind, Randomised Controlled Trial, Egypt." *British Journal of Nutrition* 114, no. 2 (July 2015): 274–285.

Office of Dietary Supplements, National Institutes of Health. "Zinc." January 1, 2018. https://ods.od.nih.gov/factsheets/Zinc-Consumer/.

Olza, Josune, Javier Aranceta-Bartrina, Marcela González-Gross, et al. "Reported Dietary Intake and Food Sources of Zinc, Selenium, and Vitamins A, E and C in the Spanish Population: Findings from the ANIBES Study." *Nutrients* 9, no. 7 (July 2017): 697+.

Rerksuppaphol, Sanguansak and Lakkana Rerksuppaphol. "Effect of Zinc plus Multivitamin Supplementation on Growth in School Children." *Pediatrics International* 58 (2016): 1193–1199.

Wong, Carmen P., Kathy R. Magnusson, and Emily Ho. "Increased Inflammatory Response in Aged Mice Is Associated with Age-Related Zinc Deficiency and Zinc Transporter Dysregulation." *Journal of Nutritional Biochemistry* 24 (2013): 353–359.

Appendix

Recommended Intake Levels of Key Vitamins and Minerals for Different Populations

Source: https://ods.od.nih.gov/Health_Information/Dietary_Reference_Intakes.aspx.

Recommended Dietary Allowance (RDA) and adequate intake (AI) for vitamins and minerals

Life Stage Group	Vitamin A (mcg per day)	Vitamin C (mg per day)	Vitamin D (mcg per day)	Vitamin E (mg per day)	Vitamin K (mcg per day)	Thiamin (mg per day)	Riboflavin (mg per day)	Niacin (mg per day)	Vitamin B6 (mg per day)	Folate (mcg per day)	Vitamin B12 (mcg per day)	Pantothenic Acid (mg per day)	Biotin (mcg per day)	Choline (mg per day)
Infants														
0–6 mo	400*	40*	10*	4*	2.0*	0.2*	0.3*	2*	0.1*	65*	0.4*	1.7*	5*	125*
6–12 mo	500*	50*	10*	5*	2.5*	0.3*	0.4*	4*	0.3*	80*	0.5*	1.8*	6*	150*
Children														
1–3 y	300	15	15	6	30*	0.5	0.5	6	0.5	150	0.9	2*	8*	200*
4–8 y	400	25	15	7	55*	0.6	0.6	8	0.6	200	1.2	3*	12*	250*
Males														
9–13 y	600	45	15	11	60*	0.9	0.9	12	1.0	300	1.8	4*	20*	375*
14–18 y	900	75	15	15	75*	1.2	1.3	16	1.3	400	2.4	5*	25*	550*
19–30 y	900	90	15	15	120*	1.2	1.3	16	1.3	400	2.4	5*	30*	550*
31–50 y	900	90	15	15	120*	1.2	1.3	16	1.3	400	2.4	5*	30*	550*
51–70 y	900	90	15	15	120*	1.2	1.3	16	1.7	400	2.4	5*	30*	550*
More than 70 y	900	90	20	15	120*	1.2	1.3	16	1.7	400	2.4	5*	30*	550*

Females														
9–13 y	600	45	15	11	60*	0.9	0.9	12	1.0	300	1.8	4*	20*	375*
14–18 y	700	65	15	15	75*	1.0	1.0	14	1.2	400	2.4	5*	25*	400*
19–30 y	700	75	15	15	90*	1.1	1.1	14	1.3	400	2.4	5*	30*	425*
31–50 y	700	75	15	15	90*	1.1	1.1	14	1.3	400	2.4	5*	30*	425*
51–70 y	700	75	15	15	90*	1.1	1.1	14	1.5	400	2.4	5*	30*	425*
More than 70 y	700	75	20	15	90*	1.1	1.1	14	1.5	400	2.4	5*	30*	425*
Pregnancy														
14–18 y	750	80	15	15	75*	1.4	1.4	18	1.9	600	2.6	6*	30*	450*
19–30 y	770	85	15	15	90*	1.4	1.4	18	1.9	600	2.6	6*	30*	450*
31–50 y	770	85	15	15	90*	1.4	1.4	18	1.9	600	2.6	6*	30*	450*
Lactation														
14–18 y	1,200	115	15	19	75*	1.4	1.6	17	2.0	500	2.8	7*	35*	550*
19–30 y	1,300	120	15	19	90*	1.4	1.6	17	2.0	500	2.8	7*	35*	550*
31–50 y	1,300	120	15	19	90*	1.4	1.6	17	2.0	500	2.8	7*	35*	550*

Life Stage Group	Calcium (mg per day)	Chromium (mcg per day)	Copper (mcg per day)	Fluoride (mg per day)	Iodine (mcg per day)	Iron (mg per day)	Magnesium (mg per day)	Manganese (mg per day)	Molybdenum (mcg per day)	Phosphorus (mg per day)	Selenium (mcg per day)	Zinc (mg per day)	Potassium (g per day)	Sodium (g per day)	Chloride (g per day)
Infants															
0–6 mo	200*	0.2*	200*	0.01*	110*	0.27*	30*	0.003*	2*	100*	15*	2*	0.4*	0.12*	0.18*
6–12 mo	260*	5.5*	220*	0.5*	130*	11	75*	0.6*	3*	275*	20*	3	0.7*	0.37*	0.57*
Children															
1–3 y	700	11*	340	0.7*	90	7	80	1.2*	17	460	20	3	3.0*	1.0*	1.5*
4–8 y	1,000	15*	440	1*	90	10	130	1.5*	22	500	30	5	3.8*	1.2*	1.9*
Males															
9–13 y	1,300	25*	700	2*	120	8	240	1.9*	34	1,250	40	8	4.5*	1.5*	2.3*
14–18 y	1,300	35*	890	3*	150	11	410	2.2*	43	1,250	55	11	4.7*	1.5*	2.3*
19–30 y	1,000	35*	900	4*	150	8	400	2.3*	45	700	55	11	4.7*	1.5*	2.3*
31–50 y	1,000	35*	900	4*	150	8	420	2.3*	45	700	55	11	4.7*	1.5*	2.3*
51–70 y	1,000	30*	900	4*	150	8	420	2.3*	45	700	55	11	4.7*	1.3*	2.0*
More than 70 y	1,200	30*	900	4*	150	8	420	2.3*	45	700	55	11	4.7*	1.2*	1.8*

Females

Age															
9–13 y	1,300	21*	700	2*	120	8	240	1.6*	34	1,250	40	8	4.5*	1.5*	2.3*
14–18 y	1,300	24*	890	3*	150	15	360	1.6*	43	1,250	55	9	4.7*	1.5*	2.3*
19–30 y	1,000	25*	900	3*	150	18	310	1.8*	45	700	55	8	4.7*	1.5*	2.3*
31–50 y	1,000	25*	900	3*	150	18	320	1.8*	45	700	55	8	4.7*	1.5*	2.3*
51–70 y	1,200	20*	900	3*	150	8	320	1.8*	45	700	55	8	4.7*	1.3*	2.0*
More than 70 y	1,200	20*	900	3*	150	8	320	1.8*	45	700	55	8	4.7*	1.2*	1.8*

Pregnancy

Age															
14–18 y	1,300	29*	1,000	3*	220	27	400	2.0*	50	1,250	60	12	4.7*	1.5*	2.3*
19–30 y	1,000	30*	1,000	3*	220	27	350	2.0*	50	700	60	11	4.7*	1.5*	2.3*
31–50 y	1,000	30*	1,000	3*	220	27	360	2.0*	50	700	60	11	4.7*	1.5*	2.3*

Lactation

Age															
14–18 y	1,300	44*	1,300	3*	290	10	360	2.6*	50	1,250	70	13	5.1*	1.5*	2.3*
19–30 y	1,000	45*	1,300	3*	290	9	310	2.6*	50	700	70	12	5.1*	1.5*	2.3*
31–50 y	1,000	45*	1,300	3*	290	9	320	2.6*	50	700	70	12	5.1*	1.5*	2.3*

Note: RDAs are in bold type and AIs in ordinary type followed by an asterisk (*).
Note: y, years; mo, months.

Tolerable upper intake level for vitamins and minerals

Life Stage Group	Vitamin A (mcg per day)	Vitamin C (mg per day)	Vitamin D (mcg per day)	Vitamin E (mg per day)	Vitamin K	Thiamin	Riboflavin	Niacin (mg per day)	Vitamin B6 (mg per day)	Folate (mcg per day)	Vitamin B12	Pantothenic Acid	Biotin	Choline (g per day)	Carotenoids
Infants															
0–6 mo	600	n.d.	25	n.d.	n.d.	n.d.	n.d.	n.d.	n.d.	n.d.	n.d.	n.d.	n.d.	n.d.	n.d.
6–12 mo	600	n.d.	38	n.d.	n.d.	n.d.	n.d.	n.d.	n.d.	n.d.	n.d.	n.d.	n.d.	n.d.	n.d.
Children															
1–3 y	600	400	63	200	n.d.	n.d.	n.d.	10	30	300	n.d.	n.d.	n.d.	1.0	n.d.
4–8 y	900	650	75	300	n.d.	n.d.	n.d.	15	40	400	n.d.	n.d.	n.d.	1.0	n.d.
Males															
9–13 y	1,700	1,200	100	600	n.d.	n.d.	n.d.	20	60	600	n.d.	n.d.	n.d.	2.0	n.d.
14–18 y	2,800	1,800	100	800	n.d.	n.d.	n.d.	30	80	800	n.d.	n.d.	n.d.	3.0	n.d.
19–30 y	3,000	2,000	100	1,000	n.d.	n.d.	n.d.	35	100	1,000	n.d.	n.d.	n.d.	3.5	n.d.
31–50 y	3,000	2,000	100	1,000	n.d.	n.d.	n.d.	35	100	1,000	n.d.	n.d.	n.d.	3.5	n.d.
51–70 y	3,000	2,000	100	1,000	n.d.	n.d.	n.d.	35	100	1,000	n.d.	n.d.	n.d.	3.5	n.d.
More than 70 y	3,000	2,000	100	1,000	n.d.	n.d.	n.d.	35	100	1,000	n.d.	n.d.	n.d.	3.5	n.d.

Females

9–13 y	1,700	1,200	100	600	n.d.	n.d.	20	60	600	n.d.	n.d.	2.0	n.d.
14–18 y	2,800	1,800	100	800	n.d.	n.d.	30	80	800	n.d.	n.d.	3.0	n.d.
19–30 y	3,000	2,000	100	1,000	n.d.	n.d.	35	100	1,000	n.d.	n.d.	3.5	n.d.
31–50 y	3,000	2,000	100	1,000	n.d.	n.d.	35	100	1,000	n.d.	n.d.	3.5	n.d.
51–70 y	3,000	2,000	100	1,000	n.d.	n.d.	35	100	1,000	n.d.	n.d.	3.5	n.d.
More than 70 y	3,000	2,000	100	1,000	n.d.	n.d.	35	100	1,000	n.d.	n.d.	3.5	n.d.

Pregnancy

14–18 y	2,800	1,800	100	800	n.d.	n.d.	30	80	800	n.d.	n.d.	3.0	n.d.
19–30 y	3,000	2,000	100	1,000	n.d.	n.d.	35	100	1,000	n.d.	n.d.	3.5	n.d.
31–50 y	3,000	2,000	100	1,000	n.d.	n.d.	35	100	1,000	n.d.	n.d.	3.5	n.d.

Lactation

14–18 y	2,800	1,800	100	800	n.d.	n.d.	30	80	800	n.d.	n.d.	3.0	n.d.
19–30 y	3,000	2,000	100	1,000	n.d.	n.d.	35	100	1,000	n.d.	n.d.	3.5	n.d.
31–50 y	3,000	2,000	100	1,000	n.d.	n.d.	35	100	1,000	n.d.	n.d.	3.5	n.d.

Life Stage Group	Boron (mg per day)	Calcium (mg per day)	Chromium	Copper (mcg per day)	Fluoride (mg per day)	Iodine (mcg per day)	Iron (mg per day)	Magnesium (mg per day)	Manganese (mg per day)	Molybdenum (mcg per day)	Nickel (mg per day)	Phosphorus (g per day)	Selenium (mcg per day)	Zinc (mg per day)	Sodium (g per day)	Chloride (g per day)
Infants																
0–6 mo	n.d.	1,000	n.d.	n.d.	0.7	n.d.	40	n.d.	n.d.	n.d.	n.d.	n.d.	45	4	n.d.	n.d.
6–12 mo	n.d.	1,500	n.d.	n.d.	0.9	n.d.	40	n.d.	n.d.	n.d.	n.d.	n.d.	60	5	n.d.	n.d.
Children																
1–3 y	3	2,500	n.d.	1,000	1.3	200	40	65	2	300	0.2	3	90	7	1.5	2.3
4–8 y	6	2,500	n.d.	3,000	2.2	300	40	110	3	600	0.3	3	150	12	1.9	2.9
Males																
9–13 y	11	3,000	n.d.	5,000	10	600	40	350	6	1,100	0.6	4	280	23	2.2	3.4
14–18 y	17	3,000	n.d.	8,000	10	900	45	350	9	1,700	1.0	4	400	34	2.3	3.6
19–30 y	20	2,500	n.d.	10,000	10	1,100	45	350	11	2,000	1.0	4	400	40	2.3	3.6
31–50 y	20	2,500	n.d.	10,000	10	1,100	45	350	11	2,000	1.0	4	400	40	2.3	3.6
51–70 y	20	2,000	n.d.	10,000	10	1,100	45	350	11	2,000	1.0	4	400	40	2.3	3.6
More than 70 y	20	2,000	n.d.	10,000	10	1,100	45	350	11	2,000	1.0	3	400	40	2.3	3.6

Females												
9–13 y	11	3,000	n.d.	5,000	10	600	40	350	6	1,100	0.6	4	280	23	2.2	3.4
14–18 y	17	3,000	n.d.	8,000	10	900	45	350	9	1,700	1.0	4	400	34	2.3	3.6
19–30 y	20	2,500	n.d.	10,000	10	1,100	45	350	11	2,000	1.0	4	400	40	2.3	3.6
31–50 y	20	2,500	n.d.	10,000	10	1,100	45	350	11	2,000	1.0	4	400	40	2.3	3.6
51–70 y	20	2,000	n.d.	10,000	10	1,100	45	350	11	2,000	1.0	4	400	40	2.3	3.6
More than 70 y	20	2,000	n.d.	10,000	10	1,100	45	350	11	2,000	1.0	3	400	40	2.3	3.6
Pregnancy												
14–18 y	17	3,000	n.d.	8,000	10	900	45	350	9	1,700	1.0	3.5	400	34	2.3	3.6
19–30 y	20	2,500	n.d.	10,000	10	1,100	45	350	11	2,000	1.0	3.5	400	40	2.3	3.6
61–50 y	20	2,500	n.d.	10,000	10	1,100	45	350	11	2,000	1.0	3.5	400	40	2.3	3.6
Lactation												
14–18 y	17	3,000	n.d.	8,000	10	900	45	350	9	1,700	1.0	4	400	34	2.3	3.6
19–30 y	20	2,500	n.d.	10,000	10	1,100	45	350	11	2,000	1.0	4	400	40	2.3	3.6
31–50 y	20	2,500	n.d.	10,000	10	1,100	45	350	11	2,000	1.0	4	400	40	2.3	3.6

Note: n.d., not determined; y, years; mo, months.

Glossary

Absorption in nutrition, the process of moving nutrients from the digestive system into the bloodstream. This mostly takes place in the small intestine.

Acne vulgaris the common form of acne in teens and young adults that is caused by overactivity of the oil glands in the skin. The skin pores become plugged and inflamed.

Adenoma noncancerous tumor.

Adiponectin a protein hormone that regulates the metabolism of lipids and glucose, and it influences the body's response to insulin.

Amino acid an organic compound that serves as a building block for protein.

Anemia a condition in which the number of red blood cells or the amount of hemoglobin in them is lower than normal.

Apoptosis cell death.

Atherosclerosis hardening and narrowing of the arteries.

Atrial fibrillation an irregular, often faster, heartbeat that may be associated with a stroke.

Attention deficit hyperactivity disorder (ADHD) a neurodevelopmental disorder characterized by hyperactivity, impulsivity, and/or inattention.

Autism spectrum disorder a group of neurodevelopmental disorders characterized by social and language deficits, stereotypic behavior, and abnormalities in motor functions.

Bariatric surgery surgery that helps to facilitate weight loss.

Binge eating disorder the consumption of an unusually large amount of food coupled with a feeling of the loss of control over eating.

Body mass index (BMI) a measure based on height and weight that applies to adult men and women and children.

Cancer a number of diseases in which cells divide abnormally and without control and may spread to nearby tissues and other parts of the body.

Carnosine a protein building block naturally produced in the body.

Catabolism the breakdown of complex molecules into simpler ones.

Cataract the clouding of the normally clear lens of the eye.

Cell the individual unit that makes up the tissues of the body.

Cheilitis cracking in the corners of the mouth.

Coronary heart disease a disease in which the blood vessels that carry blood and oxygen to the heart are narrowed or blocked, which may trigger chest pain, a shortness of breath, and a heart attack.

Deficiency an amount that is not enough, a shortage.

Depression a serious medical condition that may include feelings of sadness and despair, loss of energy, and the loss of interest in activities that were previously enjoyable. People who are depressed may have problems sleeping or sleep too much, and they sometimes consider suicide.

Dermatitis skin inflammation.

Diastolic blood pressure the bottom number of a blood pressure reading, which measures the pressure in the arteries between heart contractions.

Dietary supplement a product that is designed to supplement the diet. It may contain one or more ingredients.

Disorder in medicine, a disorder is a disturbance in the functioning of the body.

Dose the amount of medicine taken over a specific period of time.

Dyslipidemia elevated total or low-density lipoprotein (LDL) cholesterol levels, low levels of high-density lipoprotein (HDL), or elevated triglycerides.

Endothelial function the functioning of the thin layers of cells that line blood vessels.

Enrichment in food, enrichment is the replacement of nutrients that have been lost during processing or storage.

Fatigue extreme tiredness and the impairment of the ability to function.

Fortify the addition of nutrients to a food during processing to replace nutrients that have been lost.

Geometric mean central number in geometric progression.

Glossitis a tongue that is swollen, painful, and magenta in color.

Gluconeogenesis the conversion of substances like amino acids and organic acids into sugar.

Glycemic status blood sugar levels.

Graves' disease an autoimmune disorder that leads to an overactive thyroid gland.

Heart palpitation irregular beating of the heart.

Homocysteine an amino acid. When it is at higher levels in the blood, it increases the risk of a number of medical problems, including coronary artery disease, heart attack, stroke, osteoporosis, bone fractures, and Alzheimer's disease.

Hypercalcemia excessively high levels of calcium in the blood.

Glossary

Hypertension elevated blood pressure.

Hypothyroidism abnormally low activity of the thyroid gland.

IQ intelligence quotient.

Ischemic heart disease also known as coronary artery disease, it is a condition that affects the supply of blood to the heart muscle.

Ischemic stroke this usually occurs when a blood clot blocks a blood vessel in the brain, preventing the flow of blood to the brain.

Metabolic syndrome a clustering of metabolic traits, including abdominal obesity, glucose intolerance, hypertension, and elevated cholesterol.

Microgram (mcg) a unit of weight in the metric system that is equal to one-millionth of a gram. A gram is about one-thirtieth of an ounce.

Micronutrients substances needed only in small amounts for normal body functioning.

Mineral in nutrition, minerals are inorganic substances that are required to maintain health. They are found in the earth.

Multiple sclerosis an autoimmune disorder of the central nervous system that is characterized by neurological disability.

Myocardial infarction the death of heart muscle caused by a lack of oxygen.

Nerve a bundle of microscopic fibers that carry messages to and from the brain or spinal cord to other parts of the body.

Neural tube defect a disorder in which the brain, spinal cord, or the tissues protecting the brain and spine do not develop properly during pregnancy.

Nutrient a chemical compound in food that is used by the body.

Nyctalopia loss of night vision or the ability to see well when it is dark outside.

Osteoarthritis when cartilage in the joints breaks down, there may be stiffness, pain, and swelling.

Osteopenia bone mineral density that is lower than normal, but not sufficiently low to be classified as osteoporosis.

Osteoporosis a condition in which the body's bones become increasingly more porous.

Parkinson's disease a progressive disease of the nervous system marked by tremors, muscular rigidity, and slow imprecise movements.

Phonophobia hypersensitivity to sound.

Phosphate a salt that contains phosphorus.

Photophobia hypersensitivity to light.

Polycystic ovary syndrome an endocrine disorder among women of reproductive age that has symptoms such as infrequent or prolonged menstrual periods, excessive weight, and increased hair.

Preeclampsia a pregnancy complication characterized by high blood pressure and damage to another organ system, often the kidneys.

Premenstrual syndrome one of the most common disorders in women, it includes a variety of physical and psychological symptoms such as breast tenderness, abdominal cramps, bloating, crying, mood swings, and irritability.

Prenatal during pregnancy.

Primigravid pregnant for the first time.

Prophylaxis prevention.

Stroke a loss of blood flow to part of the brain. Strokes are caused by blood clots or broken blood vessels in the brain.

Systolic blood pressure the top number, which measures the pressure in the arteries when the heart contracts.

Teratology the study of malformations in developing organisms.

Type 1 diabetes an autoimmune condition in which the pancreas produces no insulin.

Index

Absorption: calcium, 6, 7, 56, 182; chromium, 20; copper, 27, 207; Crohn's disease and, xvi; iron, 47, 48–49, 51, 126; magnesium, 56; manganese, 62; probiotics and, 48–49; vitamin B1 (thiamin) and, 115, 116; vitamin B2 (riboflavin), 126; vitamin B7 (biotin), 154; vitamin K, 202. *See also* Malabsorption

Academic performance of children, manganese and, 63

Acceptable macronutrient distribution range (AMDR), xviii

ACE inhibitors. *See* Angiotensin-converting enzyme (ACE) inhibitors

Acne vulgaris, vitamin B5 (pantothenic acid) and, 139–40

Acta Obstetricia et Gynecologica Scandinavica (journal), 48

Adenoma, 10

Adequate intakes (AIs): acceptable macronutrient distribution range and, xviii; calcium, 218–19; chart, 216–19; chloride, 218–19; choline, 14, 216–17; chromium, 20, 218–19; copper, 27, 218–19; defined, xvii, xviii; fluoride, 34, 218–19; iodine, 218–19; iron, 46–47, 218–19; magnesium, 54–55, 218–19; manganese, 62, 218–19; minerals, 216–19; molybdenum, 70, 218–19; phosphorus, 75, 218–19; potassium, 86, 218–19; prevalence of, estimating, xix; selenium, 90, 218–19; sodium, 218–19; vitamin A, 216–17; vitamin B1 (thiamin) and, 216–17; vitamin B2 (riboflavin), 216–17; vitamin B3 (niacin), 131, 216–17; vitamin B5 (pantothenic acid), 138–39, 216–17; vitamin B6 (pyridoxine), 146, 216–17; vitamin B7 (biotin), 154, 216–17; vitamin B9 (folate), 158, 216–17; vitamin B12 (cobalamin), 165, 216–17; vitamin C (ascorbic acid), 174, 216–17; vitamin D, 216–17; vitamin E, 194, 216–17; vitamin K, 202, 216–17; vitamins, 216–19; zinc, 207, 218–19

Adolescents: bone mineral density in, vitamin D and, 185–86; externalizing behaviors in, magnesium and, 59; potassium and, 85, 87; psychiatric and behavior problems, vitamin B2 (riboflavin) and, 127–28; vitamin D and, 185

Advances in Nutrition (journal), xix, 85, 118
Alimentary Pharmacology & Therapeutics (journal), 189
All-cause mortality: phosphorus and, 76–77; vitamin E and, 195
Allergies, vitamin D and, 189
Allergy, Asthma & Immunology (journal), 178
Alzheimer's disease, copper and, 30–31
American Dental Association, 33, 34–35
American Heart Journal, 179–80
American Journal of Clinical Nutrition, xviii, 11, 16, 51, 58, 90–91, 125, 128, 160–61, 162, 170, 176, 185, 197, 198, 209–91
American Journal of Emergency Medicine, 115–16
American Journal of Epidemiology, 170
American Journal of Hypertension, 99
American Journal of Kidney Diseases, 77, 78
American Journal of Medicine, The, 76
American Journal of Psychiatry, 15–16
American Journal of Public Health, 35
Amino acid: homocysteine, 145–46, 158, 164; manganese and, 62; methionine, 127; molybdenum and, 62; tryptophan and, 130; vitamin B2 (riboflavin) and, 127; vitamin B3 (niacin) and, 130
Anemia: pernicious, vitamin B12 (cobalamin) and, 169–70; vitamin B2 (riboflavin) and, 126
Angiotensin 2 receptor blockers, 82
Angiotensin-converting enzyme (ACE) inhibitors: phosphorus levels and, 75; potassium levels and, 82
Animal flesh consumption, iron and, 48
Annals of Pharmacotherapy (journal), 176, 197
Antacids: magnesium in, 54; phosphorus levels and, 75; sodium in, 75
"Anthropometry, Intake and Energy Balance in Spain" (ANIBES) study, 211
Anticoagulants: vitamin E and, xv; vitamin K and, 202, 203

Antidepressants, zinc levels and, 210
Antioxidant supplements: chemotherapy and, xv; manganese, 61; vitamins C, xv; vitamins E, xv
Anti-seizure medications, vitamin B7 (biotin) levels and, 154
Antitumor necrosis factor-α, vitamin D and, 189
Apoptosis, 4
Appetite (journal), 28–29
Applied Physiology, Nutrition & Metabolism (journal), 166–67
Archives of Gynecology and Obstetrics (journal), 126–27
Ascorbic acid. See Vitamin C (ascorbic acid)
Asia Pacific Journal of Clinical Nutrition, 72, 127
Asthma, vitamin D and, 189
Atherosclerosis (journal), 8, 175
Atherosclerosis, phosphorus and, 77
Atherosclerosis, subclinical later in life, vitamin D and, 189–90
Athletic performance, sodium and, 100
Atrial fibrillation, calcium and, 8
Attention and working memory of nonhuman primates, manganese and, 66–67
Attention deficit hyperactivity disorder (ADHD): in hair, manganese and, 63–64; vitamin B2 (riboflavin) and, 125–26
Attention in children, manganese and, 63
Autism-spectrum disorders: copper and, 28; vitamin D and, 190

Bariatric surgery: chromium and, 21; vitamin A and, 111–12; vitamin B1 (thiamin) and, 115, 118; vitamin K and, 204
Behavior: adverse childhood, vitamin A and, 108; in children, manganese and, 63; externalizing, in adolescents, magnesium and, 59; neurobehavioral functioning of school-age children, manganese and, 66; problems in adolescents, vitamin B2 (riboflavin) and, 127–28

INDEX 231

Benign breast disease, carotenoid and, 110
Beriberi, xiv
Beverages, phosphorus in, 78
Binge eating disorder, chromium and, 22
Biological Trace Element Research (journal), 3, 37–38, 56–57, 64, 71–72
BioMed Research International (journal), 167
Biotin. *See* Vitamin B7 (biotin)
Birth weight: iron and, 50–51; newborn, manganese and, 67; preterm birth/low birth weight, vitamin B12 (cobalamin) and, 170; very low-birth-weight infants, vitamin A and, 109
BJOG (journal), 9
BJPsych Open (journal), 125–26
Blood donors, iron and, 49–50
Blood glucose levels, chromium for normalizing, xiv
Blood pressure: Systolic blood pressure; diastolic, calcium and, 7–8; hypertension, fluoride and, 37; magnesium and, 55; manganese and, 65; medications, phosphorus and, 75; potassium and, 82; in rats with metabolic syndrome, phosphorus and, 78–79; sodium and, 99, 102, 103; sodium-to-potassium ratio and, 83; vitamin C (ascorbic acid) and, 176. *See also* Hypertension
Blood sugar levels, prediabetes and, vitamin K and, 204
Blood thinners. *See* Anticoagulants
BMC Endocrine Disorders (journal), 65
BMC Pregnancy & Childbirth, 150–51
BMC Psychiatry (journal), 186–87
BMC Public Health (journal), 67
BMJ (journal), 196
BMJ Case Reports (journal), 211–12
BMJ Open Diabetes Research & Care (journal), 93–94
BMJ Open Gastroenterology (journal), 185–86
Body cells and structures, minerals that support, xiv
Body mass index (BMI): calcium and, 11–12; iron and, 51; vitamin B12 (cobalamin) and, 169

Body processes, minerals that regulate, xiv
Body weight: weight control, calcium and, 11–12; weight loss, chromium and, 22–23. *See also* Overweight and obesity
Bone growth, magnesium and, 56
Bone mineral density: in aging men, selenium and, 95; in healthy children and adolescents, vitamin D and, 185–86; vitamin K and, 204–5
Boric acid, 1, 2, 3
Boron, 1–5; deficiency and excess, 2; dysmenorrhea (menstrual cramps) and, 2–3; food sources, 1; intake recommendations, 1–2; knee discomfort and, 4; osteoarthritis and, 3–4; prostate cancer cells and, 4; Recommended Dietary Allowances, 2; reductions in body weight and, 3; research findings, 2–4; supplements, 1; tolerable upper intake levels, 222–23
Brazilian Journal of Epidemiology (Revista Brasileira de Epidemiologia), 107–8
Breast cancer: choline and, 16–17; manganese and, 65–66; selenium and, 92; vitamin B2 (riboflavin) and, 126–27; vitamin B6 (pyridoxine) and, 150
Breast Cancer Research and Treatment (journal), 92
Breast milk, pasteurized, molybdenum and, 72–73
British Journal of Nutrition, 9, 48–49, 50, 56, 67, 91, 117, 148, 155, 159, 188, 209
British Journal of Psychiatry, 184–85

Calcium, 6–12; absorption, 6, 7, 56, 182; adequate intakes, 218–19; body mass index (BMI) and, 11–12; colorectal adenomas and, 10; constipation and, 8; deficiency and excess, 7; diastolic blood pressure and, 7–8; food sources, 6; fractures and, 11; function of, in body, xiv; intake recommendations, 7; intensive care unit patients and, 10; iron status and, 9–10; lung cancer and,

11; as macromineral, xiii; myocardial infarction and, 8; osteoporosis and, 9; osteoporosis medications and, 7; preeclampsia and, 9; Recommended Dietary Allowances, 7, 218–19; research findings, 7–12; subclinical cardiovascular disease and, 8; tolerable upper intake levels, 222–23; weight control and, 11–12

Canadian Journal of Dietetic Practice and Research (journal), 8

Cancer: basal-cell carcinoma, 132; colorectal, vitamin B2 (riboflavin) and, 125; esophageal, molybdenum and, 71; gastrointestinal surgery for, vitamin B1 and, 119; lung cancer, calcium and, 11; nonmelanoma skin cancers, vitamin B3 (niacin) and, 132; pancreatic cancer, choline and, 18; pre-cervical cancer, selenium and, 91; site-specific, vitamin B9 (folate) and, 161–62; squamous-cell carcinoma, 132; vitamin B6 (pyridoxine) and, 149; vitamin B9 (folate) and, 160–61; vitamin E and, 198. *See also* Breast cancer; Liver cancer; Prostate cancer

Cancer Causes & Control (journal), 127

Cancer Epidemiology, Biomarkers & Prevention (journal), 18

Cancer Science (journal), 16

Cardiovascular disease: and all-cause mortality, phosphorus and, 76–77; of people with diabetes and kidney problems, potassium and, 84; of people with/without chronic kidney disease, phosphorus and, 77–78; in rats with metabolic syndrome, phosphorus and, 78–79; sodium and, 99–100; vitamin B3 (niacin) and, 133; vitamin B5 (pantothenic acid) and, 139; vitamin B12 (cobalamin) and, 168; vitamin E and, 196

Cardiovascular Pathology (journal), 78–79

Caries (cavities), fluoride and, 34–35

Carnosine, 23–24

Carotenoid: benign breast disease in adolescents and, 110; type 2 diabetes and, 110–11

Catabolism, 197

Cataracts, vitamin C (ascorbic acid) and, 177

Cephalalgia (journal), 124

Cheilitis, 123, 154

Children: adverse behavior in, vitamin A and, 108; attention, cognition, behavior, and academic performance, manganese and, 63; bone growth, magnesium and, 56; bone mineral density in, vitamin D and, 185–86; cognitive development, fluoride and, 37; fortifying bread with iodized salt for school children, iodine and, 43–44; neurobehavioral functioning of school-age children, manganese and, 66; neuro-intellectual outcomes of, iodine and, 41–42; picky eaters, copper and, 28–29; preschool, potassium and, 85–86; Puerto Rican, vitamin B5 (pantothenic acid) and, 141; in school, zinc and, 208; toddlers, potassium and, 85; younger, vitamin D and, 188–89

Chloride: adequate intakes, 218–19; intake recommendations, 98; Recommended Dietary Allowances, 218–19; tolerable upper intake levels, 222–23

Cholesterol levels: in overweight women, iodine and, 43; vitamin B3 (niacin) and, 134

Cholesterol-reducing medications: niacin levels and, 135; vitamin B3 (niacin) and, 135; vitamin B5 levels and, 139

Choline, 14–18; adequate intakes, 216–17; breast cancer and, 16–17; cardiovascular disease mortality and, 15; deficiency and excess, 15; dyslipidemia and, 18; food sources, 14; intake recommendations, 14–15; memory and, 16, 17; nonalcoholic fatty liver disease and, 17–18; pancreatic cancer and, 18; Recommended Dietary Allowances, 216–17; research findings, 15–18; schizophrenia and, 15–16; tolerable upper intake levels, 15, 220–21

Chromium, 20–25; absorption, 20; adequate intakes, 218–19; bariatric surgery and, 21; binge eating disorder and, 22; cognitive functioning and, 23; deficiency and excess, 21; food sources, 20; intake recommendations, 20–21; morbid obesity and, 21; psychiatric problems and, 22; Recommended Dietary Allowances, 218–19; research findings, 21–25; supplements, 20; tolerable upper intake levels, 222–23; weight loss and, 22–23

Chronic low back pain, craniosacral therapy in patients with, potassium and, 83–84

Chronic stable heart failure, copper and, 30

Circulation (journal), 102–3

Circulation: Cardiovascular Quality and Outcomes (journal), 135–36

Circulation: Heart Failure (journal), 179, 199

Clinica Chimica Acta (journal), 76

Clinical Cases in Mineral and Bone Metabolism (journal), 29

Clinical Interventions in Aging (journal), 4

Clinical Journal of the American Society of Nephrology, 84

Clinical Nutrition Research (journal), 134

Cobalamin. *See* Vitamin B12 (cobalamin)

Cognitive decline: fluoride and, 37–38; vitamin B6 (pyridoxine) and, 148–49; vitamin B12 (cobalamin) and, 170–71; vitamin D and, 187; vitamin E and, 197–98

Cognitive functioning: childhood cognitive development, fluoride and, 37; in children, manganese and, 63; chromium and, 23; iron and, 50; vitamin C (ascorbic acid) and, 176

Colorectal adenomas, calcium and, 10

Colorectal cancer, vitamin B2 (riboflavin) and, 125

Community Dentistry and Oral Epidemiology (journal), 35

Complementary Therapies in Clinical Practice (journal), 2

Constipation, calcium and, 8

Contact Dermatitis (journal), 142–43

Copper, 26–31; absorption, 27, 207; adequate intakes, 218–19; Alzheimer's disease and, 30–31; autism spectrum disorder and, 28; chronic stable heart failure and, 30; deficiency and excess, 27–28; food sources, 27; herbal infusions and, 31; intake recommendations, 27; osteopenia and, 29; osteoporosis and, 29; picky eaters and, 28–29; Recommended Dietary Allowances, 27, 218–19; research findings, 28–31; supplements, 27; tolerable upper intake levels, 27, 222–23; ultra-processed foods and, 29–30; zinc and, 29; zinc supplements and, 29

Copper deficiency myelopathy, zinc and, 211–12

Coronary artery disease, vitamin B6 (pyridoxine) and, 148

Coronary Artery Risk Development in Young Adults (study), 77

Coronary heart disease: atherosclerosis, phosphorus and, 77; chronic stable heart failure, copper and, 30; mortality, choline and, 15; subclinical, calcium and, 8

Coronary stenosis, vitamin B6 (pyridoxine) and, 148

Coumadin, xvi, 202. *See also* Anticoagulants

Craniosacral therapy in patients with chronic low back pain, potassium and, 83–84

Crohn's disease: absorption and, xvi; vitamin A and, 111

Current Aging Science (journal), 195

Deficiencies: amount of vitamins body needs to prevent, xvii; boron, 2; choline, 15; chromium, 21; copper, 27–28; fluoride, 34; iodine, 40–41; iron, 47; magnesium, 55; manganese, 62–63; molybdenum, 70–71; people considered to be at higher risk for, xvi; phosphorus, 75–76; potassium, 81–82; research on problems associated with, xiv; selenium, 90; sodium, 98–99; vitamin A, 106–7; vitamin B1 (thiamin), xiv, 115–16; vitamin B2 (riboflavin), 123; vitamin B3 (niacin), 131–32; vitamin B5 (pantothenic acid), 138–39; vitamin B6 (pyridoxine), 146–47; vitamin B7 (biotin), 154; vitamin B9 (folate), 158–59; vitamin B12 (cobalamin), 165–66; vitamin C, xiv; vitamin C (ascorbic acid), 174–75; vitamin D, 183; vitamin E, 194; vitamin K, 202–3; zinc, 207–8

Dementia, vitamin E and, 198

Depression: depressive moods, selenium and, 95–96; magnesium and, 58–59; postpartum, iron and, 51–52; vitamin B3 (niacin) and, 134; vitamin B6 (pyridoxine) and, 147; vitamin B12 (cobalamin) and, 167

Depressive moods, selenium and, 95–96

Depressive symptoms: vitamin B5 (pantothenic acid) and, 141; vitamin D and, 184–85; in women, zinc and, 210

Dermatitis, vitamin B5 (pantothenic acid) and, 142–43

Dermatology and Therapy (journal), 139–40

Diabetes: gestational, vitamin B9 (folate) and, 160; inflammation and, vitamin C (ascorbic acid) and, 178; magnesium and, 59; medication, vitamin C (ascorbic acid) and, 179; premenopausal women with prediabetes, blood sugar levels in, vitamin K and, 204; selenium and, 93–94; type 1, vitamin B2 (riboflavin) and, 127; vitamin B7 (biotin) and, 155. *See also* Type 2 diabetes

Diabetes Care (journal), 160

Diastolic blood pressure, calcium and, 7–8

Diet, health associated with, xiv

Dietary Approaches to Stop Hypertension (DASH) diet, 99

Dietary References Intakes (DRIs): defined, xvii–xviii; determining, xvii–xix; on food labels, xviii, xix; history of, xviii–xix; iron, 46–47; nutrient reference values, xvii–xviii. *See also* Adequate intakes (AIs);
Estimated average requirements (EARs); Recommended Dietary Allowances (RDAs); Tolerable upper intake levels (ULs)

Dietary supplements: boron, 1; calcium, 6; chart, 216–23; choline, 14; chromium, 20; copper, 27; defined, xv, xvii; of fat-soluble vitamins, avoiding, xiii; fluoride, 33; history of, xvi, xviii–xix; iodine, 40; iron, 46; magnesium, 54; manganese, 62; molybdenum, 70; people who benefit from, xiv; phosphorus, 74–75; potassium, 81; reacting with other supplements and/or prescription medications, xvi; safety and regulation of, xv–xvi; selenium, 89–90; sodium, 98; as substitute for healthful diet, xvi; vitamin A, 105–6; vitamin B1 (thiamin), 114; vitamin B2 (riboflavin), 122; vitamin B3 (niacin), 131; vitamin B5 (pantothenic acid), 138; vitamin B6 (pyridoxine), 146; vitamin B7 (biotin), 154; vitamin B9 (folate), 158; vitamin B12 (cobalamin), 164–65; vitamin C (ascorbic acid), 173–74; vitamin D, 182–83; vitamin E, 193–94; vitamin K, 202; zinc, 206–7

Diuretics: magnesium levels and, 55; phosphorus levels and, 75; potassium levels and, 82; vitamin B1 (thiamin) levels and, 116

Drug and Alcohol Dependence (journal), 118–19

Drug Design, Development and Therapy (journal), 178

Dyslipidemia, choline and, 18

Dysmenorrhea (menstrual cramps), boron and, 2–3

Eating disorders: binge eating disorder, chromium and, 22; vitamin B5 (pantothenic acid) and, 140

Eczema, vitamin D and, 189

Elderly. *See* Older adults

Endothelial function, vitamin C (ascorbic acid) and, 175

Endurance training, vitamin C (ascorbic acid) and, 176–77

INDEX 235

Enrichment, 115
Enteral nutrition, molybdenum and, 72
Environmental Health Perspectives (journal), 64–65, 66
Environmental Research (journal), 63, 65
Esophageal cancer, molybdenum and, 71
Estimated average requirements (EARs), xvii
European Journal of Clinical Nutrition, 51, 55, 147, 166, 167–68
European Journal of Nutrition, 51–52, 59
European Prospective Investigation into Cancer and Nutrition study (EPIC), 90–91
Excesses: boron, 2; choline, 15; chromium, 21; copper, 27–28; fluoride, 34; iodine, 40–41; iron, 47; magnesium, 55; manganese, 62–63; molybdenum, 70–71; phosphorus, 75–76; potassium, 81–82; selenium, 90; sodium, 98–99; vitamin A, 106–7; vitamin B1 (thiamin), 115–16; vitamin B2 (riboflavin), 123; vitamin B3 (niacin), 131–32; vitamin B5 (pantothenic acid), 138–39; vitamin B6 (pyridoxine), 146–47; vitamin B7 (biotin), 154; vitamin B9 (folate), 158–59; vitamin B12 (cobalamin), 165–66; vitamin C (ascorbic acid), 174–75; vitamin D, 183; vitamin E, 194; vitamin K, 202–3; zinc, 207–8
Exercise: athletic performance, sodium and, 100; breathing problems after, vitamin C (ascorbic acid) and, 178; endurance training, vitamin C (ascorbic acid) and, 176–77; higher-fat diets and, vitamin B5 (pantothenic acid) and, 143; molybdenum and, 72; physical performance of older adults, magnesium and, 58
Experimental Gerontology (journal), 187, 197–98
Externalizing behaviors in adolescents, magnesium and, 59

FASEB Journal, 17
Fatigue: inflammatory bowel disease and, vitamin B1 (thiamin) and, 116; vitamin D and, 183–84

Fat-soluble vitamins: vitamin A, 105–12; vitamin D, 182–90; vitamin K, 201–5
Federal Trade Commission, xvi
Fluoride, 32–38; adequate intakes, 218–19; adult tooth loss and, 35–36; caries (cavities) and, 34–35; childhood cognitive development and, 37; cognitive health in elderly and, 37–38; deficiency and excess, 34; food sources, 33; hypertension and, 37; hypothyroidism and, 36; intake recommendations, 34; IQ and, 37; Recommended Dietary Allowances, 218–19; research findings, 34–38; supplements, 33; tea drinkers and, 36; tolerable upper intake levels, 34, 222–23
Folate. *See* Vitamin B9 (folate)
Folic acid. *See* Vitamin B9 (folate)
Food Additives & Contaminants (journal), 71
Food and Nutrition Board of the Institute of Medicine, 14, 81, 90, 98, 207
Food and Nutrition Board of the National Academy of Sciences, xvii, 70
Food & Drug Administration (FDA), xvi
Food labels. *See* Labeling information
Food & Nutrition Research (journal), 87
Food prepared outside the home, sodium in, 102–3
Fortifying bread with iodized salt for school children, 43–44
Fractures: calcium and, 11; hip, in elderly, vitamin K and, 205; vitamin B12 (cobalamin) and, 168
Funk, Casimir, xiv

Gastrointestinal surgery for cancer, vitamin B1 (thiamin) and, 119
Gender: intake levels determined by, xiii, xvii; iron and, 50–51; magnesium and, 54–55; sodium and high blood pressure, 102; vitamin A and primary liver cancer, 110; vitamin A intake and, 106; vitamin B6 and, 146; vitamin B12 (cobalamin) and morbid obesity, 169; vitamin C and risk of heart failure, 179–80; vitamin K and bone mineral

density, 204–5; vitamin K and risk for hip fractures in elderly, 205; vitamin K intake recommendations, 202
Geometric mean, 65
Gestational diabetes, vitamin B9 (folate) and, 160
Global Journal of Health Science, 71, 72
Glossitis, vitamin B7 (biotin) and, 154
Gluconeogenesis, manganese and, 61–62
Glycemic status, vitamin K and, 204
Graves' disease, selenium and, 94–95

Headache (journal), 116–17
Health, diet associated with, xiv
Heart attack, vitamin E and, 196–97
Heart disease: ischemic, manganese and, 65; mortality from, sodium and, 101
Heart failure: in older men, vitamin C (ascorbic acid) and, 179; vitamin B1 (thiamin) and, 116; vitamin E and, 199; in women, vitamin C (ascorbic acid) and, 179–80
Heart medication. *See* Angiotensin-converting enzyme (ACE) inhibitors
Heart palpitation, vitaminB9 (folate) and, 159
Heart rate, potassium and, 84
Heavy menstrual bleeding, iron and, 48
Herbal infusions, copper and, 31
Hip fractures in elderly, vitamin K and, 205
Homocysteine, 145–46, 158, 164
Household food expenditures, vitamin A and, 109
Hypercalcemia, vitamin D and, 183
Hypertension: fluoride and, 37; inflammation in, vitamin C (ascorbic acid) and, 178; sodium-to-potassium ratio and, 83. *See also* Blood pressure
Hypothyroidism: fluoride and, 36; in newborns, iodine and, 42

Immunity markers in elderly, zinc and, 209–10
Infant formula: molybdenum in, 71–72; vitamin B7 (biotin) in, 155
Inflammation in hypertensive and/or diabetic obese adults, vitamin C (ascorbic acid) and, 178

Inflammatory bowel diseases (IBD): fatigue and, vitamin B1 (thiamin) and, 116; vitamin D and, 189
Intake recommendations: boron, 1–2; chart, 216–23; choline, 14–15; chromium, 20–21; copper, 27; fluoride, 34; iodine, 40; iron, 46–47; magnesium, 54–55; manganese, 62; molybdenum, 70; phosphorus, 75; potassium, 81; selenium, 90; sodium, 98; vitamin A, 106; vitamin B1 (thiamin), 114–15; vitamin B2 (riboflavin), 122–23; vitamin B3 (niacin), 131; vitamin B5 (pantothenic acid), 138; vitamin B6 (pyridoxine), 146; vitamin B7 (biotin), 154; vitamin B9 (folate), 158; vitamin B12 (cobalamin), 165; vitamin C (ascorbic acid), 174; vitamin D, 183; vitamin E, 194; vitamin K, 202; zinc, 207. *See also* Adequate intakes (AIs); Estimated average requirements (EARs); Recommended Dietary Allowances (RDAs); Tolerable upper intake levels (ULs)
Intensive care unit patients, calcium and, 10
Internal Medicine (journal), 167
International Journal for Vitamin and Nutrition Research, 141, 195
International Journal of Cancer, 125
International Journal of Clinical Practice, The, 204
International Journal of Endocrinology & Metabolism, 41
International Journal of Environmental Research and Public Health, 36, 141
International Journal of Epidemiology, 159–60
International Journal of Food and Nutritional Sciences, 169
International Journal of Food Sciences and Nutrition, 31
International Journal of Medical Sciences, 3
International Ophthalmology (journal), 111
International Wound Journal, 141–42
Iodine, 39–44; adequate intakes, 218–19; cholesterol levels in overweight women

and, 43; deficiency and excess, 40–41; food sources, 40; fortifying bread with iodized salt for school children, 43–44; hypothyroidism in newborns and, 42; intake recommendations, 40; IQ and, 41; on labeling information, 40; neuro-intellectual outcomes of children and, 41–42; pasteurized milk and, 41; pregnancy outcomes and, 44; Recommended Dietary Allowances, 40, 218–19; requirements for pregnant women, 43; research findings, 41–44; supplements, 40; thyroid disorders and, 43; tolerable upper intake levels, 40, 222–23

IQ: fluoride and, 37; iodine and, 41

Iranian Journal of Allergy, Asthma and Immunology, 107

Iron, 46–52; absorption, 47, 48–49, 51, 126; adequate intakes, 218–19; animal flesh consumption and, 48; blood donors and, 49–50; body mass index (BMI) and, 51; calcium and, 9–10; cognition and, 50; deficiency and excess, 47; food sources, 46; heavy menstrual bleeding and, 48; infant birth weight and, 50–51; intake recommendations, 46–47; overweight women and, 51; postpartum depression and, 51–52; probiotics and, 48–49; Recommended Dietary Allowances, 47, 218–19; red blood cells and, xiv; research findings, 48–52; supplements, 46; tolerable upper intake levels, 47, 222–23

Irritable bowel syndrome (IBS), vitamin D and, 185

Ischemic heart disease, manganese and, 65

Ischemic stroke, potassium and, 86

JAMA (journal), 49, 101, 199
JAMA Neurology (journal), 198
JAMA Pediatrics (journal), 85
Journal of the Academy of Nutrition and Dietetics, 99, 101–2
Journal of Affective Disorders, 210
Journal of Allergy and Clinical Immunology, 189

Journal of Alternative and Complementary Medicine, The, 22, 83–84, 116
Journal of Alzheimer's Disease, 187
Journal of the American College of Cardiology, 133
Journal of the American College of Nutrition, 156–57
Journal of the American Dental Association, 34–35
Journal of the American Dietetic Association, xix
Journal of the American Society of Nephrology, 77, 79, 84
Journal of Applied Physiology, 133
Journal of Cardiac Failure, 116
Journal of Cardiovascular Nursing, 30
Journal of Caring Sciences, 150
Journal of Clinical and Experimental Medicine, 65–66
Journal of Clinical Biochemistry and Nutrition, 204–5
Journal of Clinical Endocrinology & Metabolism, 42, 94–95, 187–88, 189–90
Journal of Clinical Lipidology, 134
Journal of Clinical Pathology, 29
Journal of Cosmetic Science, 142
Journal of Diabetes & Metabolic Disorders, 140, 204
Journal of Education and Health Promotion, 7
Journal of Epidemiology, 150
Journal of Epidemiology and Community Health, 36
Journal of Headache and Pain, The, 123–24
Journal of Human Hypertension, 82
Journal of Human Nutrition and Dietetics, 186
Journal of Hypertension, 82, 102
Journal of the National Cancer Institute, 92–93, 149
Journal of Nutrition, Health & Aging, The, 168
Journal of Nutrition, The, 15, 17–18, 43, 95–96, 118, 119–20, 155–56, 203
Journal of Nutritional Biochemistry, 208
Journal of Nutritional Science and Vitaminology, 143

Journal of Perinatology, 72–73
Journal of Pharmacy & Pharmaceutical Sciences, 23
Journal of Physiology, 176–77
Journal of Psychosomatic Research, 22
Journal of Science and Medicine in Sport, 100
Journal of Sports Science & Medicine, 100
Journal of the American Heart Association, 177
Journal of the Royal Society of Medicine Open, 210
Journal of the Science of Food and Agriculture, 208–9

Kidney disease: cardiovascular systems of people with diabetes and, potassium and, 84; chronic, cardiovascular events in people with/without, phosphorus and, 77–78; magnesium and, 58; phosphorus and, 76; type 2 diabetes and, manganese and, 65
Kidney International (journal), 58
Kidneys, water-soluble vitamins regulated by, xiii
Knee discomfort, boron and, 4

Labeling information: Dietary References Intakes (DRI or DRIs) on, xviii, xix; Federal Trade Commission and, xvi; Food & Drug Administration and, xvi; iodine on, 40; manufacturer claims on, xvi; phosphorus on, 78; "Supplement Facts" panel on, xv; vitamin A on, 106
Lancet (journal), 161–62
Lipid levels in people with type 2 diabetes, vitamin C (ascorbic acid) and, 178–79
Liver cancer: primary, vitamin A and, 110; selenium and, 90–91
Lozenges for common cold, zinc, 210
Lung cancer, calcium and, 11

Macrominerals, xiii
Magnesium, 53–59; absorption, 56; adequate intakes, 218–19; in antacids, 54; blood pressure and, 55; childhood bone growth and, 56; deficiency and excess, 55; depression and, 58–59; diabetes and, 59; diuretics and, 55; externalizing behaviors in adolescents and, 59; food sources, 54; intake recommendations, 54–55; kidney disease and, 58; metabolic syndrome and, 56–57; migraine headaches and, 57; physical performance of elderly and, 58; Recommended Dietary Allowances, 54–55, 56, 218–19; research findings, 55–59; supplements, 54; systolic blood pressure and, 55; tolerable upper intake levels, 222–23
Malabsorption: phosphorus, 75; selenium, 90; vitamin B12 (cobalamin), 165; vitamin C, 174. *See also* Absorption
Manganese, 61–67; absorption, 62; adequate intakes, 218–19; amino acid and, 62; attention and working memory of nonhuman primates and, 66–67; blood pressure and, 65; breast cancer and, 65–66; children's attention, cognition, behavior, and academic performance and, 63; deficiency and excess, 62–63; food sources, 62; in hair and attention deficit hyperactivity disorder and, 63–64; intake recommendations, 62; metabolic syndrome and, 67; neurobehavioral functioning of school-age children and, 66; newborn birth weight and, 67; preeclampsia and, 64; Recommended Dietary Allowances, 218–19; research findings, 63–67; sex hormones and, 61; supplements, 62; tolerable upper intake levels, 62, 222–23; type 2 diabetes and, 64–65; type 2 diabetes and renal dysfunction and, 65
Maternal & Child Nutrition (journal), 44
Medical Archives (journal), 111
Medications. *See* Over-the-counter medications; Prescription medications
Medicine (journal), 183–84
Mediterranean diet, zinc and, 211
Memory: Alzheimer's disease, copper and, 30–31; attention and working memory of nonhuman primates, manganese and, 66–67; choline and, 16, 17; dementia, vitamin E and, 198

Menstrual bleeding, heavy, iron and, 48
Metabolic benefits, of selenium, 91
Metabolic syndrome: blood pressure and cardiac problems in rats with, phosphorus and, 78–79; magnesium and, 56–57; manganese and, 67; vascular disease in people with, vitamin B3 (niacin) and, 132–33; vitamin D and, 187–88; vitamin E and, 197
Metformin, vitamin C levels and, 179
Methionine, 127
Microgram (mcg), 90
Micronutrients: ultra-processed foods and, 29–30; vitamin B1 (thiamine) deficiency in elderly, 117; vitamin B2 (riboflavin) and, 127; vitamin B6 (pyridoxine) and, 127
Migraine headaches: magnesium and, 57; vitamin B1 (thiamin) and, 117; vitamin B2 (riboflavin) and, 123–24
Minerals: adequate intakes, 216–19; body processes regulated by, xiv; boron, 1–5; calcium, 6–12; choline, 14–18; chromium, 20–25; classifying, xiii–xiv; copper, 26–31; deficiencies, research on problems associated with, xiv; fluoride, 32–38; function of, in body, xiv; intake levels of, determining, xvii–xix; iodine, 39–44; iron, 46–52; magnesium, 53–59; manganese, 61–67; molybdenum, 69–73; phosphorus, 74–79; potassium, 80–87; Recommended Dietary Allowances, 216–19; selenium, 89–96; sodium, 98–103; tolerable upper intake levels, 220–23; zinc, 206–12. *See also individual minerals*
Molecular Psychiatry (journal), 190
Molybdenum, 69–73; adequate intakes, 218–19; amino acid and, 62; deficiency and excess, 70–71; esophageal cancer and, 71; exercise and, 72; food sources, 70; in infant formulas, 71–72; intake recommendations, 70; parenteral and enteral nutrition and, 72; pasteurization of breast milk and, 72–73; Recommended Dietary Allowances, 218–19; research findings, 71–73; supplements, 70; tolerable upper intake levels, 222–23
Morbid obesity, chromium and, 21
Mortality risk, vitamin K and, 203–4
Mothers and newborns, vitamin A and, 107–8
Multiple sclerosis: progressive, vitamin B7 (biotin) and, 156; vitamin A and, 107
Multiple Sclerosis (journal), 156
Myocardial infarction: calcium and, 8; vitamin B3 (niacin) and, 135; vitamin E and, 197

National Health and Nutrition Examination Survey (NHANES), 56, 58–59, 83, 85, 160, 162, 195–96
Nausea and vomiting associated with pregnancy, vitamin B6 (pyridoxine) and, 150–51
Neural tube defect, vitamin B9 (folate) and, 158, 159
Neurobehavioral functioning of school-age children, manganese and, 66
Neuro-intellectual outcomes of children, iodine and, 41–42
Neurological benefits of vitamin B12 (cobalamin), 170–71
Neurology (journal), 170–71
NeuroReport (journal), 28
NeuroToxicology (journal), 66
Neurotoxicology and Teratology (journal), 37
Newborns, vitamin A and, 107–8
New England Journal of Medicine, The, 10, 132, 135
Niacin. *See* Vitamin B3 (niacin)
Niacinamide, 130
Nicotinamide adenine dinucleotide (NAD), 131
Nicotinamide adenine dinucleotide phosphate (NADP), 131
Nigerian Journal of Clinical Practice, 169
Night blindness, vitamin A and, 111
Nonalcoholic fatty liver disease, choline and, 17–18
Nonmelanoma skin cancers, vitamin B3 (niacin) and, 132

Nonprescription medications. *See* Over-the-counter medications
Nutrición Hospitalaria (journal), 112
Nutrients (journal), 43–44, 48, 83, 85–86, 110, 124–25, 148–49, 151, 162, 166, 175–76, 211
Nutrition, Metabolism & Cardiovascular Diseases (journal), 84, 110–11, 196–97
Nutritional Neuroscience (journal), 17, 23
Nutritional Research (journal), 109
Nutrition Journal, 50, 93
Nutrition Research (journal), 109, 148
Nyctalopia, vitamin D and, 111

Obesity. *See* Overweight and obesity
Obesity Surgery (journal), 21
Obstetrics and Gynaecology Research (journal), 24–15
Older adults: cognitive decline, vitamin B6 (pyridoxine) and, 148–49; cognitive decline in, vitamin C (ascorbic acid) and, 176; cognitive decline in, vitamin E and, 197–98; cognitive function in, vitamin D and, 187; heart failure in men, vitamin C (ascorbic acid) and, 179; immunity markers in, zinc and, 209–10; neurological or cognitive benefits of vitamin B12 (cobalamin), 170–71; physical performance of, magnesium and, 58; postmenopausal women, vitamin B5 (pantothenic acid) and, 140; vitamin B1 (thiamin) and, 117–18; vitamin B12 (cobalamin) and, 166–68
Open-label studies, 111, 156, 178
Ophthalmology (journal), 177
Oral contraceptives: side effects from, vitamin B6 (pyridoxine) and, 151; vitamin B6 (pyridoxine) and, 146–47, 151; vitamin B6 levels and, 146–47, 151; vitamin B12 levels and, 166
Osteoarthritis, boron and, 3–4
Osteopenia, copper and, 29
Osteoporosis: calcium and, 9; copper and, 29; medications, calcium and, 7; potassium and, 86
Osteoporosis International (journal), 11, 168, 205

Over-the-counter medications: antacids, 54, 75; sodium in, 98, 103; zinc in, 207
Overweight and obesity: cholesterol levels in overweight women, iodine and, 43; in Mexican American children, vitamin B1 (thiamin) and, 119–20; morbid obesity, chromium and, 21; morbid obesity, vitamin K and, 204; reductions in, boron and, 3; vitamin B1 (thiamin) and, 118; vitamin B12 (cobalamin) and, 169; vitamin D and, 186; women, and iron, 51
Oxidative DNA damage, vitamin B6 (pyridoxine) and, 149

Pain Physician (journal), 57
Pancreatic cancer, choline and, 18
Panthenol, adverse reactions to, 142–43
Pantothenic acid. *See* Vitamin B5 (pantothenic acid)
Parenteral nutrition, molybdenum and, 72
Parkinson's disease: medications, vitamin B6 levels and, 147; vitamin B6 (pyridoxine) and, 148
Pasteurized milk: breast milk, molybdenum and, 72–73; iodine and, 41
Patient Preference and Adherence (journal), 9
Pediatrics (journal), 103, 110, 188
Pediatrics International (journal), 108, 155, 208
Pernicious anemia, vitamin B12 (cobalamin) and, 169–70
Pharmacology Research & Perspectives (journal), 132–33
Phosphate: calcium and, 6; phosphorus and, 77–78, 79
Phosphorus, 74–79; ACE inhibitors and, 75; adequate intakes, 218–19; antacids and, 75; in beverages, 78; blood pressure and cardiac problems in rats with metabolic syndrome and, 78–79; blood pressure medications and, 75; cardiovascular and all-cause mortality and, 76–77; cardiovascular events in people with/without chronic kidney disease and, 77–78; coronary atherosclerosis and, 77; deficiency

and excess, 75–76; diuretics and, 75; food sources, 74–75; function of, in body, xiv; intake recommendations, 75; interacting with over-the-counter medications, 75; kidney problems and, 76; on labeling information, 78; as macromineral, xiii; malabsorption, 75; phosphate and, 77–78, 79; Recommended Dietary Allowances, 218–19; research findings, 76–79; socioeconomic status and, 79; supplements, 74–75; tolerable upper intake levels, 75, 222–23

Physical performance of elderly, magnesium and, 58

Picky eaters, copper and, 28–29

Placenta (journal), 57

PLoS ONE (journal), 23–24, 77–78, 83, 95, 126, 160, 195–96

Polycystic ovary syndrome, chromium and, 24

Postmenopausal women, vitamin B5 (pantothenic acid) and, 140

Postpartum depression, iron and, 51–52

Potassium, 80–87; ACE inhibitors and, 82; adequate intakes, 218–19; adolescents and, 85, 87; blood pressure and, 82; craniosacral therapy in patients with chronic low back pain and, 83–84; deficiency and excess, 81–82; diuretics and, 82; food sources, 81; heart rate and, 84; intake recommendations, 81; kidneys and cardiovascular systems of people with diabetes and, 84; osteoporosis and, 86; preschool children and, 85–86; Recommended Dietary Allowances, 218–19; research findings, 82–87; sodium-to-potassium ratio and high blood pressure and, 83; stroke and, 86; supplements, 81; systolic blood pressure and, 82, 85; toddlers and, 85

Pre-cervical cancer, selenium and, 91

Prediabetes and blood sugar levels, vitamin K and, 204

Preeclampsia: calcium and, 9; manganese and, 64; selenium and, 91–92

Pregnancy: body mass index (BMI), iron and, 51; gestational diabetes and, 160; iodine and, 44; nausea and vomiting associated with, vitamin B6 (pyridoxine) and, 150–51; neural tube defect and, vitamin B9 (folate) and, 158, 159; zinc and, 209

Premenopausal women with prediabetes, blood sugar levels in, vitamin K and, 204

Premenstrual syndrome: vitamin B2 (riboflavin) and, 128; vitamin B6 (pyridoxine) and, 150

Prenatal supplements: choline, 17; vitamin A, 108; vitamin B9 (folate), 159–60

Prescription medications: ACE inhibitors, 75, 82; antacids, 75; antibiotics, 147, 154, 202–3; anticoagulants, xv, 202–3; antidepressants, 210; anti-seizure, 154; antitumor necrosis factor-α, 189; blood pressure, 75; cholesterol-reducing, 135, 139; diabetes, 179; diuretics, 55, 75, 82, 116; for migraines, 123; oral contraceptives, 146–47, 151, 166; for osteoporosis, 7; for Parkinson's disease, 147; sodium in, 98; steroids, 147; supplements interacting with, overview of, xv, xvi; thyroid, 41–42; vitamin A in, vitamin A toxicity and, 107; zinc-induced copper deficiency and, 29. *See also individual medications*

Preventive Medicine (journal), 127–28

Primary liver cancer, vitamin A and, 110

Primigravid, selenium and, 92

Probiotics, iron and, 48–49

Proceedings of the National Academy of Sciences (journal), 30–31

Product labels. *See* Labeling information

Prostate, The (journal), 93, 161

Prostate cancer: boron and, 4; selenium and, 92–93; vitamin B9 (folate) and, 161; vitamin E and, 199

Protein, fat-soluble vitamins and, xiii

Psychiatric problems: in adolescents, vitamin B2 (riboflavin) and, 127–28; chromium and, 22

Psychiatry Investigation (journal), 63–64

Psychiatry Research (journal), 184

Psychogeriatric patients, vitamin D and, 186–87

Psycho-Oncology (journal), 116–17
Pteroylglutamic acid. *See* Vitamin B9 (folate)
Public Health Nutrition (journal), 59, 140, 211
Puerto Rican children, vitamin B5 (pantothenic acid) and, 141
Pyridoxine. *See* Vitamin B6 (pyridoxine)

Reactions, adverse: to panthenol, 142–43; taking supplements with other supplements, xvi; taking supplements with prescription medications, xv, xvi; to vitamin B6, 147
Recommended Dietary Allowances (RDAs): boron, 2; calcium, 7, 218–19; chart, 216–19; chloride, 218–19; choline, 216–17; chromium, 218–19; copper, 27, 218–19; defined, xvii; determining, xvii–xix; for different populations, 216–20; fluoride, 218–19; history of, xviii–xix; iodine, 40, 218–19; iron, 47, 218–19; magnesium, 54–55, 56, 218–19; manganese, 218–19; minerals, 216–19; molybdenum, 218–19; phosphorus, 218–19; potassium, 218–19; selenium, 90, 218–19; sodium, 218–19; vitamin A, 216–17; vitamin B1 (thiamin), 118, 216–17; vitamin B2 (riboflavin), 216–17; vitamin B3 (niacin), 216–17; vitamin B5 (pantothenic acid), 140, 216–17; vitamin B6 (pyridoxine), 146, 216–17; vitamin B7 (biotin), 154, 216–17; vitamin B9 (folate), 158, 216–17; vitamin B12 (cobalamin), 165, 216–17; vitamin C (ascorbic acid), 174, 216–17; vitamin D, 216–17; vitamin E, 194, 216–17; vitamin K, 216–17; vitamins, 216–19; zinc, 207, 218–19
Red blood cells, iron and, xiv
Reduced-sodium meals, 101–2
Renal dysfunction. *See* Kidney disease
Research findings: boron, 2–4; choline, 15–18; chromium, 21–25; copper, 28–31; fluoride, 34–38; iodine, 41–44; iron, 48–52; magnesium, 55–59; manganese, 63–67; molybdenum, 71–73; phosphorus, 76–79; potassium, 82–87; selenium, 90–96; sodium, 99–103; vitamin A, 107–12; vitamin B1 (thiamin), 116–20; vitamin B2 (riboflavin), 123–28; vitamin B3 (niacin), 132–36; vitamin B5 (pantothenic acid), 139–43; vitamin B6 (pyridoxine), 147–51; vitamin B7 (biotin), 155–57; vitamin B9 (folate), 159–62; vitamin B12 (cobalamin), 166–71; vitamin C (ascorbic acid), 175–80; vitamin D, 183–90; vitamin E, 195–99; vitamin K, 203–5; zinc, 208–12
Revista Brasileira de Epidemiologia (Brazilian Journal of Epidemiology), 107–8
Revista de Saúde Pública (journal), 29–30
Rheumatoid arthritis and smoking, sodium and, 101
Rheumatology (journal), 101
Riboflavin. *See* Vitamin B2 (riboflavin)
Rice, vital amine in, xiv
Roczniki Państwowego Zakładu Higieny (journal), 86

Schizophrenia: choline and, 15–16; vitamin B3 (niacin) and, 134–35
Science of the Total Environment (journal), 37
Scientific Reports (journal), 11
Scurvy, xiv
Selective serotonin reuptake inhibitor, zinc levels and, 210
Selenium, 89–96; adequate intakes, 218–19; bone mineral density in aging men and, 95; breast cancer and, 92; deficiency and excess, 90; depressive moods and, 95–96; diabetes and, 93–94; food sources, 89–90; Graves' disease and, 94–95; intake recommendations, 90; liver cancer and, 90–91; malabsorption, 90; metabolic benefits, 91; pre-cervical cancer and, 91; preeclampsia and, 91–92; prostate cancer and, 92–93; Recommended Dietary Allowances, 90, 218–19; research findings, 90–96; supplements, 89–90; thyroid gland and, 94; tolerable upper intake levels, 222–23

Sex. *See* Gender
Sex hormones: boron deficiency and imbalance of, 2; manganese and, 61; phosphorus levels and, 77
Sickle cell disease, zinc and, 207
Skin inflammation, vitamin B5 (pantothenic acid) and, 142–43
Skin moisture, vitamin B5 (pantothenic acid) and, 142
Smoking and rheumatoid arthritis, sodium and, 101
Socioeconomic status: phosphorus and, 79; vitamin D and, 186
Sodium, 98–103; adequate intakes, 218–19; in antacids, 75; athletic performance and, 100; blood pressure and, 99, 102, 103; cardiovascular disease and, 99–100; DASH diet and, 99; deficiency and excess, 98–99; in food prepared outside the home, 102–3; food sources, 98; intake recommendations, 98; mortality from heart disease, stroke, and type 2 diabetes and, 101; Recommended Dietary Allowances, 218–19; reduced-sodium meals, 101–2; research findings, 99–103; smoking and rheumatoid arthritis and, 101; supplements, 98; systolic blood pressure and, 103; tolerable upper intake levels, 98, 222–23
SpringerPlus (journal), 10
Squamous-cell carcinoma, 132
Steroids, vitamin B6 (pyridoxine) and, 147
Stroke: mortality from, sodium and, 101; potassium and, 86; vitamin C (ascorbic acid) and, 177–78
Stroke (journal), 86
Subclinical atherosclerosis later in life, vitamin D and, 189–90
Subclinical cardiovascular disease, calcium and, 8
"Supplement Facts" panel, xv
Supplement industry, history and reputation of, xvi
Supplements. *See* Dietary supplements

Support Care Cancer (journal), 119
Systolic blood pressure: magnesium and, 55; potassium and, 82, 85; sodium and, 103; vitamin C and, 176

Taiwanese Journal of Obstetrics and Gynecology, 91–92
Taste sensation, and vitamin B7 (biotin), 156–57
Tea drinkers, fluoride and, 36
Thiamin. *See* Vitamin B1 (thiamin)
Thyroid (journal), 41–42
Thyroid disorders, iodine and, 43
Thyroid gland, selenium and, 94
Thyroid medications, maternal iodine supplementation and, 41–42
Toddlers, potassium and, 85
Tolerable upper intake levels (ULs): boron, 222–23; calcium, 222–23; chart, 220–23; chloride, 222–23; choline, 15, 220–21; chromium, 222–23; copper, 27, 222–23; defined, xviii; fluoride, 34, 222–23; iodine, 40, 222–23; iron, 47, 222–23; magnesium, 222–23; manganese, 62, 222–23; minerals, 220–23; molybdenum, 222–23; phosphorus, 75, 222–23; selenium, 222–23; sodium, 98, 222–23; vitamin A, 106, 220–21; vitamin B1 (thiamin), 115, 220–21; vitamin B2 (riboflavin), 123, 220–21; vitamin B3 (niacin), 220–21; vitamin B5 (pantothenic acid), 138, 220–21; vitamin B6 (pyridoxine), 220–21; vitamin B7 (biotin), 220–21; vitamin B9 (folate), 158, 162, 220–21; vitamin B12 (cobalamin), 220–21; vitamin C (ascorbic acid), 174; vitamin D, 220–21; vitamin E, 220–21; vitamin K, 220–21; vitamins, 220–21; zinc, 207, 222–23
Tooth loss in adults, fluoride and, 35–36
Trace minerals, xiii–xiv; iron, 46–52; zinc, 206–12
Transfusion (journal), 49–50
Tryptophan, 130
Tumour Biology (journal), 4
Type 1 diabetes, vitamin B2 (riboflavin) and, 127

Type 2 diabetes: lipid levels in people with, vitamin C (ascorbic acid) and, 178–79; manganese and, 64–65; mortality from, sodium and, 101; renal dysfunction, manganese and, 65; vitamin A and, 110–11

Ultra-processed foods, copper and, 29–30

Vascular health: disease in people with metabolic syndrome, vitamin B3 (niacin) and, 132–33; vitamin B3 (niacin) and, 133
Vascular Health and Risk Management (journal), 139
Vegetarian diets: vitamin B12 (cobalamin) and, 166, 168; zinc and, 208–9
Vitamin A, 105–12; acne and, 111; adequate intakes, 216–17; adverse childhood behavior and, 108; bariatric surgery and, 111–12; carotenoid and benign breast disease and, 110; Crohn's disease and, 111; deficiency and excess, 106–7; food sources, 105–6; household food expenditures and, 109; intake recommendations, 106; on labeling information, 106; for mothers and newborns, 107–8; multiple sclerosis and, 107; night blindness and, 111; primary liver cancer and, 110; Recommended Dietary Allowances, 216–17; research findings, 107–12; supplements, 105–6; tolerable upper intake levels, 106, 220–21; type 2 diabetes and, 110–11; very low-birth-weight infants and, 109
Vitamin B1 (thiamin): 114–20; absorption, 115, 116; adequate intakes, 216–17; adiposity in Mexican American children and, 119–20; alcohol addiction and, 118–19; bariatric surgery and, 115, 118; beriberi and, xiv; cancer and, 116–17; deficiency and excess, 115–16; diuretics and, 116; fatigue associated with inflammatory bowel disease and, 116; food sources, 114; gastrointestinal surgery for cancer and, 119; heart failure and, 116; intake recommendations, 114–15; migraine headaches and, 117; obesity and, 118; older adults and, 117–18; Recommended Dietary Allowances, 118, 216–17; research findings, 116–20; supplements, 114; tolerable upper intake levels, 115, 220–21
Vitamin B2 (riboflavin): 122–28; absorption, 126; adequate intakes, 216–17; adolescent psychiatric and behavior problems and, 127–28; amino acid and, 127; anemia and, 126; attention deficit hyperactivity disorder (ADHD), 125–26; breast cancer and, 126–27; colorectal cancer and, 125; deficiency and excess, 123, 124–25; food sources, 122; intake recommendations, 122–23; migraine headaches and, 123–24; premenstrual syndrome and, 128; Recommended Dietary Allowances, 216–17; research findings, 123–28; supplements, 122; tolerable upper intake levels, 123, 220–21; type 1 diabetes and, 127
Vitamin B3 (niacin): 130–36; adequate intakes, 216–17; amino acid and, 130; cardiovascular disease and, 133; cholesterol levels and, 134; cholesterol-reducing medications and, 135; deficiency and excess, 131–32; depression and, 134; food sources, 131; intake recommendations, 131; myocardial infarction and, 135; nonmelanoma skin cancers and, 132; people who should avoid, 135–36; Recommended Dietary Allowances, 216–17; research findings, 132–36; schizophrenia and, 134–35; supplements, 131; tolerable upper intake levels, 220–21; vascular disease in people with metabolic syndrome and, 132–33; vascular health and, 133
Vitamin B5 (pantothenic acid): 137–43; acne and, 139–40; adequate intakes, 216–17; cardiovascular health and,

139; cholesterol-reducing medications and, 139; deficiency and excess, 138–39; depressive symptoms and, 141; dermatitis or skin inflammation and, 142–43; eating disorders and, 140; exercise and higher-fat diets and, 143; food sources, 138; intake recommendations, 138; postmenopausal women and, 140; Puerto Rican children and, 141; Recommended Dietary Allowances, 140, 216–17; research findings, 139–43; skin moisture and, 142; supplements, 138; tolerable upper intake levels, 138, 220–21; wound-healing properties in, 141–42

Vitamin B6 (pyridoxine): 145–51; adequate intakes, 216–17; adverse reactions to, 147; antibiotics and, 147; breast cancer and, 150; cancer risk and, 149; cognitive decline and, 148–49; coronary artery disease and, 148; deficiency and excess, 146–47; depression and, 147; food sources, 146; intake recommendations, 146; nausea and vomiting associated with pregnancy and, 150–51; oral contraceptives and, 146–47, 151; oxidative DNA damage and, 149; Parkinson's disease and, 148; premenstrual syndrome and, 150; Recommended Dietary Allowances, 146, 216–17; research findings, 147–51; side effects from oral contraceptives and, 151; steroids and, 147; supplements, 146; tolerable upper intake levels, 220–21

Vitamin B7 (biotin): 153–57; absorption, 154; adequate intakes, 216–17; antibiotics and, 154; antidiabetic properties of, 155; anti-seizure medications and, 154; deficiency and excess, 154, 155–56; food sources, 154; in infant formula, 155; intake recommendations, 154; progressive multiple sclerosis and, 156; Recommended Dietary Allowances, 154, 216–17; research findings, 155–57; supplements, 154; taste sensation and, 156–57; tolerable upper intake levels, 220–21

Vitamin B9 (folate): 157–62; adequate intakes, 216–17; cancer risk and, 160–61; deficiency and excess, 158–59; food sources, 158; gestational diabetes and, 160; intake recommendations, 158; prenatal benefits, 159–60; prostate cancer and, 161; Recommended Dietary Allowances, 158, 216–17; research findings, 159–62; site-specific cancer and, 161–62; supplements, 158; tolerable upper intake levels, 158, 162, 220–21

Vitamin B12 (cobalamin): 164–71; acid-lowering agents and, 167; adequate intakes, 216–17; body mass index (BMI) and, 169; cardiovascular health and, 168; deficiency and excess, 165–67; depression and, 167; elderly and, 166–68; food sources, 164–65; fractures and, 168; intake recommendations, 165; malabsorption, 165; neurological or cognitive benefits to elderly, 170–71; obesity and, 169; oral contraceptives and, 166; pernicious anemia and, 169–70; preterm birth/low birth weight and, 170; Recommended Dietary Allowances, 165, 216–17; research findings, 166–71; supplements, 164–65; tolerable upper intake levels, 220–21; vegetarians and, 166, 168

Vitamin C: malabsorption, 174; systolic blood pressure and, 176

Vitamin C (ascorbic acid), 173–80; adequate intakes, 216–17; blood pressure and, 176; breathing problems after exercise and, 178; cataracts and, 177; cognitive decline and, 176; deficiency and excess, 174–75; diabetes medication and, 179; endothelial function and, 175; endurance training and, 176–77; food sources, 173–74; heart failure in older men and, 179; heart failure in women and, 179–80; inflammation in hypertensive and/or diabetic obese adults and, 178; intake recommendations, 174; lipid levels in people with type 2 diabetes and, 178–79; Recommended Dietary Allowances, 174, 216–17; research findings, 175–80; scurvy and, xiv; stroke and, 177–78; supplements, 173–74; tolerable upper intake levels, 174; tolerable upper level for, 220–21; younger men with marginal vitamin C status and, 175–76

Vitamin D, 182–90; adequate intakes, 216–17; adolescents and, 185; antitumor necrosis factor-α and, 189; asthma, allergies, and eczema and, 189; autism-spectrum disorders and, 190; bone mineral density in healthy children and adolescents and, 185–86; cognition and, 187; cognitive function in older adults and, 187; deficiency and excess, 183; depressive symptoms and, 184–85; fatigue and, 183–84; food sources, 182–83; inflammatory bowel diseases and, 189; intake recommendations, 183; irritable bowel syndrome and, 185; metabolic syndrome and, 187–88; obesity and socioeconomic status and, 186; overweight/obese children and, 188; psychogeriatric patients and, 186–87; Recommended Dietary Allowances, 216–17; research findings, 183–90; subclinical atherosclerosis later in life and, 189–90; supplements, 182–83; tolerable upper intake levels, 220–21; younger children and, 188–89

Vitamin E, 193–99; adequate intakes, 216–17; all-cause mortality and, 195; anticoagulants and, xv; cancer risk and, 198; cardiovascular disease and, 196; cognitive decline in older people and, 197–98; deficiency and excess, 194, 195–96; dementia and, 198; food sources, 193–94; heart attack and, 196–97; heart failure and, 199; intake recommendations, 194; metabolic syndrome and, 197; myocardial infarction and, 197; prostate cancer and, 199; Recommended Dietary Allowances, 194, 216–17; research findings, 195–99; supplements, 193–94; tolerable upper intake levels, 220–21

Vitamin K, 201–5; absorption, 202; adequate intakes, 216–17; antibiotics and, 202–3; anticoagulants and, 202, 203; bariatric surgery and, 204; blood sugar levels in premenopausal women with prediabetes and, 204; bone mineral density and, 204–5; deficiency and excess, 202–3; food sources, 202; hip fractures in elderly and, 205; intake recommendations, 202; morbid obesity and, 204; mortality risk and, 203–4; Recommended Dietary Allowances, 216–17; research findings, 203–5; supplements, 202; tolerable upper intake levels, 220–21

Vitamins: adequate intakes, 216–19; classifying, xiii; deficiencies, research on problems associated with, xiv; defined, xiii; intake levels of, determining, xvii–xix; minerals distinguished from, xiii; Recommended Dietary Allowances, 216–19; recommended intake levels of, for different populations, 216–20; tolerable upper intake levels, 220–21; vitamin A, 105–12; vitamin B1 (thiamin), 114–20; vitamin B2 (riboflavin), 122–28; vitamin B3 (niacin), 130–36; vitamin B5 (pantothenic acid), 137–43; vitamin B6 (pyridoxine), 145–51; vitamin B7 (biotin), 153–57; vitamin B9 (folate), 157–62; vitamin B12 (cobalamin), 164–71; vitamin C (ascorbic acid), 173–80; vitamin D, 182–90; vitamin E, 193–99; vitamin K, 201–5. *See also individual vitamins*

Water-soluble vitamins, xiii; choline and, 14; vitamin B3 (niacin), 130–36; vitamin B9 (folate), 157–62
Weight control, calcium and, 11–12
Weight loss, chromium and, 22–23

INDEX 247

Weight problems. *See* Overweight and obesity
Wound-healing properties, in vitamin B5 (pantothenic acid), 141–42

Zinc, 206–12; ability to absorb, as people age, 208; adequate intakes, 218–19; copper deficiency and, 29; copper deficiency myelopathy and, 211–12; deficiency and excess, 207–8; depressive symptoms in women and, 210; food sources, 206–7; immunity markers in elderly and, 209–10; intake recommendations, 207; lozenges for common cold, 210; Mediterranean diet and, 211; pregnancy outcomes and, 209; Recommended Dietary Allowances, 207, 218–19; research findings, 208–12; schoolchildren and, 208; sickle cell disease and, 207; Spanish ANIBES population and, 211; supplements, 206–7; tolerable upper intake levels, 207, 222–23; vegetarian diets and, 208–9

About the Authors

MYRNA CHANDLER GOLDSTEIN, MA, has been a freelance writer and independent scholar for more than 25 years. She is the author of Greenwood's *The 50 Healthiest Habits and Lifestyle Changes*, *Healthy Oils: Fact versus Fiction*, *Healthy Herbs: Fact versus Fiction*, and *Healthy Foods: Fact versus Fiction*.

MARK A. GOLDSTEIN, MD, is founding chief of the Division of Adolescent and Young Adult Medicine at Massachusetts General Hospital and associate professor of pediatrics at Harvard Medical School. He is author or editor of numerous professional and lay publications. His research interests include studying the effects of eating disorders and malnutrition on bone mineralization in adolescents and young adults.

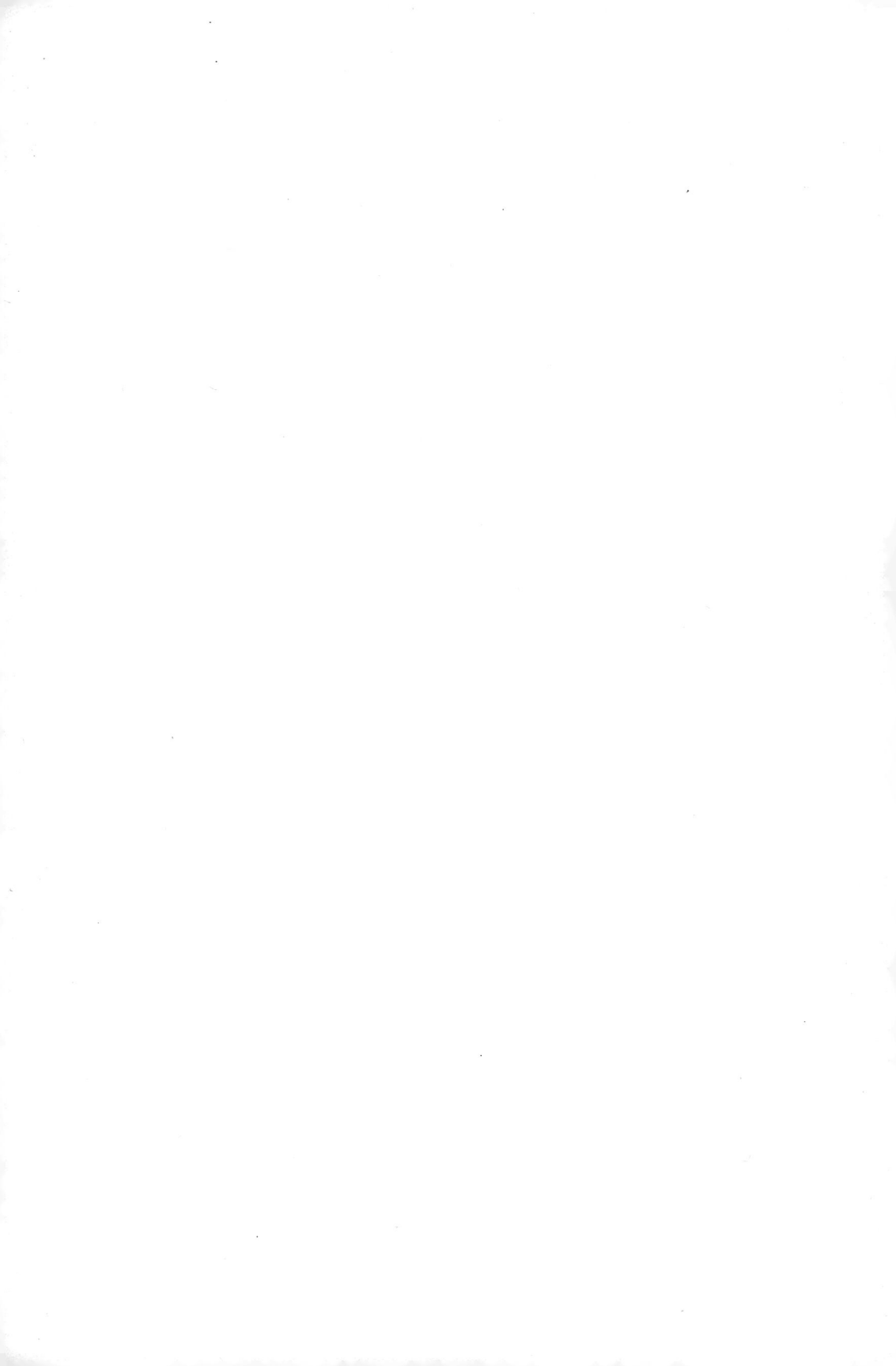